MENTAL HEALTH OF A NATION

MENTAL HEALTH OF A NATION

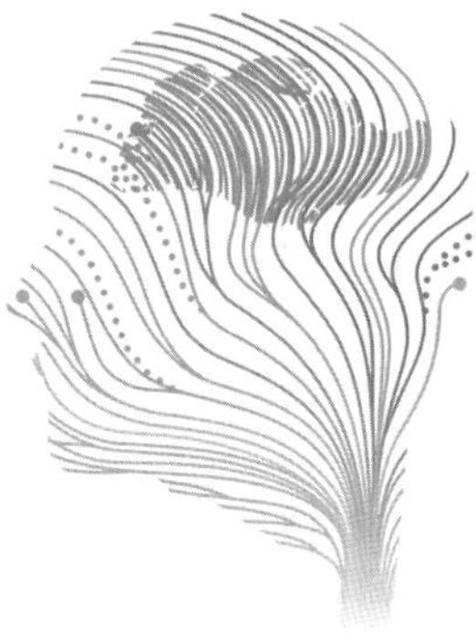

Editors

A/Prof. Ng Beng Yeong
Ng Beng Yeong Psych Medicine Clinic
Mount Elizabeth Medical Centre
Adjunct Associate Professor, Duke-NUS Medical School
Yong Loo Lin School of Medicine, NUS
Singapore

A/Prof. Daniel Fung
Institute of Mental Health
Yong Loo Lin School of Medicine, NUS
Duke-NUS Medical School
Lee Kong Chian School of Medicine, NTU
Singapore

World Scientific

NEW JERSEY • LONDON • SINGAPORE • BEIJING • SHANGHAI • HONG KONG • TAIPEI • CHENNAI • TOKYO

Published by

World Scientific Publishing Co. Pte. Ltd.

5 Toh Tuck Link, Singapore 596224

USA office: 27 Warren Street, Suite 401-402, Hackensack, NJ 07601

UK office: 57 Shelton Street, Covent Garden, London WC2H 9HE

Library of Congress Cataloging-in-Publication Data
Names: Ng, Beng Yeong, editor. | Fung, Daniel, editor.
Title: Mental health of a nation / edited by Ng Beng Yeong & Daniel Fung.
Description: New Jersey : World Scientific, 2016. | Includes bibliographical references.
Identifiers: LCCN 2016045199| ISBN 9789813206908 (hardcover : alk. paper) |
ISBN 9789813206915 (pbk. : alk. paper)
Subjects: | MESH: Mental Health Services | Mental Health | Mental Disorders--therapy |
Psychiatry--education | Health Policy | Singapore
Classification: LCC RC455 | NLM WM 30 JS6 | DDC 362.2--dc23
LC record available at https://lccn.loc.gov/2016045199

British Library Cataloguing-in-Publication Data
A catalogue record for this book is available from the British Library.

Printed in Singapore

A recent survey by the World Psychiatric Association countries showed that nearly half of the countries belonging to the British Commonwealth do not have a mental health policy. Some of the reasons include colonial influences and others include stigma and a clear discrimination and lack of equity between mental and physical health. Cartesian mind-body dualism has unwittingly led to a deep division between physical and mental health and in many countries specialists in mental and physical health do not communicate effectively with each other. Furthermore a lack of integration between different age groups can lead to artificial barriers which patients and their carers may find difficult to navigate.

This volume describes not only the state of psychiatry in Singapore but also explains different subspecialties. The descriptions are by academics, clinicians and others making the story of Singapore psychiatry become vivid in the reader's mind's eye. There are innovative services for example early intervention service working with children and young people. Subspecialities are described both in the historical context and also in the present making it easy for the reader to understand challenges, issues and examples of good practice. In addition the book has contributions from other disciplines and their development in the country which contributes a holistic approach to mental health care and delivery. This is a welcome addition to the field and hopefully will be read widely as there are lessons to be learnt by other countries in planning and delivering services.

Prof. Dinesh Bhugra, CBE
MA, MSc, MPhil, MBBS, FRCP, FRCPE, FRCPsych, FFPHM, PhD, FRCPsych(Hon), FACP(Hon), FHKCPsych(Hon), FAMS(Sing), FRSA, FAcad Med Ed
Emeritus Professor of Mental Health and Cultural Diversity
Institute of Psychiatry, Psychology and Neuroscience
King's College London
President, World Psychiatric Association 2014–2017

Beng Yeong and Daniel have done the Singapore mental healthcare community a great service by bringing together in one volume a comprehensive collection of papers documenting the recent history of developments in the treatment and care of persons with mental health conditions seen from a broad spectrum of players — clinicians, allied health professionals, social workers, academics etc. This will certainly serve as a must-have reference for all organisations involved in mental health work for many years to come!

Dr. Francis Yeoh
President, Singapore Association for Mental Health

I heartily congratulate the authors for their excellent portrayal of the way mental health care has developed in Singapore, as our sciences advance and social perceptions change. Mental health is both an art and a science, and delivery of care continues to evolve. This book chronicles in detail the development of our community of health professionals committed to improving care for mental health within Singapore and our region. Rightly so, it is a collaborative effort of psychiatrists, psychologists and other allied healthcare professionals who have played key roles in the exponential growth mental health care landscape within Singapore. This book serves as a good read for psychiatrists and non-psychiatrists alike to appreciate how our community of health professionals dedicated to mental health care together with healthcare models have developed steadily over the years. From psychiatry education to the growth of new fields of psychiatry and allied health professions focused on mental health, there is really a wealth of knowledge within this book which everyone can learn from. I strongly encourage all to pick up this book!

Dr. Selan Sayampanathan, PBM
MB,BS (S'pore), FRCS (Edin), FAMS (Orth)
Master (2016–2018)
Academy of Medicine, Singapore

Preface

Under the supervision and guidance from Professor Chee Kuan Tsee, the first author Ng Beng Yeong traced and chronicled the historical developments of psychiatry and mental health services in Singapore from 1841 to 1993. The documentation ended in 1993 as in April 1993, Woodbridge Hospital moved to its new premises in Hougang, and the Institute of Mental Health was established. For many years after the book *Till the Break of Day: A History of Mental Health Services in Singapore, 1841–1993* was published, it has been our cherished dream that a sequel can be written to update readers on the developments in the mental health scene following 1993. The idea to have this second book was largely the second author Daniel Fung's brainchild and it is indeed very different from the first one. This second book is written by many authors, so that readers will gain a broader perspective from different individuals, who helped to create and developed the mental health services that we have today.

In 2005, the Ministry of Health (MOH) appointed a National Mental Health Committee to propose a National Mental Health Policy for Singapore. The committee, made up of public and private psychiatrists as well as MOH administrators, collaborated with other mental health professionals and representatives from non-governmental organisations to draw up the policy. The committee followed the guidelines of the World Health Organisation (WHO) in identifying the aims, the values that underpin the policy and the strategic focus for the following 10 years. The aims of Singapore's National Mental Health Policy are essentially twofold: to promote mental health and, where possible, prevent the development of mental health problems and disorders; and to reduce the impact of mental disorders. Acting on the National Mental Health Policy, the committee drew up the National Mental Health Blueprint (NMHB), which highlights the strategic focus for the next five years from 2007 to 2011 as follows: Mental Health Education and Promotion; Integrated Mental Health Care; Developing Mental Health Professionals; and Developing Mental Health Research. All these efforts are chronicled in this book.

NMHBP led to projects totalling S$180 million including the Singapore Mental Health Study (completed in 2010). The Community Mental Health Masterplan was developed in 2012 and the estimated budget for this Masterplan was S$237 million. Taken together, these two plans focus on strengthening the core mental health services for the detection, intervention and rehabilitation of mental health patients, especially in the community. Important progress has since been made in the key areas, and it is hence timely for us to document the milestones that we have achieved.

In 2014, a 127-year-old boundary wall of a defunct lunatic asylum was unearthed in the heart of the Singapore General Hospital (SGH). The wall is significant as it was part of the 1887 New Lunatic Asylum. Asia Paranormal Investigators co-founder Charles Goh had alerted the National Heritage Board (NHB) to the 3 m-high, 75 m-long wall in September 2014. Mr Goh, a heritage enthusiast, had stumbled upon the wall while exploring the old forested area near Macalister Road. The NHB then embarked on a three-month research project. The New Lunatic Asylum was revolutionary for its time as its practices demonstrated humanity; for instance, it stopped using straitjackets. The only mechanical restraint used at the asylum was locked gloves which consisted of two small padded canvas bags tied around the wrists to prevent self-injury or destructive behaviour. The treatment of the inmates at the new asylum was holistic and included 'kindness, freedom from restraint, regular hours, good food, open air exercise and occupation' (cited from the Straits Settlements records). It is hoped that various agencies can work towards protecting the wall so that we will have something historic to show future generations.

Over the years, important changes have also taken place in the way in which we train our next generation of psychiatrists. We have switched from the British-based basic and advanced traineeship system to the American-based Residency Programme. Inevitably, there are challenges to the existing healthcare system and it is important to document the switch and transitions that have occurred. An important milestone in the history of local psychiatry was achieved on 5 November 2014 when the College of Psychiatrists was officially formed. Also, we now have three medical schools in Singapore and there is an increasing need to harmonise the training programmes for psychiatry in the three schools. It is hoped that this second book will be a useful guide for mental health professionals and be an important tool in the training of psychiatrists, medical students, psychologists, social workers, nurses, counsellors and other healthcare professionals.

A/Prof. Ng Beng Yeong
Consultant Psychiatrist
Ng Beng Yeong Psych Medicine Clinic
Mount Elizabeth Medical Centre
Adjunct Associate Professor, Duke-NUS Medical School
Past President, College of Psychiatrists
Singapore

and

A/Prof. Daniel Fung
Chairman, Medical Board
Institute of Mental Health
Yong Loo Lin School of Medicine, NUS
Duke-NUS Medical School
Lee Kong Chian School of Medicine, NTU
Singapore

Foreword

The history of psychiatry has been one which is fraught with more misses than hits in terms of helping the mentally ill. More often than not, because of the stigma and myths of mental illness, the story of the development of mental health services are often hidden or untold. The Institute of Mental Health (IMH) has been the main provider of mental health services in Singapore and its history until Dr Ng Beng Yeong's *Till the Break of Day* was never told in a systematic way. Yet that first systematic account is now over 20 years old and the progress that mental health services have made demands an update. The stigma of mental illness is still prevalent. Psychiatry is still very much disconnected from mainstream health services. But the tide is changing. As governments realise that acute medical care is becoming too expensive to sustain and as most services start to focus on the Institute of Healthcare Improvement's Triple Aim of Population Health, Cost Effective Care and a better Experience of Care, the importance of mental health in health becomes increasingly important. The need to integrate mental health and health means that the development of all medical services must consider the development of mental health services. There is no better time to tell the story of how mental health and IMH have moved in these last 23 years since 1993, when IMH relocated to its present premises and heralded the development of psychiatric services in every general hospital. Like many stories, this is an ongoing journey and I am glad that unlike the first account, it is one told from multiple viewpoints, psychiatrists as well as other members of the multidisciplinary team. I must congratulate the authors for making the effort to bring this chapter in the development of mental health services in Singapore to life.

A/Prof. Chua Hong Choon
Chief Executive Officer
Institute of Mental Health, Singapore

Contents

Preface vii

Foreword xi

Development of Services

Child and Adolescent Psychiatry 1
TOR Phern Chern, Daniel FUNG and ONG Say How

Children and Psychiatry 1
Child Psychiatry in Singapore 2
Research and Education 5
Specialised Services 7
Development of Child Mental Health Services 8
References 9

Early Psychosis Intervention Programme 11
Swapna VERMA, Sujatha RAO, Helen LEE,
POON Lye Yin and CHONG Siow Ann

Psychosis and the Need for Early Intervention 11
Duration of Untreated Psychosis 12
Development of a New System of Care 13
Public Education 14
Networking with Primary Healthcare Providers 15
Clinical Services 17
Moving Towards Indicated Prevention 18
Peer Support Movement in EPIP 20
Recognition of the Work 20
New Initiatives Moving Forward 23

EPIP Inpatient Centre 24
References 26

Addiction Medicine 29
Suresh ANANTHA

Alcohol, Addiction and Mental Health 29
Other Addictions 30
Alcohol Treatment Centre at the New Woodbridge Hospital 31
Community Addictions Management Programme (CAMP) 32
CAMP and the Buprenorphine Years 36
Treatment for Special Populations and Helpline 37
Other Community-Based Services 38
Inpatient Programme 39
The Transformation of CAMP to NAMS 40
NAMS and Problem Gambling 41
Specialist Outpatient Clinic C 42
Development of New Clinical Services 42
Research in Addictions 45
The Future 47
References 49

Geriatric Psychiatry 51
NG Li Ling and SENG Kok Han

Development of Services for the Elderly 51
Aged Psychiatry Community and Treatment Service (APCATS) 52
Dementia-Friendly Ward and Memory Clinic 53
References 54

Community Psychiatry 55
LEE Cheng

Mental Health Services in the Community 55
Community Psychiatric Services in Singapore 57
Community Clinics 58
Community Psychiatric Nursing (CPN) Service 59

Assertive Community Treatment (ACT) 60
Mobile Crisis Team (MCT) 61
Community Mental Health Team (CMHT) 63
Mental Health Helpline 67
Community Psychiatry of the Future 68
References 69

Military Psychiatry 71
SOH Teck Hwee and Christopher CHEOK

Psychiatrists in the Military 71
The Early Years 72
Evolving Needs in Operations 72
Increasing Capacity 74
Part of the National Mental Health System 77
Reference 79

Forensic Psychiatry 81
Jerome GOH, Kenneth KOH, Stephen PHANG and ONG Say How

Introduction 81
Forensic Subspecialisation 82
Adult Psychiatry Services in IMH 82
Child and Adolescent Forensic Psychiatry Services in IMH 87
Conclusions and Future Plans 90
References 92

Suicide in Singapore 93
CHIA Boon Hock

Introduction 93
Suicide Rates 94
Singapore's Suicide Rate 95
Ethnic Differences 97
Elderly Suicide Rates 97
Gender Differences 99
Protective Factors 99

Risk Factors 100
Identifying Suicidality 106
Methods of Suicide 111
The Role of the Media 113
Conclusion 114
References 115

Mental Health Professions

Psychotherapy Movement 119
GWEE Kok Peng

Introduction 119
Universal Historical Development 120
The Development of Therapies in Singapore 121
The New Millennium — Back to the Beginning 124
The 2010s and Beyond — Facing the Future 126
Giving Back 128
References 130

The Development of Psychiatric Nursing 133
Samantha ONG

The Pioneering Years 133
Beginning of a New Era 134
Psychiatric Nursing in the New Millennium 139
Patient Safety and Quality Improvement 141
Advanced Practice Nursing 142
Mental Health Nursing Education 143
Centre for Mental Health Education 144
JIBI — IMH Attliate Centre for Mental Health Care 145
American Nurses Credentialing Center Accreditation with Distinction 145
National Resuscitation Council Accreditation 146
Management of Aggression and Violence Training 146
Nursing Research and Evidence Based Practice 147

Community Psychiatric Nursing Services 149
Nursing Projects 150
Awards 151
Conclusion 152
Acknowledgement 153
Reference 153

Allied Health Professionals in Psychiatry Care

Psychiatric Social Work in Singapore 155
Lilian MARK and Siti Sohanah Binte KASMANI

How the Past Has Shaped the Future 155
A New Era 157
A Renewed Focus: Towards Advanced Practice in Psychiatric Social Work 159
Conclusion 163
References 163

The Growth and Development of the Psychological Services in IMH 165
Clare YEO, Carolyn KEE, Kala MEHROTRA, GOH Tze Jui, ONG Lue Ping, Jolly CHUA, Nikki LIM, ONG Li Min, GWEE Kenji, HUANG Wanping, Chermain WONG, Siva PENCHALIAH, Haanusia Prithivi RAJ, Matthew WOO, Ann-Marie LO CASTRO, Shannon PEH, Jade JANG, WONG Chin Meng, Clare KWAN and KOK Yun Fern

Early Years 165
1993–2000 166
2000–Present 167
Clinical Units and Services 168
Intervention Programmes and Interest Groups 178
Training and Supervision 183
Mental Health Education Initiatives 185
Future Direction of the Psychological Services at IMH 187
References 188

Psychological Services in Other Hospitals 189
Jimmy YAP

Introduction 189
Tan Tock Seng Hospital 189
National University Hospital 191
Singapore General Hospital 194
Changi General Hospital 196
Khoo Teck Puat Hospital 199
KK Women's and Children's Hospital 200
Acknowledgement 204

Occupational Therapists 205
TAN Bhing Leet, HO Soo Fung, IBRAHIM Kamaldin, SIM So Sin, ANN Esther and Jovin HO

Moving into New Premises 205
Rehabilitation in Occupational Therapy Workshops 206
Activities and Events 207
Vocational Rehabilitation in the 1990s 211
Developing Vocational Rehabilitation in Mental Health (2003–2013) 212
Rehabilitating Patients with Psychiatric Disorders 218
Specialised Occupational Therapy Services 222
OT Services in Restructured Hospitals 227
OT Services in Voluntary Welfare Organisations 228
Conclusion 230
References 230

Case Managers 231
Margaret HENDRICKS

Introduction 231
Definition of Case Management, the Model We Use and What Do We Do 232
Training 233
What We Have Achieved 235

Awards 237
How Do Our Patients View Our Services 240
What Our Team Members Think of the Case Managers 242
Case Managers at Work 243
Conclusion 244
References 244

Psychiatric Services in General Hospitals

Changi General Hospital: From Service to Department 245
YAP Hwa Ling and TAN Sheng Neng

About Changi General Hospital 245
Facilities 245
Staffing 246
Range of Services 246
Teaching, Training and Research 247
The Future 248

National University Hospital System: The Journey of Academic Psychiatry in a University Hospital 249
TENG Jia Ying and John Chee Meng WONG

Founding of the Department (1979–1994) 249
Education and Training 251
Research 252
Development of Clinical Services (1995–2016) 255
Specialised Clinical Services 256
Improving Clinical Services and Teaching at Ward 33 256
Compassion for our Patients 257
Integrated Care in the Community 257
Further Development of Research, Training and Education 261
Nurturing the Next Generation 261
The Way Forward 261
Acknowledgement 262
References 262

Khoo Teck Puat Hospital 263
Chris CHEOK and CHAN Keen Loong

Pioneering Care in the North 263
Community Programmes 263
Manpower Resources 265
Conclusions 265

Jurong Health Services: Psychiatry for the West 267
Michael YONG Kian Hui

The Birth of Psychiatry in Singapore General Hospital 271
WAN Yi Min and Leslie LIM

Conclusion 278
Acknowledgements 278
References 279

A Brief History of the Department of Psychological Medicine, Tan Tock Seng Hospital 283
Aaron ANG Lye Poh

In the Beginning 283
Developing Services 285
Severe Acute Respiratory Syndrome 287
Mental Health Blueprint and Other Programmes 289
The Next Lap 290
Acknowledgements 292
References 292

Psychiatry Services at KK Women's and Children's Hospital 293
Helen CHEN Yu

Introduction of Psychiatry to KKH 293
KKH Mental Wellness Service (2006-2012) 294
Mental Wellness Service — Pop or Real? 295
Becoming Department of Psychological Medicine, KKH 299
Conclusion 302
References 302

Education in Mental Health

Training for Undergraduates 303
Roger HO, Melvyn ZHANG, Aaron TIONG and Joel WONG

The Experiences at Yong Loo Lin School of Medicine, National University of Singapore: 1990–2015 303
Education Direction for the Future 304
Undergraduate Research Opportunity Programme 310
Conclusion 315

Academic Psychiatry 317
Rathi MAHENDRAN

Introduction 317
Psychiatry Education 317
Research 319
Clinical Service 320
The Growth of Academic Psychiatry 320
The Future 321
References 323

Psychiatry Specialist Training 325
CHIAM Peak Chiang

Introduction 325
Seamless Training 326
Residency Training 326
Evolving Specialist Training 329
References 329

Mental Health Research 331
CHONG Siow Ann

Definition of Research 331
Development of Research in IMH 331
Cognition and Biomarkers 333
Mental Health Policy 333

Addictions 334
Children and Adolescents 335
Ethics 336
Notable Achievements 336
Acknowledgements 338

Mental Health of the Nation

Developing a National Mental Health Blueprint 339
Daniel FUNG and CHUA Hong Choon

Strategic Initiatives 343
Focus Area 1: Primary Prevention and Health Promotion 344
Focus Area 2: Provision and Coordination of Services 345
Focus Area 3: Mental Health Professionals 347
Focus Area 4: Monitoring 348
Focus Area 5: Research 348
Cost of Initiatives 349
Indicators and Targets Used 349
Conclusions 350
Moving Ahead 351
References 352

Samaritans of Singapore 353
Arnab Kumar GHOSH, KHOO Hui Leng and Christine WONG

Introduction 353
History 353
Key Milestones 354
24-Hour Hotline Service 355
Email Befriending 357
Specialist Counselling 357
Local Outreach to Suicide Survivors (LOSS) 357
Healing Bridge 358
Crisis Support 358
Referral and Case Consultations 359

Professional Training 359
Community Awareness and Outreach 360
Conclusion 360
References 361

The Development of Mental Health Services by VWOs 363
TAN Weng Mooi and Elaine SOH

Moving from Custodial Care to Community Support Care 363
Community Support Care 365
Paradigm Shift to Community Therapeutic Care 369
Caregiver' Mental Well-Being is Equally Important as the Clients' 372
Destigmatisation 374
Not Forgetting Development of Support for Dementia Clients and Caregivers 375
National Mental Health Blueprint 377
Community Mental Health Masterplan Towards a Community-Based Population Health Approach 378
With HEART, We Can Achieve "Integrated Community Living, Ageing in Place' 383
References 384

Child and Adolescent Psychiatry

TOR Phern Chern, Daniel FUNG and ONG Say How

Children and Psychiatry

A child in Singapore as defined by the Children and Young Person's Act is someone under the age of 14. Worldwide definitions for age of majority when children become adults by law differ country to country, ranging from 15 (e.g. Indonesia) to 21 (e.g. Singapore), and is complicated by the period that defines adolescence. While it remains debatable whether adolescence should start at age 13 (*Psychology Today*, 2017) and ends at age 19 or even as high as 25 (Arnone, 2014) in current developmental psychology, the World Health Organization defines adolescence as a period between 10 and 19 years of age. The development of the discipline of child psychiatry emerged from research surrounding child development and that of emotional disturbance and disabilities. Adolescent psychiatry is that aspect of child psychiatry that focuses on mental health issues arising or presenting typically during the adolescence phase. For convenience and practicality, child and adolescent psychiatry is considered together here as a single 'child psychiatry' entity. Child psychiatry is a subspecialty of psychiatry while psychiatry is a medical specialty. There is much public confusion of this as many professionals, including doctors, think that psychiatrists and psychologists are interchangeable terms. The reality is that psychiatrists are medical doctors while psychologists are not, and only clinical psychologists work in clinical settings like clinics and hospitals. This confusion is made worse in child psychiatry where most of the work does not involve medications which only the medical doctor can prescribe. In the English-speaking world, most psychiatrists will agree that child psychiatry started at the turn of the 19th century and became popularised through the child guidance clinic movement in the 1920s. Its goal was to prevent juvenile delinquency but it also saw the importance of fostering educational interventions and protecting the child from abuse. The first textbook of child psychiatry was published in 1935 by Leo Kanner (Kanner 1935, 1943) (who was also credited with describing autism in 1943) and the first Chair of Child Psychiatry was established in Missouri, USA, occupied by E. James Anthony.

Child Psychiatry in Singapore

Child psychiatry in Singapore officially began on 7 April 1970 under Dr Wong Sze Tai, when the Ministry of Health (MOH) opened the Child Guidance Clinic (CGC) at the Outram Road General Hospital (now known as the Singapore General Hospital) in a bungalow originally occupied by the medical superintendent. The groundwork for establishing CGC was undertaken by Dr Ho Eng Siong (a Senior Registrar psychiatrist) and Mr Fred Long (psychologist) under the leadership of Dr Yap Meow Foo (the medical superintendent of Woodbridge Hospital, WH) between 1967 and 1969. CGC operated initially on the equivalent of two days a week. Less than a year after starting the service, the roof of the clinic collapsed as a supporting beam broke. The building was declared unsafe for occupation and the clinic moved to the Kallang Maternal and Child Health Clinic and resumed services on 17th Mar 1971 with the equivalent of three days a week after the addition of a medical officer and social worker. CGC stayed in Kallang for two years and was providing full-time services from 1972.

CGC subsequently moved to a pre-war nurse's hostel (Annexe building) at Russel Road at Alexandra Park and stayed there for the next 10 years. Patients were charged $1 for subsidised referrals and $35 for named referrals. Despite the multiple logistical and manpower challenges at the time, the mood was described as "exciting, with time for tea between cases" and "one of hope amidst great struggling". From the beginning a team approach was adopted with all cases seen by the psychiatrist, psychologist, social worker, nurse, occupational therapist, a trained child therapist from Australia and even a remedial teacher from the Ministry of Education. New cases were discussed by the multidisciplinary team (MDT) during memorable lunchtime meetings to establish a management plan.

Under Dr Wong Sze Tai's leadership, CGC was renamed Child Psychiatry Clinic (CPC) in 1972 to reflect that the clinic provided more services than ''mere guidance''. It moved in 1982 to a more conveniently located and expanded facility at the Institute of Health in Outram Road. An observation room with a one-way mirror was set up in CPC that allowed trainees and staff to observe assessments and therapy sessions. The sessions could also be recorded for teaching and evaluation purposes. In 1993 the clinic went back to being called the Child Guidance Clinic in line with the establishment of the Department of Child and Adolescent Psychiatry (DCAP) and in 1998 it moved to its current location at the Health Promotion Board (HPB) building in the Outram Park campus.

There was simultaneously a clear need for an inpatient Child Psychiatry service. Children and adolescents that required psychiatric admission were admitted to the adult wards in WH. This situation was far from ideal due to the custodial nature of WH at that time and there were efforts to have a Child Psychiatry inpatient unit at St Andrew's Hospital in Siglap in collaboration with Dr Stephanie Leonard, before the Child Psychiatry Inpatient Unit (CPIU) (*The Straits Times, 1981*) was established in WH in 1980 initially under Dr Goh Choo Woon and then under Dr Pushpa Bose for the next 10 years.

The CPIU was an 18-bed unit converted from the old Matrons quarters and enjoyed a more homely atmosphere than the rest of WH. It was moved to the basement of Block 3 in the new WH in 1993 and called the Child and Adolescent Inpatient Unit (CAIU) led by Dr Aw Soh Choo. In 2005 the inpatient ward was reorganised to allow for graded levels of care to allow disturbed patients and recovered patients to be at different ends of the ward with space set aside for sports and recreation. The new ward was renamed Sunrise Wing and had 20 beds catering to the most severely ill children and adolescents with mental disorders.

In 1993 the new WH was opened after years of planning (*The Straits Times*, 1989) and the Department of Child and Adolescent Psychiatry was formed and headed by Dr Cai Yiming. Over the years, the Department developed various services to address specific needs such as Children's One-Stop Psycho-Educational Service (COPES) which was led by Dr Daniel Fung.

Table 1: Heads of Department of Child and Adolescent Psychiatry.

Year	Head	Service/Department
1970	Dr Wong Sze Tai	Child Psychiatric Clinic
1993	Dr Cai Yiming	Child and Adolescent Psychiatry
2006	Dr Daniel Fung	Child and Adolescent Psychiatry
2011	Dr Ong Say How	Child and Adolescent Psychiatry

Source: Department of Child & Adolescent Psychiatry Statistics (2014), Institute of Mental Health.

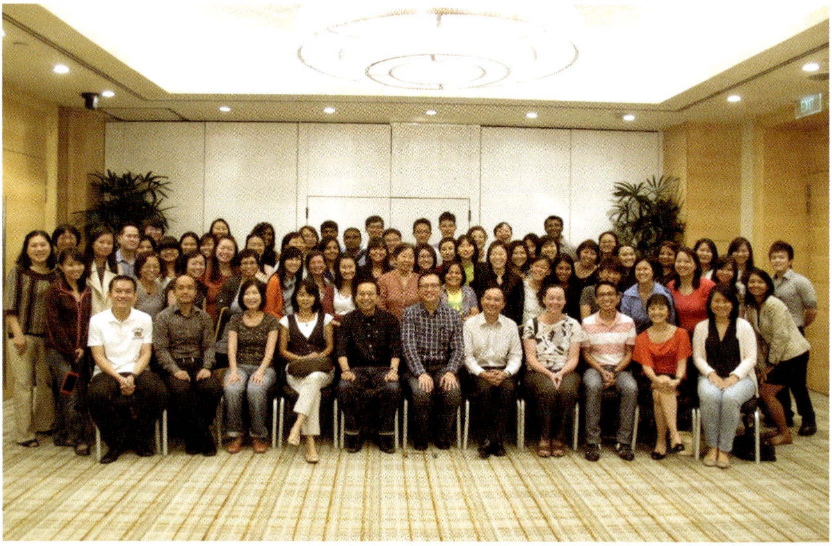

Institute of mental health child psychiatry departmental retreat held in 2012.

'I remember how Dr Cai as he assumed the headship of the Child Psychiatric Clinic and the setting up of the Department of Child and Adolescent Psychiatry in 1993, started a practice of reviewing work output on little charts at the front of the clinic. Every clinician's monthly workload was reflected and it made me as a medical officer, rather conscious of the number of new patients I saw. This was my introduction to regular feedback

and accountability of work which is the hallmark of my personal practice. Today, our hospital is focused on measuring, not only output, but outcomes and providing individual accountability for our work.'

Daniel Fung

Research and Education

Despite heavy clinical and teaching loads, CGC had a clear research agenda right from its inception. Dr Wong encouraged multisectoral research well before it was popular to do so. One example was the work with the Ministry of Community Development on a prospective four-year study of the effects of kindergarten versus home care for children as the government was encouraging women to go to work. The 1979 report was entitled 'The Child and Changing Family Patterns in Singapore' and stated that children in kindergarten did better in mathematics and children at home had better language development, but these effects were temporary. This research led to a white paper that went up to then Prime Minister Goh Chok Tong and that later led to the development of the National Family Council. It also received prominent attention in the mainstream media. CGC also collaborated with Dr Aileen Wong (later Senior Minister of State for Health) on research on low-cost housing and children. A 1994 interview with the then president of Singapore Association for Mental Health (SAMH), Dr Ang Peng Chye, highlighted the increasing demand for mental healthcare for children (*The Straits Times*, 1994). This increase in number of children being brought by their parents to see psychiatrists for stress-related problems was reported in another article in *The Straits Times* (*The Straits Times*, 1999). Recognizing the need to reach out to the public to correct their misconceptions about mental illnesses, an open house with a Youth Carnival theme was organised by WH in June 2000 (*The Straits Times*, 2000) to encourage teens to seek help early as many psychological problems take root in teenage years.

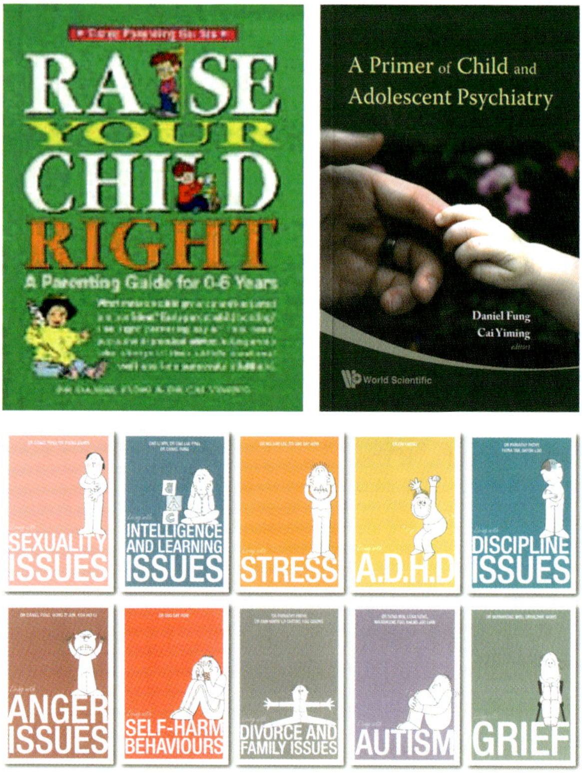

Some books on child mental health.

A well-received series of books on issues in child mental health was published from 1998 by Times Books International with titles like *Help Your Child to Cope: Understanding Childhood Stress* and *Raise Your Child Right: A Parenting Guide for 0–6 Years*. In 2008 the first local textbook on child psychiatry, *A Primer of Child and Adolescent Psychiatry*, was published by World Scientific (Fung and Cai, 2008). Other books published include the well-reviewed *Living with* series covering 10 topics ranging from attention deficit hyperactivity disorder and autism to self-harm and grief. These books have since been updated in 2015.

Table 2: Patients seen in the outpatient clinics, 2007–2014.

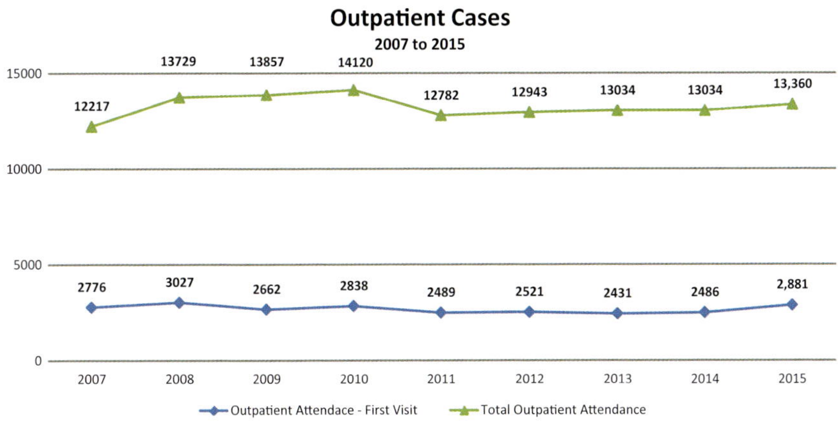

Sources: http://www.singstat.gov.sg/publications/publications-and-papers/population-and-population-structure/population-trends

Department of Child & Adolescent Psychiatry Statistics (2014), Institute of Mental Health.

Specialised Services

Child psychiatry in Singapore has grown from an ad hoc, part-time service to a full department with 12 consultants, six medical officers, six clinical psychologists and three medical social workers with a full complement of nurses and administrative staff. From 550 children and families a year in 1980, CGC now sees just under 3000 a year in 2011. The Autism Clinic was set up in 2006 to deal with behavioural and emotional problems in autism and led by Dr Sung Min. With National Mental Health Blueprint (NMHBP), community teams were developed over five years from 2007, spearheaded by the department but working across three hospitals: Institute of Mental Health, Kandang Kerbau Hospital Women's and Children's Hospital (KKH) and National University Hospital System (NUHS). The programme is named REACH (Response, Early Intervention and Assessment in Community Mental Health) which clearly emphasises its objectives to reach out to all the schoolgoing children through working with their school counsellors. Further subspecialisation of child psychiatry services was conducted to better reflect the tertiary nature of the work in 2010–2011: Neurobehavioural Clinic (NBC), Mood and Anxiety Clinic (MAC) and Child Forensic Services (FRIENDS, Forensic Rehabilitation, Intervention, Evaluation & Network Development Services). Each team is fully supported by child psychiatrists and multidisciplinary allied health staff.

Development of Child Mental Health Services

The plans going forward are to continue integration of services in KKH and NUHS, and to strengthen links with community agencies to enhance mental healthcare for the future of our nation. NUHS has since developed a full-fledged service while specialist clinics have also began to operate in Singapore General Hospital (for eating disorders), Changi General Hospital (for adolescent services) and Khoo Teck Puat Hospital (outpatient child psychiatry services). Additionally, collaboration with several key players such as HPB, Ministry of Social and Family Development (MSF), Voluntary Welfare Organizations (VWOs) and Ministry of Education (MOE) are ongoing in several projects and programmes. The main focus presently is to target the younger population further upstream so as to reduce psychiatric and psychological problems as they grow up to be adolescents and young adults. One example of such initiatives include setting up a community-based programme for all preschoolers like that of the REACH programme which is accessible by all public and special education schools. Closer collaboration in research locally and internationally has also taken flight over the last five years with inter-ministerial collaborations and multinational research with overseas universities and hospitals.

Improving existing medical education and cultivating the younger generation of doctors and psychiatrists have also been the mission of the department. With the recent addition of a third medical school, Lee Kong Chian School of Medicine (the others being NUS Yong Loo Lin School of

Medicine and DUKE-NUS Medical School), there would be challenges ahead in terms of coordination and organisation of teaching and curriculum development to meet the unique needs of the different groups of medical students. Likewise, with the implementation of the National Psychiatry Residency Programme and upcoming child psychiatry residency in the elective year, the medical education landscape is set to change. What one would expect would be a more integrated and concerted effort in curriculum development, greater use of innovative and effective teaching methods and benchmarking local training against international standards.

Changes in the landscape of child psychiatry in Singapore have indeed become more rapid and observable over the past 10 years especially in the form of shaping mental health policies, improving medical education, intensifying research collaborations and developing new clinical services. With certainty, these will be met with great anticipation by all child mental health professionals and workers now and in the future.

References

Arnone JM (2014). Adolescents may be older than we think: Today 25 is the new 18, or is it? *J Celiac Dis* **2**(2): 47–48. DOI: 10.12691/ijcd-2-2-4.

Fung D, Cai Y, eds. (2008). *A Primer of Child and Adolescent Psychiatry*. World Scientific Publishing Company, Singapore.

Kanner L (1935). *Child Psychiatry*. Chas. C. Thomas, Springfield.

Kanner L (1943). Autistic disturbances of affective contact. *Nerv Child* **2**: 217–250.

Protection of Children in Singapore: An Overview. Research and Advocacy Standing Committee, Singapore Children's Society. https://www.childrensociety.org.sg/resources/front/template/scs/.../child-protection.pdf

Teenagers — Adolescence. *Psychology Today*. Retrieved 19 June 2017 from https://www.psychologytoday.com/basics/adolescence.

The Straits Times, 23 May 1981. 'New Unit for Young Patients'.

The Straits Times, 11 Jun 1989. 'New Name, New Facilities for Woodbridge Hospital'.

The Straits Times, 24 Oct 1994. 'More Children Receiving Psychiatry Care'.
The Straits Times, 11 Oct 1999. 'More Parents Taking Kids to Psychiatrists'.
The Straits Times, 11 Jun 2000. 'Open House to Encourage Teens to Seek Help'.
Thirumoorthy T, Loke P. (August 2013). Consent in Medical Practice 3. SMA Centre for Medical Ethics & Professionalism, *SMA News*.

Early Psychosis Intervention Programme

Swapna VERMA, Sujatha RAO, Helen LEE,
POON Lye Yin and CHONG Siow Ann

'We should remember that the alternative to early, optimal intervention is delayed and substandard treatment with all its consequences.'

Lieberman and Fenton (2000)

Psychosis and the Need for Early Intervention

Psychosis is a serious and potentially chronic mental disorder with a profound impact on patients and their families and on society. The World Health Organization's Global Burden of Disease lists schizophrenia among the top 10 contributors to health burden and disability worldwide (Murray and Lopez, 1996). A study carried out within the United Kingdom's National Health Service (NHS) revealed that the annual expenditure for chronic diseases is the highest for psychosis (NHS Executive, 1996). The cost of treatment for schizophrenia is estimated to be as much as £397 million, and the indirect cost of schizophrenia is estimated to be as much as £1.76 billion per annum (Sainsbury Centre for Mental Health, 1998). The concept of early intervention had been around for decades but did not become of popular opinion until the publication of some key research studies (e.g. Falloon 1992; Loebel *et al.*, 1992; McGlashan, 1996; McGorry, 1998) and a rapid growth of enthusiasm during the 1990s. Several countries had begun to develop national mental health strategies or frameworks to guide major reform in mental healthcare and encourage a preventative approach. This blend of science and social movement led to a substantial change in the way mental illnesses were managed.

Duration of Untreated Psychosis

The growing body of evidence showed that early treatment could result in a significant reduction in morbidity (i.e. reduction in disabilities, hospitalisation, disruption in the family, suicides and costs), and a better quality of life for patients and their families (McGlashan, 1996, Larsen *et al.*, 1998). Table 1 shows the potential benefits of early intervention. By reducing the duration of untreated psychosis (DUP) — defined as the time between the onset of the first psychotic symptoms and the first adequate treatment — the outcome of schizophrenia could potentially be changed. A review reported that approximately two-thirds of the 25 studies on DUP have shown a significant association between shorter DUP and better outcome (Lieberman *et al.*, 2001). The average DUP in most Western countries is between one and two years (Johnstone *et al.*, 1986). In Singapore, we found that the average DUP of patients with first-episode psychosis was 33 months (Chong *et al.*, 2005a).

There may be several factors that contribute to a long DUP, including: ignorance, stigma, denial, lack of motivation, absence of information about early psychosis and lack of access to appropriate interventions. In Singapore the manifestations of psychosis are often attributed to supernatural causes. It was found that around 24% of patients with first-episode psychosis had sought the help of traditional healers at the first

Table 1: Potential benefits of early intervention.

- Reduced morbidity.
- More rapid recovery.
- Better prognosis.
- Preservation of psychosocial skills.
- Preservation of family and social supports.
- Decreased need for hospitalisation.
- Early detection of new cases.
- Shortening the delays to effective treatment.
- Provision of optimal and sustained treatment in the early ‘critical period’.

onset of symptoms (Chong *et al.*, 2001). Studies have also shown that the 'critical period' follows recovery from a first episode of psychosis and extends for up to five years subsequently, and it is a phase of high vulnerability (Birchwood *et al.*, 1998). It has been shown that the level of disability attained within the first two years or so after entry to treatment, strongly predicts the level of disability many years later. Also, the delay in treatment actually contributes to a worse outcome, or is the link due to a common underlying factor such as a more severe form of the illness, a more insidious onset, more negative symptoms, more paranoid ideation, less salience and awareness of change or less willingness to seek and accept treatment. Reducing the burden of disease during this crucial period is worthwhile even if it does not influence the ultimate level of disability. Table 2 shows the factors associated with delay of treatment.

Table 2: Factors associated with treatment delay.

- Difficulties in recognition: general practitioners' lack of experience and training in psychiatric interviewing can mean that important features of mental state go unrecognised.
- Misinterpretation by families i.e. attributed to supernatural causes.
- Reluctance to seek help: poor knowledge of the features of mental disorders and their treatability.
- The stigma and shame associated with mental disorders.
- Denial that a problem exists.
- Lack of confidence in the health professionals and the treatments they provide.
- Lack of access to effective interventions.

Development of a New System of Care

The alarmingly long DUP in Singapore, its possible consequences and the lack of appropriate and effective interventions for psychotic disorders, were the impetus for establishing the Early Psychosis Intervention Programme (EPIP). The programme was initiated in April 2001 under the auspices of the Health Services Development Programme of the Singapore Ministry of Health.

epip
early
psychosis
intervention
programme

The aims of EPIP are to:

- Raise awareness of the early signs and symptoms of psychosis.
- Reduce the stigma associated with psychosis.
- Establish strong links with primary healthcare providers and collaborate in the detection, referral, and management of those with psychosis.
- Detect and manage psychosis early through screening and continuous monitoring of those with a 'high risk' of developing psychosis.
- Improve the outcome and quality of life of those with psychosis and reduce the burden of care for their families.

With these aims in mind, EPIP embarked on engaging the different stakeholders using a variety of strategies.

Public Education

The aim of providing the public with information on the manifestation of psychosis and the importance of early treatment is to encourage help-seeking behaviour, thereby increasing self/family referrals and reducing police referrals as well as increasing the number of individuals screened for psychosis, hence reducing the duration of untreated psychosis. Public education campaigns include the following:

- A series of English and Mandarin public forums were held around Singapore, some of which involved local celebrities to aid in the campaigns.

- Regularly scheduled interviews with a psychiatrist were aired on radio stations, providing the public with opportunities to call in to have their questions answered.
- Numerous articles on psychosis and the services of the programme have been published in national newspapers and magazines since the programme's inception.
- An easy-to-read, psychosis-specific book was published for patients, families and care providers.
- Posters were displayed at Mass Rapid Transit stations.

A website (www.epip.org.sg) and a hotline telephone service were set up to provide information on the programme and to facilitate inquiries from the public.

Networking with Primary Healthcare Providers

The majority of the people approach primary healthcare providers before they seek help from psychiatrists. It was found that around 24% of patients

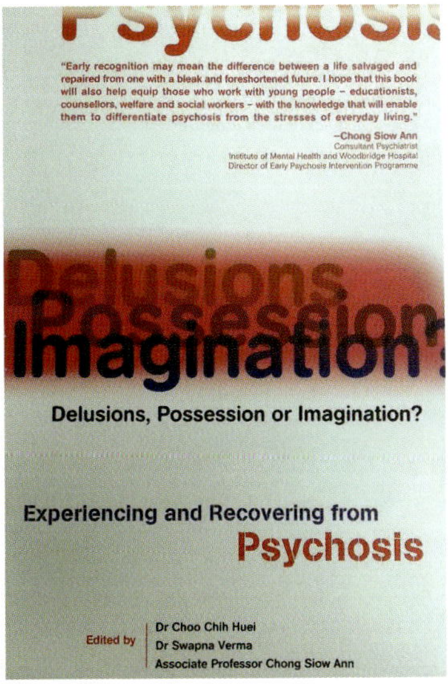

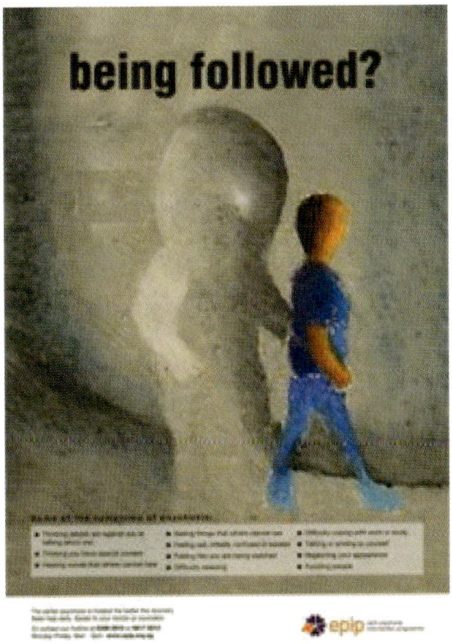

Posters displayed in MRT stations.

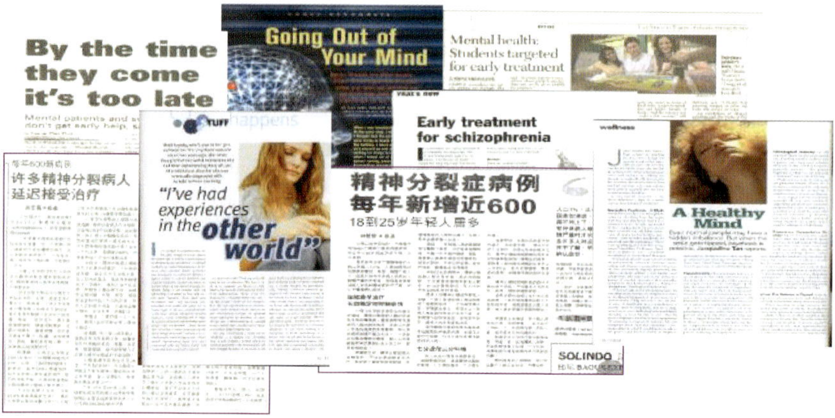
By the time they come it's too late
Going Out of Your Mind
Mental health: Students targeted for early treatment
Early treatment for schizophrenia
许多精神分裂病人延迟接受治疗
"I've had experiences in the other world"
精神分裂症病例每年新增近600
18到25岁年轻人居多
A Healthy Mind
SOLINDO

Articles on psychosis and EPIP in mass media.

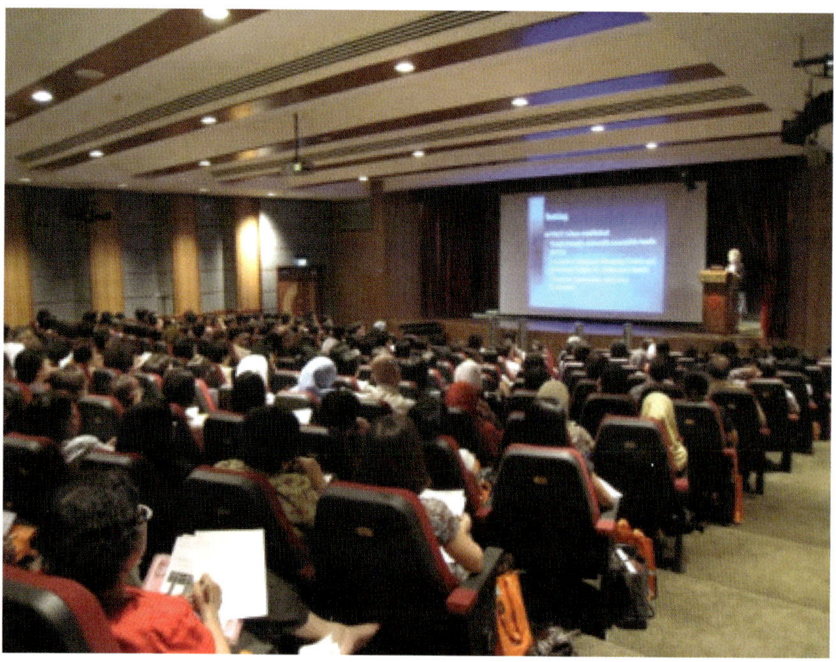

Training workshop for counselors from Institutes of Higher Learning.

with first-episode psychosis had sought the help of traditional healers at the first onset of symptoms (Chong *et al.*, 2005a). Primary healthcare providers included private and polyclinic general practitioners (GPs), counsellors from the various tertiary institutions, counsellors/professionals of social and welfare services as well as the Singapore Armed Forces (SAF). Training and networking with primary healthcare providers are essential to meet the aim of increasing the number of professionals who are educated and trained in the early detection of psychosis, in turn increasing referrals from this sector. To make the treatment continuous and seamless, it is vital for primary healthcare workers and other service providers to be engaged in the programme — not just in detecting unwell individuals early, but also to collaborate in the management of these patients.

Clinical Services

The clinical service of EPIP offers comprehensive, integrated and patient-centred care by a multidisciplinary team of psychiatrists, case managers, psychologists, medical social workers, nurses, occupational therapists and family therapists. Each team member complements one another and each has a significant role to play in the patients' lives.

The clinical service of EPIP provides phase-specific treatment to all patients with first-episode psychosis (FEP) between the ages of 16 and 40 years. Patients in whom the psychotic symptoms are secondary to organic etiology or are substance-induced are not treated by EPIP and are referred to other appropriate services. Assessment and treatment constitute the core of early intervention. Ongoing and comprehensive bio-psychosocial assessments are a prerequisite to accurate case formulation and help in setting treatment goals and management plans. Intervention is customised according to patients' needs and the phases of recovery. These consist of three main phases. In the **acute phase**, the focus is on assessment and diagnosis, initiating anti-psychotic treatment with an emphasis on starting low and going slow. The team builds a therapeutic alliance with the patients and families with early intensive engagement, and by coordinating services and providing supportive counselling. Patients and caregivers are educated, if possible, on the illness, the symptoms, medication for treatment and side effects. In the **stabilisation phase**, the team works on re-integration back to school/work and community, while at the same time ensuring medication adherence, and monitoring for psychiatric and/or medical co-morbidities including metabolic side effects. The patients and caregivers are taught to identify strengths, resources and improving coping skills with an emphasis on stress management. Finally, in the **stable phase**, patients' goals are revisited with an emphasis on maintaining a healthy lifestyle and on relapse prevention by going through symptoms and early warning signs.

Moving Towards Indicated Prevention

> *'The best hope now for the prevention of schizophrenia lies with indicated preventive interventions targeted at individuals manifesting precursor signs and symptoms who have not yet met full criteria for diagnosis. The identification of individuals at this early stage, coupled with the introduction of pharmacological and psychosocial interventions, may prevent the development of the full-blown disorder.'*
>
> Mrazek and Haggerty (1994)

It has been shown that psychotic disorders are generally preceded by a prodromal phase, which presents as changes in a person's well-being and psychosocial functioning. This prodromal phase is a period of progressive cognitive and functional deterioration and at times occurs concurrently with the emergence of sub-threshold psychotic symptoms. The term 'At Risk Mental State' (ARMS) was coined by Yung *et al.* (1996) to describe this prodromal phase whereby an individual is at increased risk of developing a psychotic disorder. It was found that about 40% made the transition from ARMS to psychosis within a year of identification (Yung *et al.*, 2003). Other clinics around the world have found incidence rates of conversion to psychosis that vary in a range of 6–50% (Miller *et al.*, 2002; Skeate *et al.*, 2004).

The **Support for Wellness Achievement Programme (SWAP)** was first established in Singapore, in April 2008 to provide a treatment service for those experiencing ARMS. This programme was initiated within the remit of EPIP to target individuals with ARMS. SWAP offers its service to help-seeking individuals between the ages of 16 and 30. Phillips *et al.* (2000) have defined an operational set of clinical features that can be used to identify individuals presenting with ARMS and this criterion has been adopted by SWAP.

An individual is deemed to have ARMS if they fulfill the criteria for any of the three groups in addition to a decline in functioning over the preceding one year. The groups are as follows:

- Vulnerability Group: this includes individuals with a family history of a psychotic disorder in a first-degree relative or a diagnosis of Schizotypal Personality Disorder in these individuals.
- Attenuated Symptom Group: this consists of individuals with attenuated or low-grade psychotic symptoms that are deemed to be of sub-threshold frequency or intensity.
- Brief Limited Intermittent Psychotic Symptoms (BLIPS): This consists of individuals that have experienced a frank psychotic episode that resolved spontaneously within a week.

SWAP also uses a multidisciplinary team approach, and management is based on a bio-psychosocial model of care. Psychotropic medication is prescribed for any existing co-morbid mental disorders but anti-psychotic medication is not routinely prescribed for individuals with ARMS unless the individual is extremely distressed by the attenuated symptoms or if the individual requests for it.

Peer Support Movement in EPIP

EPIP started to organise client-professional facilitated peer support groups in 2008. This led to the formalisation of peer support within EPIP in 2009. This was to foster collaboration between the EPIP professionals and EPIP clients (patients and families), in promoting recovery-oriented messages and advocacy of mental health issues, and supported by the Woodbridge Hospital Charity Fund.

Since then, we have named it Peers4Rs (Peers Remembering Respect, Resilience and Recovery). Peers4Rs consists of initiatives involving patients-in-recovery and caregivers who are actively involved in supporting other patients and families, collectively known as peer support specialists (PSS). Our PSS are an integral part of EPIP's holistic service delivery, delivering messages of hope through their 'lived experience'. The programme also looks into sustaining the efficacy of the PSS' efforts through training and development.

Our PSS provide a varied range of services such as co-facilitating in peer support groups, social skills groups or outings, conducting phone support or face-to-face sessions as well as speaking in mental health campaigns or symposiums. As for our caregiver PSS, they provide one-to-one phone and/or face-to-face support (i.e. psychoeducation, self-care, behavioural management and resource management) and sharing of their experiences. The caregiver PSS also contribute actively to outreach events organised by EPIP. For their time and efforts, our PSS receive hourly-rated reimbursements funded by the Woodbridge Hospital Charity Fund.

Recognition of the Work

In recognition of our outstanding contribution to research in health promotion, EPIP was awarded the inaugural State of Kuwait Health Promotion (Chong *et al.*, 2005b) for 2005 by the World Health Organisation (WHO).

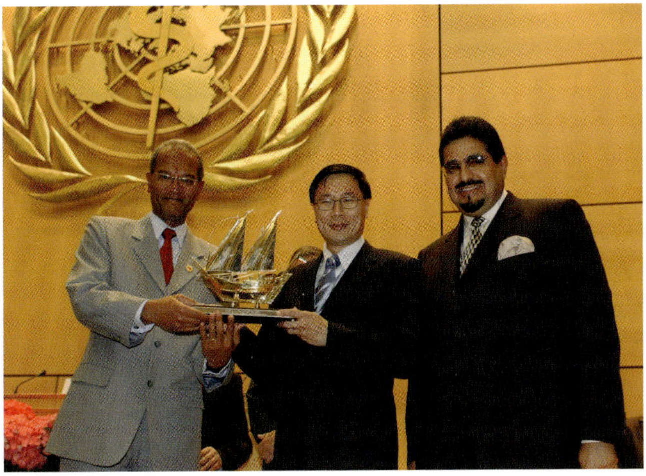

EPIP wins the WHO State of Kuwait Award for Research in Health Promotion.

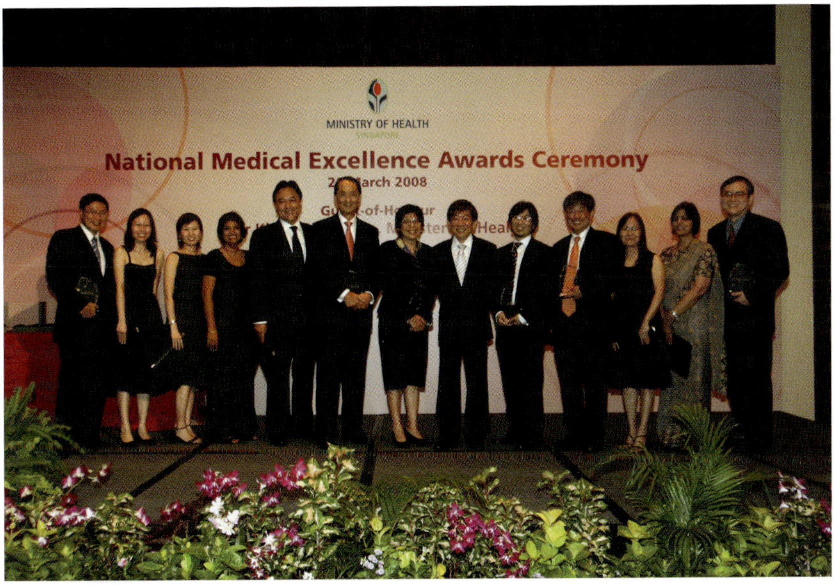

EPIP wins the inaugural National Excellence Award in the Team category.

EPIP was also awarded the inaugural National Medical Excellence Team Award in March 2008. This award recognises individuals and teams who have contributed significantly in clinical work and research, leading to positive outcomes in healthcare delivery that have benefited patient care.

In 2015, EPIP was one of the award recipients of the Inaugural Singapore Patient Action Awards. EPIP's psychosocial interventions incorporating Club EPIP and Peers4Rs won the category of the Singapore Patient Engagement Initiative (Team-Based).

While the former focuses on function and psychosocial recovery, the latter leverages on the lived experience of persons-in-recovery and caregivers to provide support to other patients with early psychosis and their caregivers. The two are synergistic in creating collaborations among various parties for the benefit of EPIP patients and families:

- Our psychosocial interventions identify patients for leadership roles during Club EPIP groups and involve them in planning activities, and interest them in providing peer support.
- Peer support specialists and staff are involved in co-running groups for other patients and caregivers leading to patients feeling they are heard and being more willing to engage in EPIP services.
- Such relationships also help with identifying different systems that are in place for patients as staff and PSS work together to help patients familiarise themselves and work with different community systems.
- As part of their ongoing professional development, PSS undergo certification courses, incorporating their learning in group and individual sessions.

The Awards Ceremony took place on 30 October 2015 at the 2015 Singapore Patient Conference in the Theatrette at Tan Tock Seng Hospital.

The Abilympics is an annual international skills competition for people with disabilities and special needs contesting in areas such as vocational, leisure and living skills. For the Seventh International

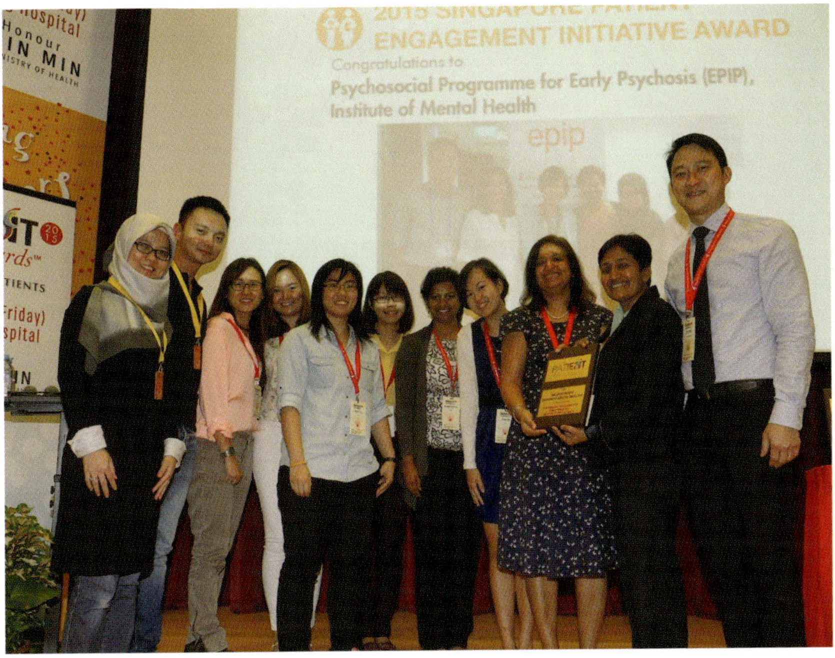
ENGAGEMENT INITIATIVE AWARD
Congratulations to
Psychosocial Programme for Early Psychosis (EPIP),
Institute of Mental Health
epip

EPIP wins the Singapore Patient Action Award in the Team category.

Abilympics in Japan in 2007, Institute of Mental Health (IMH) successfully trained recovering patients who bagged silver and bronze medals in the photography and architectural categories. They were the only Singaporeans who won medals for the competition and both were from IMH, EPIP. IMH was again invited to participate in the Ninth International Abilympics in 2016. Three patients participated in the local selection and all of them were chosen to represent Singapore to compete internationally in France, for the photography and poster design categories.

New Initiatives Moving Forward

Under the National Mental Health Blueprint (NMHBP), EPIP has expanded its services to a broader scope of youth mental health promotion

Community Health
Assessment Team

by setting up the Community Health Assessment Team (CHAT) in April 2009. CHAT aims to increase awareness of youth mental health issues, and increase and streamline access to mental health resources and services. CHAT has identified the following target customers and uses a multipronged approach to engage them:

1. Young people between the ages of 16 and 30 in distress: information, resources and a free mental health assessment are available at our CHAT Hub located at a youth-friendly and non-traditional mental health centre in the heart of town.
2. Community partners who work with young people: CHAT provides training to counsellors, teachers and students in institutes of higher learning on detecting early signs and symptoms of youth mental health issues and how to advise young people to seek help.
3. General public: CHAT provides information and resources on youth mental health through our website (www.chat.mentalhealth.sg) and Facebook page (www.facebook.com/chatfans) and through events and talks.

EPIP Inpatient Centre

With the support of the Singapore Ministry of Health, EPIP extended our service provision with the opening of a dedicated inpatient centre. Renovation of the centre commenced on 4 September 2015 and it became

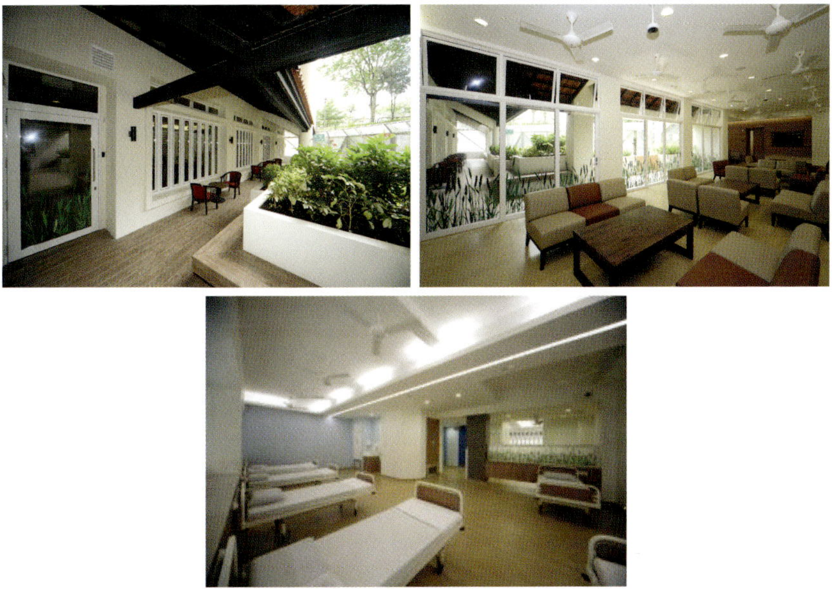

The EPIP inpatient centre.

operational from 1 February 2016. This 20-bed mixed-gender facility is dedicated to the care of early psychosis in Singapore and helmed by a specialised inter-professional team comprising recovered patients and healthcare professionals to support our clients across inpatient, outpatient and community settings.

Designed to facilitate therapeutic work and recovery, it boasts of features such as an open pantry, a night lounge and an outdoor garden. To complement the facility, we have specially designed programmes and activities for meaningful engagement, and to promote and support recovery. We will continue to engage our patients and caregivers in the development and provision of services within our ward.

In preparation for our specialised inpatient centre, the EPIP team involved our stakeholders in various improvement initiatives to streamline our processes and identify processes that add more value for our clients. In addition, patient focus groups were conducted and the team also visited the inpatient units of other hospitals to learn from best practices. We also had a chance to pilot some new processes that will be incorporated into this new inpatient centre.

While introducing new processes and facilities in the ward, the team engaged in various quality improvement discussions to pro-actively ensure that workflow and ward designs are safe for patients and staff.

References

Bertolote J, McGorry P (2005). Early intervention and recovery for young people with early psychosis: Consensus statement. *Br J Psychiatry* **187**: s116–119.

Birchwood M, Todd P, Jackson C (1998). Early intervention in psychosis: The critical period hypotheses. *Br J Psychiatry* **172**: 53–59.

Chong SA, Verma SK, Lee C (2001). Psychosis — Everyone's concern: The Early Psychosis Intervention Programme (EPIP) in Singapore. *Singapore Fam Physician* **27**: 49–52.

Chong SA, Mythily M, Lum A, Chan YH, McGorry P (2005a). Determinants of duration of untreated psychosis and the pathway to care in Singapore. *Int J Soc Psychiatry* **51**: 55–62.

Chong SA, Mythily S, Verma SK (2005b). Reducing the duration of untreated psychosis and changing help-seeking behaviour in Singapore. *Soc Psychiatry Psychiatr Epidemiol* **40**: 619–621.

Falloon IRH (1992). Early intervention for first episodes of schizophrenia: A preliminary exploration. *Psychiatry* **55**: 4–15.

Johnstone EC, Crow TJ, Johnson AL, MacMillan JF (1986). The Northwick Park Study of first episodes of schizophrenia. I. Presentation of the illness and problems relating to admission. *The Br J Psychiatry* **148**: 115–120.

Larsen TK, Johannessen JO, Opjordsmoen S (1998). First-episode schizophrenia with long duration of untreated psychosis. *Br J Psychiatry* **172**: 45–52.

Lieberman JA, Fenton WS (2000). Delayed detection of psychosis: Causes, consequences, and effects on public health. *Am J Psychiatry* **157**: 1727–1730.

Lieberman JA, Perkins D, Belger A, Chakos M, Jarskog F, Boteva K, Gilmore J (2001). The early stages of schizophrenia: Speculation on pathogenesis, pathophysiology, and therapeutic approaches. *Biol Psychiatry* **50**: 884–897.

Loebel AD, Lieberman JA, Alvir JM, Mayerhoff DI, Geisler SH, Szymanski SR (1992). Duration of psychosis and outcome in first-episode schizophrenia. *Am J Psychiatry* **149**: 1183–1188.

McGlashan T (1996). Early detection and intervention in schizophrenia: Editor's introduction. *Schizophr Bull* **22**: 197–199.

McGorry P (1998). Preventative strategies in early psychosis: Verging on reality. *Br J Psychiatry* **172**: 1–2.

Miller TJ, McGlashan TH, Rosen JL, Somjee L, Markovich PJ, Stein K, Woods SW (2002). Prospective diagnosis of the initial prodrome for schizophrenia based on the Structured Interview for Prodromal Syndromes: Preliminary evidence of interrater reliability and predictive validity. *Am J Psychiatry* **159**: 863–865.

Mrazek PJ, Haggerty RJ, eds. (1994). *Reducing Risks for Mental Disorders: Frontiers for Preventive Intervention Research.* National Academy Press.

Murray CJL, Lopez AD, eds. (1996). *The Global Burden of Disease.* Harvard University Press, Boston.

NHS Executive, Department of Health, United Kingdom (1996). Burdens of disease: A discussion document. Department of Health, London.

Phillips LJ, Yung AR, McGorry PD (2000). Identification of young people at risk of psychosis: Validation of Personal Assessment and Crisis Evaluation Clinic intake criteria. *Aust N Z J Psychiatry* **34**: S164p169.

Sainsbury Centre for Mental Health (1998). Keys to engagement. Review of care for people with severe mental illness who are hard to engage with services. Sainsbury Centre for Mental Health, London.

Skeate A, Patterson P, Birchwood M (2004). Transition to psychosis in a high-risk sample: The experience of ED:IT, Birmingham, UK. *Schizophr Res* **70**: S44.

Yung AR, McGorry PD, McFarlane CA, Jackson HJ, Patton GC, Rakkar A (1996). Monitoring and care of young people at incipient risk of psychosis. *Schizophr Bull* **22**: 283nloph

Yung AR, Phillips LJ, Yuen HP, Francey SM, McFarlane CA, Hallgren M, McGorry PD (2003). Psychosis prediction: 12-month follow up of a high-risk ('prodromal') group. *Schizophr Res* **60**: 21–32.

Addiction Medicine

Suresh ANANTHA

'I have absolutely no pleasure in the stimulants in which I sometimes so madly indulge. It has not been in the pursuit of pleasure that I have periled life and reputation and reason. It has been the desperate attempt to escape from torturing memories, from a sense of insupportable loneliness and a dread of some strange impending doom.'

Edgar Allan Poe

Alcohol, Addiction and Mental Health

Addiction is a chronic and relapsing illness that involves the compulsive use of drugs and alcohol despite adverse consequences. In recent years, at least in the past 30 years or so, non-substance-related compulsive behaviours have also been recognised as potentially addictive. For example, Pathological Gambling was added to the *Diagnostic and Statistical Manual of Mental Disorders* (DSM) in 1980, 28 years after its first publication in 1952 (National Center for Responsible Gaming, 2013). These 'behavioural addictions' include excessive online activities related to gaming, pornography and social networking. With the rise and popularity of new designer drugs, smart phones, and increased internet speeds and penetration, the rapidly evolving addiction landscape poses challenges for prevention specialists and educators, clinicians, law enforcement officials and policy makers.

Mental health and addiction overlap, and co-morbidities involving addiction and other mental health disorders (such as depression and anxiety) are common worldwide. The close relationship between mental health and addiction has long been recognised and understood by medical professionals. In 1987, Dr Aline Wong, Chair of the Government Parliamentary Committee for Health and Environment, spoke about plans to set up a 30-bed ward specifically to treat alcoholics at the new Woodbridge Hospital that was to be relocated to the present-day Buangkok Green Medical Park. The Medical Director for Woodbridge Hospital at that time, Dr Teo Seng Hock, explained that alcoholics required psychiatric assistance, as they suffered from '... disoriented thinking, delirium and bizarre behavior' (*The Straits Times*, 1987).

The new Woodbridge Hospital would also undertake research into the prevalence of alcoholism in Singapore. In 1989, the Acting Minister for Health, Mr Yeo Cheow Tong, expressed concerns that the extent of alcoholism, and whether it was similar to other developing countries, was not known (*The Straits Times*, 1989). The number of alcohol-related emergency-room presentations had been rising since 1983, and doctors had noted that the profile of help-seeking alcoholics had shifted, with more professionals seeking treatment (*The Straits Times*, 1988). Alcohol-related research was viewed as important to understanding the whole public and mental health picture in Singapore.

Other Addictions

In the 1980s and 1990s, while there were growing concerns about alcoholism as a potentially serious public health issue, drug abuse was viewed primarily as relating to the criminal justice system. However, in the mid-1990s, the Ministry of Home Affairs (MHA) introduced several schemes that emphasised a greater role for counselling and aftercare, in order to address a rising recidivism rate in prisons and drug rehabilitation centres (DRCs). These included full-time aftercare officers who provided counselling and case management, partnership with halfway houses to facilitate rehabilitation and community reintegration, and the use of Naltrexone for eligible prison and DRC inmates. In retrospect, the use of Naltrexone could be viewed as a partial but significant opening of the door to medical and pharmacological inputs into the rehabilitation of local drug offenders, particularly for those who abused heroin.

Problem gambling would not capture the public's attention until 2004, when Mr George Yeo, Minister for Trade and Industry, announced in Parliament that the government was considering having a local casino, and that there would be a '… need to put in place control measures to limit its access by Singaporeans and make sure there is no organised crime' (Da Cunha, 2010). Similarly, online addictions would become a greater concern locally in the early to mid-2000s, as a result of faster internet speeds, greater penetration into offices and homes, and disturbing reports in the media about internet addicts in South Korea and China.

Alcohol Treatment Centre at the New Woodbridge Hospital

When the new Woodbridge Hospital opened its doors in 1993, a new unit was set up to treat alcoholism. The Alcohol Treatment Centre (ATC) started operating in August 1993, headed by Dr Ong Thiew Chai. Its inpatient ward housed 38 beds. Outpatients were seen at Institute of Mental Health (IMH) Clinic B and the Alexandra Outpatient Clinic. ATC provided medical, psychiatric and psychological evaluation to patients suffering from alcoholism. Evening support groups, based on the 12 steps of Alcoholics Anonymous, were conducted at ATC on Tuesday and Thursday evenings.

ATC was instrumental in grooming local psychiatrists who would later gain prominence in the field of addiction medicine. They included Dr Lim Yun Chin, Dr Arthur Lee and Dr Munidasa Winslow. The latter, while a registrar at ATC, helped to pioneer the development of the first local certification board for substance abuse professionals in 1998. The certification board, now known as the Association of Professionals Specialising in Addictions Counselling (APSAC), was formed in 1998 to certify local substance abuse professionals. Since 2004, APSAC also provides certification to professionals who treat gambling disorders.

ATC continued to operate until 2000, when it split into two sister units, one running at Woodbridge Hospital and the other at Alexandra Hospital. Dr Arthur Lee led the Psychological Addiction Medicine Service (PAMS) at Alexandra Hospital. Dr Winslow formed the Community Addictions

Management Programme (CAMP) at Woodbridge Hospital in April 2001, through funding from the Ministry of Health (MOH) under the Health Services Development Programme (HSDP).

Community Addictions Management Programme (CAMP)

CAMP was a novel and innovative clinical venture, in that the treatment of addiction was approached differently from anything that had been done previously in Singapore.

Firstly, CAMP set out to treat *all* types of addictions, including (1) traditional substances of abuse such as alcohol, heroin and benzodiazepines; (2) emergent drugs of abuse, such as ice, ecstasy and ketamine — ice and ecstasy abuse were first detected by local enforcement agencies in 1996, while ketamine was only listed as a controlled drug in September 1999 (Central Narcotics Bureau, 2003); and (3) behavioural addictions such as problem gambling, online addictions and sex addiction.

Secondly, evidence-based treatment strategies that had worked in other jurisdictions were adopted and customised for local patients. For example, a day treatment programme called Bridge was launched in December 2001 to plug the service gap between regular inpatient and outpatient treatment services.

Patient placement criteria developed by the American Society of Addiction Medicine in the 1980s advocated a range of services, with increasing intensity of interventions to suit patients' needs. Bridge was conducted over 20 days, running from 10 am to 4 pm, as an intensive outpatient programme for patients who did not require inpatient admission. Treatment was provided in a closed group setting, combining psychoeducation, skills building, and process elements.

Recovery support groups were initiated in 2001 to provide ongoing support for patients who had either completed treatment or who were still being followed up as outpatients. The groups were run on Wednesday evenings and Saturday mornings at the seminar rooms located adjacent to the IMH auditorium.

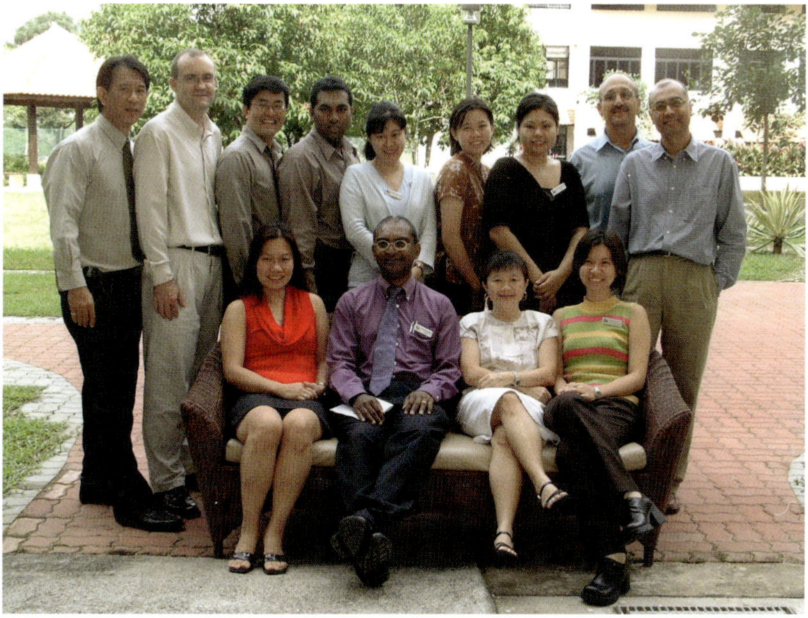

CAMP team in its early days, 2002.

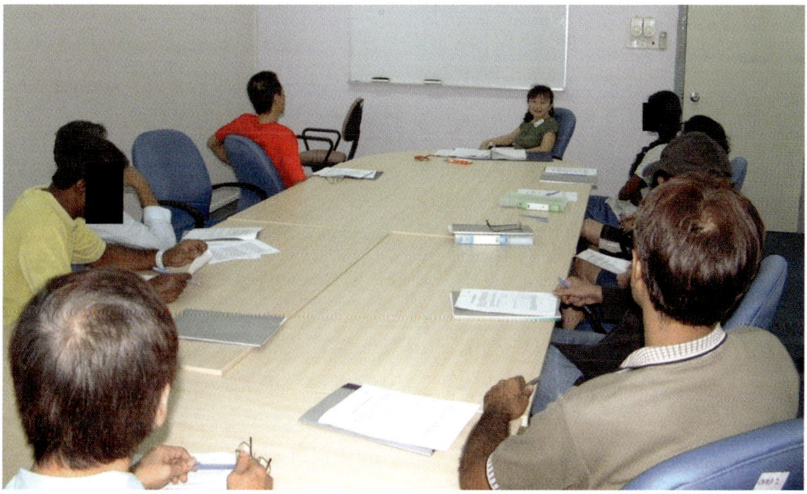

Bridge in session in 2002, conducted by Ms Treena Tan (Bridge Coordinator).

To provide a complete continuum of care, from inpatient through aftercare, CAMP set up the WE Centre for Addictions Recovery and Education (WE CARE) on 15 December 2005, at 620 Tiong Bahru Road, inside the Alexandra Day Centre. The aims of WE CARE were threefold. These included (1) to get recovering patients to help themselves through participating in self-help groups, self-learning and mentorship of persons in various stages of recovery; (2) to provide a drop-in centre for patients who had completed treatment, and needed a safe place to interact with other recovering people and addiction professionals; and (3) to be an entry point for the treatment of substance and behavioral addicts and their families, by functioning as an information, resource and referral centre.

WE CARE was supported by CAMP staff during its first year of operation. Subsequently, WE CARE would function as a voluntary welfare organisation (VWO) that would be self-sufficient in its operations. However, the relationship with IMH would continue, to the benefit of both organisations and their respective clients.

Thirdly, CAMP forged robust relationships with various community-based agencies, including the Singapore Prisons service, Singapore Corporation for Rehabilitative Enterprises (SCORE), Ministry for Community Youth and Sports (MCYS) (now Ministry for Social and Family Development, MSF), National Council on Problem Gambling (NCPG), halfway houses, family service centres and Family Courts.

Through such relationships, new initiatives that involved cooperation between medical and non-medical community-based organisations developed, such as Project SAVE with Family Courts in 2002, to treat perpetrators of domestic violence who abused alcohol. In 2004, CAMP collaborated with NCPG to develop a national training and treatment framework that included a spectrum of services, from early detection to tertiary treatment which would be provided by CAMP. Training would also be provided by CAMP to the other agencies that were part of the national framework.

Finally, CAMP set out to educate the public (including other medical and allied health professionals) on addictions. Long perceived as primarily a social and legal problem rather than a mental health concern, addicts were regarded as people with character flaws and poor self-control. Through training of its community partners, and public educational messages, CAMP sought to change the perception of addicts as 'bad' people, and represent them as people with a disorder that could be treated, like other mental health disorders.

Educational activities aimed at moderating the public's perceptions of addictions included conducting three national addictions conferences from 2001 to 2003, the First Asia Pacific Institute of Addictions (APIA) in 2004, Second APIA in 2006, and various seminars and forums.

In particular, the First APIA (29 May–4 June 2004) attracted almost 500 delegates from 26 countries. CAMP collaborated with the World Health Organisation (WHO) to sponsor 30 delegates from developing countries, including India, China, Bangladesh, Myanmar and Nepal. The conference, opened by Prof Satku K (Director, Medical Services), included a glittering array of speakers including Dr George Vaillant (Professor, Harvard Medical School), Mr Jerry Moe (National Director of Childrens' Programs, Betty Ford Centre) and Dr David Mee-Lee (American Society of Addiction Medicine).

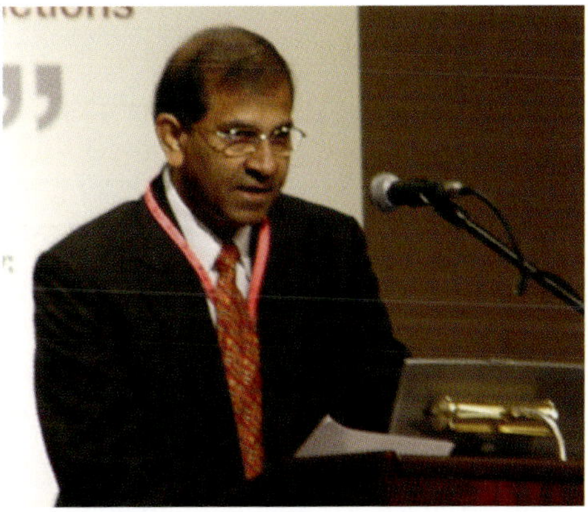

Prof Satku K delivering his opening address at the First APIA, 30 May 2004.

The First APIA had originally been planned a year earlier in 2003. However, when severe acute respiratory syndrome (SARS) reached our shores in 2003, the conference had to be put on hold until the following year.

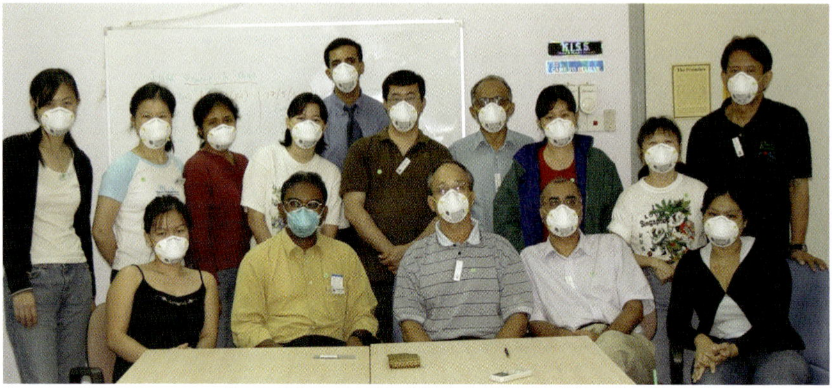

Intrepid CAMPers during SARS, 2003.

In 2006, the Second APIA (1 September–5 September 2006) was held, and close to 300 local and overseas delegates attended the conference. This would be the final APIA conference; two years later, CAMP would undergo structural changes and emerge as the National Addictions Management Service (NAMS) in 2008.

CAMP and the Buprenorphine Years

Buprenorphine, or Subutex, is a semi-synthetic opioid that was approved for use in 2002 (Chua and Lee, 2006) to treat heroin dependence. A partial agonist and antagonist, it had been successfully used to treat heroin dependence in the United States and in Europe. When used sublingually to reduce cravings and withdrawal, its abuse potential was low. However, if administered intravenously, particularly in combination with other depressant drugs, addicts reported feeling heroin-like euphoria and eventual dependence.

Despite guidelines from MOH, which included eight hours of training by CAMP and mandatory logging in of prescription details by doctors (the Central Addiction Registry System was developed to track patients and prescriptions in 2005), Buprenorphine became widely abused. In fact, because of the legal status of Buprenorphine, many former heroin addicts switched to the Buprenorphine as their drug of choice. The consequences were often devastating, both in introducing an intravenous drug culture into Singapore, and causing many users to contract blood-borne diseases and infections.

As a result, Buprenorphine was listed as a controlled drug in Aug 2006 (Central Narcotics Bureau, 2007). The penalties for trafficking and consuming Buprenorphine would be the same as for heroin. The Subutex Voluntary Rehabilitation Programme (SVRP) was conducted from 21 August to 13 October 2006, when Buprenorphine users could voluntarily be weaned off the newly controlled drug without legal consequences to them. SVRP was conducted by CAMP at the basement of Block 9. At the same time, the inpatient ward, consisting of 24 beds for detox and rehab, was increased to 42 beds to cater to the increase in patients treated during SVRP. Close to 3,000 Buprenorphine users were treated during the SVRP period.

Treatment for Special Populations and Helpline

Several treatment programmes for special populations were started during the CAMP years, which have since become key services at NAMS. These include Continuous Recovery through Education and Skill Training (CREST), Families in Recovery through Education Support and Hope (FRESH) and Gambling Addiction Management through Education (GAME).

CREST was developed in 2004 for recovering substance abusers, incorporating modules on relapse prevention, skills training and continuing recovery. Separate sessions were run in English and Mandarin. Patients who completed CREST could subsequently participate in recovery support groups.

In recognition of the importance of family involvement in a patient's therapy, FRESH was developed with family members in mind.

FRESH was started in late 2005, and taught families how they could best help the addict, and also take care of their own needs, which were often neglected.

GAME was first conducted in early 2006. A year earlier, the counsellor selected to take the lead in developing problem gambling services for CAMP was attached for three months to a gambling treatment centre at the Veterans' Hospital in Ohio. He had been sent on a Health Manpower Development Programme (HMDP) attachment to look at the type of services that were available to problem gamblers in the United States, and to identify those that could be adapted to our local context. When he returned to Singapore, he initiated GAME, which included six topics and conducted over six weeks. The current incarnation of GAME run at NAMS includes eight topics.

Other Community-Based Services

Another service that began with CAMP that has evolved, and continues to evolve, is the addictions helpline. In early 2006, two staff members were sent on a study trip to Healthlink in Australia, which ran several extensive helpline services linking patients to medical services. Following the study trip, one staff member was attached to Healthlink in early 2007 on an HMDP scholarship for three months.

Upon his return, he helped to start a helpline on addictions in July 2007. The helpline had two phone lines, one for gambling and the other for all other addictions, which operated from the IMH Call Centre. In the beginning, the number of calls was low, between 150 to 200 total calls per month for both lines.

CAMP counsellors were placed on a roster to answer calls. It was recognised very early that responding to helpline calls took specialised skills. As a result, Mr Adrian Scarfe of GAMCARE, the largest telephone helpline service in the United Kingdom, was recruited to train the counsellors. The training included role playing many scenarios typical of helpline calls, and was conducted over five days.

In November 2007, CAMP partnered with NCPG to take over the National Problem Gambling Helpline, though the all addictions helpline would continue to function. Both helplines operated from 8.30 am to 6 pm. However, after 6 pm, the calls made to the National Problem Gambling Helpline were routed to Tanjong Pagar Family Service Centre, and re-routed to NAMS the following morning. Calls made after 6 pm to the all addictions helpline would be transferred to voicemail after 6 pm.

The number of gambling-related helpline calls saw a steep increase when the two casinos started operating in 2010. From an average of 644 calls per month in 2009, the National Problem Gambling Helpline averaged around 1600 calls per month the following year.

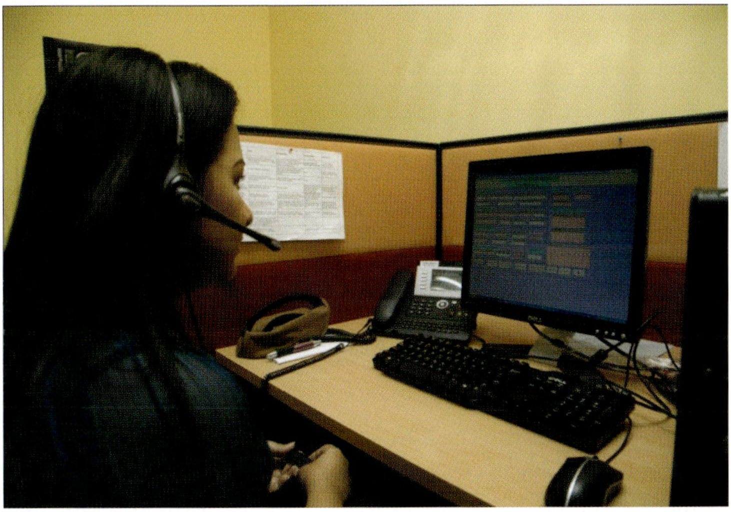

Helpline counsellor.

Inpatient Programme

When CAMP first started operating in 2001, there was no specific inpatient ward for addictions. CAMP was primarily an outpatient service. Patients seen by CAMP who required inpatient care were channelled to

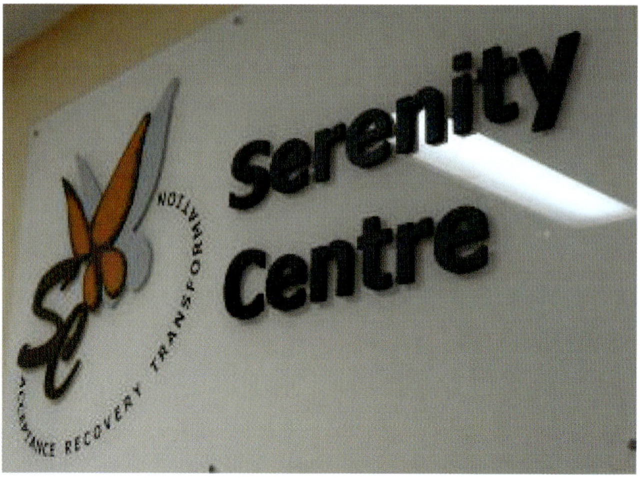

Sign outside Ward 23A, the butterfly symbolising transformation and maturity.

various other wards. Ward 23A, as a dedicated inpatient addiction ward, would only start to operate after PAMS returned to IMH from Alexandra Hospital in 2003. In 2005, Ward 23A was renamed Serenity Centre.

The Transformation of CAMP to NAMS

The five-year HSDP funding for CAMP terminated in 2006. CAMP continued to function as the outpatient arm of the Addiction Medicine Department (AMD) for the next two years. Many in the department dreamed of a national centre to treat addictions, building upon the progress that CAMP had made since 2001. In consultation with MOH, it was envisaged that it would take further capacity building before an independent, standalone centre could be constructed.

In the meantime, an addiction service located at IMH could serve the country's needs, until such time that a national centre would be appropriate. This service could lay the foundation for a future centre. Out of this idea, the National Addictions Management Service (NAMS) was born, and A/Prof Wong Kim Eng was appointed as the first clinical director in August 2008.

To provide direction and guidance for NAMS' growth, an International Advisory Panel (IAP) was set up in 2007 by MOH and MCYS (now MSF). Initially, there was a single IAP team of consultants who would provide advice and guidance to both NAMS (on treating addictions and staff training) and NCPG (on the development of national-level gambling-related services that included public safeguards, public education and treatment). The first IAP included eight members whose contracts would be renewed every two years.

The first IAP visit, with all eight members in attendance, was conducted from 5 to 7 December 2007. A subsequent visit took place on 13–14 August 2009, with six IAP members attending the two days of meetings. During the last IAP visit, on 23–24 October 2012, the IAP consisted of two teams, one to advise NCPG on broader national issues, and the other to advise NAMS on treatment. The IAP team that consulted with NAMS consisted of three members.

NAMS and Problem Gambling

By the beginning of 2009, efforts to protect Singaporeans (including Permanent Residents) from possible gambling-related harm had acquired a new sense of urgency. The two casinos would begin operating in 2010. The government introduced new schemes to protect the public, including casino self-exclusion, family exclusion and third-party exclusion. Public education messages on the ills of problem gambling increased in prominence and visibility.

NCPG collaborated with and engaged NAMS to provide training to family service centres, betting outlets and grass roots organisations. The training involved imparting knowledge and skills on recognising problem gambling behaviours and providing basic interventions such as making effective referrals. The increased publicity and training were paying off as more people came forward willingly to seek treatment.

In just five years, from FY08 to FY12, the number of new problem gamblers treated at NAMS had more than doubled, from 168 to 356, respectively.

As a result of greater awareness of problem gambling, there was also an increase in calls made to the National Problem Gambling Helpline, which NAMS helped to run in partnership with NCPG. In 2009, there was an average of 644 calls per month. The number of calls received monthly exceeded 1000 in February 2010, coinciding with the opening of the first local casino (Resorts World Sentosa). A year later, in February 2011, the National Problem Gambling Helpline received almost 2000 calls.

As the number of calls increased annually, NAMS was asked to consider increasing its helpline operating hours to 10 pm. A proposal was submitted to MOH and MSF for NAMS to employ paracounsellors to man the helpline full time. By the start of 2013, six paracounsellors had been recruited. On average, the helpline received about 1800 calls per month during the first quarter of 2013.

Specialist Outpatient Clinic C

A milestone in NAMS' development was the official opening of the Specialist Outpatient Clinic C on 14 July 2010. In the past, addiction patients were seen at outpatient clinics A and B. The new clinic separated adolescent and gambling patients from the adult substance-abusing patients. In addition to its own patient registration and pharmacy counters, Clinic C included separate stations for nursing review, data collection for treatment outcome monitoring and interviews with a medical social worker. A total of 17 consultation rooms were available to clinicians to see their patients. The official opening was attended by Prof Satku K as the Guest of Honour, guests from the National Healthcare Group and MOH, and community partners.

Development of New Clinical Services

When CAMP evolved into NAMS, new services were added, while existing ones revised. GAME went from six to eight topics/sessions, and recruited recovery peers to add depth to the sessions. Recovery peers

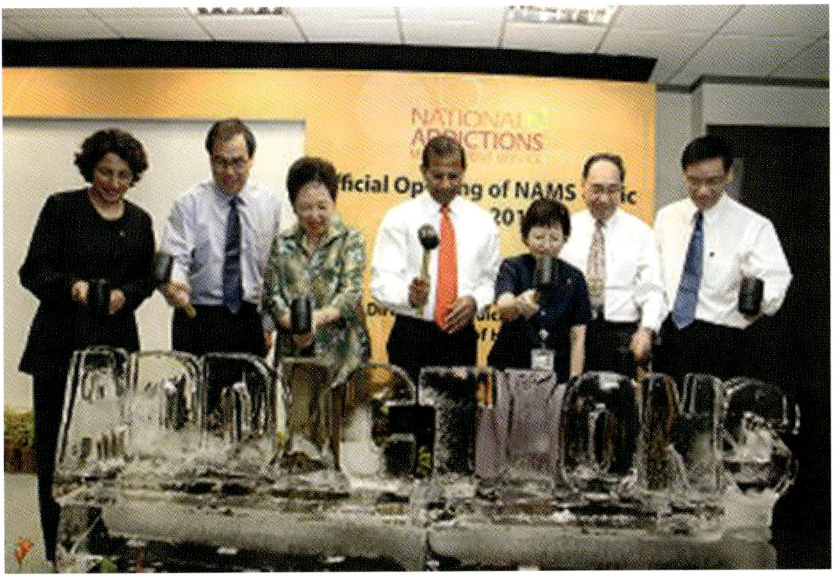

From L to R: A/Prof Rathi Mahendran (CMB, IMH), Mr Soh Gim Teik (Member, NHG Board of Directors), Madam Kay Kuok (Chairman, NHG Board of Directors), Prof Satku K (DMS). A/Prof Wong Kim Eng (Clinical Director, NAMS), Prof Goh Chee Leok (MOH), Mr Leong Yew Meng (CEO, IMH).

were patients who had been in stable recovery for at least two years, and volunteered to share their knowledge and experience during GAME sessions. While GAME was facilitated by counsellors, the recovery peers played a complementary role by injecting the sessions with their personal recovery stories.

Patients who completed GAME could continue to receive group support by participating in the GAME Recovery Support Group (GAME-RSG). A support group for family members, GAME-Family, was first run in September 2012, and was extremely well received by families. GAME, GAME-RSG and GAME-Family all run on Thursday evenings. Plans to develop recovery peers for other programmes, such as CREST, are in progress.

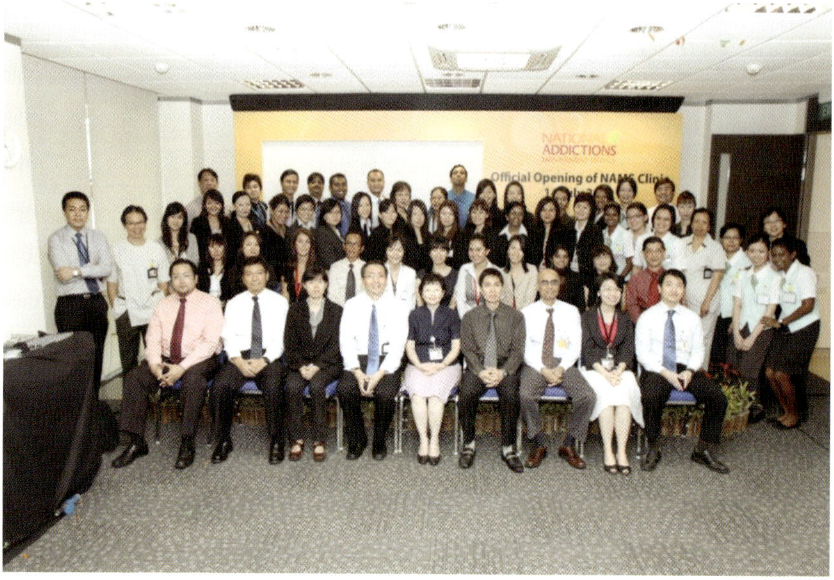

NAMS team at the official opening of specialist outpatient clinic C.

Other new services were also provided. These include Families in Recovery through Education and Empowerment (FREE), which was first run in May 2010. FREE runs twice a month during Monday evenings, and provides information to members of the public on how they could manage family members who had a gambling problem but were not in treatment.

A women-only group, Women in Recovery through Support, Education and Empowerment (WISE), was developed in 2012 to support our female patients struggling with addictions. WISE runs every Monday evening.

A group for parents of our adolescent patients, HOPE, runs on alternate Monday evenings, consisting of six topics.

Adolescent services, rebranded as RELIVE in 2011, runs services for young patients aged between 13 and 18, both at Clinic C and at various gazetted homes such as Singapore Boys' and Girls' Homes.

Public education continued to be a priority as well, particularly since addictions were so poorly understood, and often subject to misinformation and prejudice. Four public forums on problem gambling were conducted between 2010 and 2013, the first one at the Singapore Management University in 2010, the second at the HDB Hub in 2011, and the rest at the Health Promotion Board in 2012 and 2013. A public forum on alcohol abuse was also conducted at the Health Promotion Board on 24 November 2012.

The revamped NAMS website went live in Apr 2013, and included video presentations featuring staff and patients, links to social media like Facebook and Twitter, and an online gambling workbook. The latter allowed members of the public to complete a workbook which enabled the user to conduct a self-screen for problem gambling, and work on various chapters that explored the user's gambling behaviour and provided advice on lowering risk.

The online gambling workbook was conceived as a means of reaching out to problem gamblers who lacked awareness of the extent to which their gambling was causing problems and encouraging them to seek treatment, or at the very least to modify their gambling-related behavior.

As part of raising the public's awareness, NAMS also published a book entitled *Don't Gamble your Life Away: Help for Pathological Gamblers* in 2010. The book contained nine chapters (excluding the foreword and epilogue) that explored various aspects of problem and pathological gambling, including signs and symptoms, treatment and help resources in the community.

Research in Addictions

An integral part of NAMS' mission has been to increase understanding of addictions as they manifest in Singapore. So much addiction-related research is from Western countries, and most of our understanding has tended to be anecdotal or based on arrest statistics.

Since its formation in 2009, the NAMS research team has embarked on a programme of research aimed at improving our understanding of addictive disorders, their consequences and optimal treatment approaches. The team began by undertaking a series of audit and profiling studies to

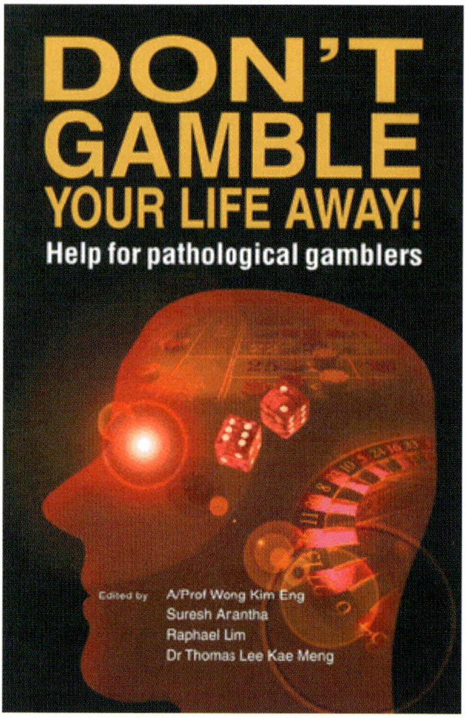

NAMS book on gambling, published in 2010.

determine the characteristics of the local addiction population, clinical needs and research priorities.

In 2010 the team completed a study examining stress-coping styles and psychological morbidity amongst family members of addiction patients, and a study of methadone-based treatment for elderly opium-dependent patients. Using data from treatment outcome monitoring protocols designed and implemented in 2009–2010, the team published papers on the effectiveness of NAMS' treatment, identifying predictors of clinically meaningful change for both alcohol patients and problem gamblers. The research team then broadened its scope to explore ways of enhancing treatment outcome through neuropsychological assessment, and psychological or pharmacological intervention studies. A series of neurocognitive studies were undertaken examining memory, executive functioning and impulsivity in recently detoxed alcohol-dependent patients and pathological gamblers. The findings of these studies led to the development of a study evaluating the effectiveness of a cognitive screening tool (MoCA) to detect cognitive impairment among substance misusers.

In 2012, the team commenced its first clinical drug trial. This principal-investigator led, double-blind, Phase-4 randomised controlled trial would examine the safety and efficacy of Lofexidine versus diazepam for the management of the opioid withdrawal syndrome. In collaboration with the local research science institute A*STAR, the team commenced an epigenetic study on addiction (pathological gambling and alcohol dependence) in 2013, as well as a clinical randomised controlled trial of NAMS' Cognitive Behavioural Therapist workbook, compared to non-workbook-based therapy for treating gambling disorders.

The Future

Our knowledge about the neurobiology of addiction has grown by leaps and bounds in the last 20 years. We have come to see that addiction may have genetic bases; we also know the regions in the brain that are implicated as a result of human neuroimaging studies, and the impact of neurotransmitters. We have also begun to understand how substances, and even certain behaviours, can change brain structure and function.

Despite the scientific evidence, the stereotypical behaviours of addicts are what get noticed most. These behaviours reinforce society's image of the addicted individual as manipulative, flawed in character, untrustworthy and even dangerous. The fact that these individuals need help, and indeed can be helped, becomes lost.

Society's perception can impede people who need help from seeking help. Early intervention is critical, but individuals suffering from addictions may delay treatment in order to hide their problem. It may take many years of unhealthy living for heart disease to develop. Addiction, on the other hand, can develop over a very short period of time. Early intervention is hence critical.

We know that the number of people seeking help is significantly much less than the actual number of people who are suffering from an addiction. A population-based survey of mental health disorders showed that alcohol abuse and alcohol dependence had a lifetime prevalence of 3.1% and 0.5%, respectively (Chong *et al.*, 2012).

However, alcohol abuse and alcohol dependence also had the highest proportion of treatment gaps among the common mental health disorders, at 96.2% and 88.3%, respectively (Chong *et al.*, 2012). Treatment gap can be defined generally as the proportion of people who require treatment or care for a particular disorder, but aren't receiving it.

A survey on Singaporeans participating in gambling activities in 2011 showed that 1.4% of the population could be classified as pathological gamblers, and 1.2% as probable problem gamblers (National Council on Problem Gambling, 2011). For a population of 5 million people, that relates to 70,000 individuals whose gambling behaviour might be classified as pathological. However, less than 400 new patients are seen at NAMS annually.

The challenge for NAMS is to work with relevant authorities to encourage those affected to seek treatment early, to minimise the treatment gap. This is not just a Singapore problem — even in the United States, only 10% of people with an addiction actually receive the treatment that they require (Open Society Foundations, 2010).

The history of addictions treatment at IMH began with the setting up of the Alcohol Treatment Centre in 1993. The world, and indeed Singapore, is a very different place now. Changes in societal norms, technology, education and politics will colour how we define and respond to addictions. NAMS will continue to evolve to meet these challenges, and operate on the conviction that everyone's life has worth and meaning, and everyone deserves help, without prejudice or shame.

References

Central Narcotics Bureau (2003). Singapore Country Report 2003. Available at: http://www.aspacngo.org/Acrobat/drug_reports/Singapore_1.PDF

Central Narcotics Bureau (2007). Drug Situation Report 2007. Available at: http://www.cnb.gov.sg/drugsituationreport/drugsituationreport2007.aspx

Chong SA, Abdin E, Vaigankaar JA, Heng D, Sherbourne C, Yap M, Lim YW, Wong HB, Ghosh-Dastidar B, Kwok KW, Subramaniam M (2012a). A population survey of mental health disorders in Singapore. *Ann Acad Med Singapore* **41**: 49–66.

Chong SA, Abdin E, Sherbourne C, Vaigankar JA, Heng D, Yap M, Subramaniam M (2012b). Treatment gap in common mental disorders: The Singapore perspective. *Epidemiol Psychiatr Sci* **21**: 195–202.

Chua SM, Lee TS (2006). Abuse of prescription Buprenorphine, regulatory controls and the role of the primary physician. *Ann Acad Med Singapore* **35**: 492–495.

Da Cunha D (2010). *Singapore Places Its Bets: Casinos, Foreign Talent and Remaking a City-State*. Straits Times Press, Singapore.

Gambling Disorders 360° (2013). Available at: http://blog.ncrg.org/issues-insights/redefining-pathological-gambling-new-research-highlights

National Council on Problem Gambling (2011). Report of Survey on Participation in Gambling Activities Among Singapore Residents. Available at: http://www.knowtheline.sg/pdf/2011_NCPG_Gambling_Participation_Survey_23_Feb_2012.pdf

Open Society Foundations (2010). Defining the Addiction Treatment Gap. Available at: http://www.opensocietyfoundations.org/sites/default/files/data-summary-20101123.pdf

The Straits Times, 23 Oct 1987. Ward for Alcoholics to be Set Up at Woodbridge.

The Straits Times, 24 Sep 1988. Hitting the Bottle: More Professionals Seek Help to Battle Drinking.

The Straits Times, 11 June 1989. New Name, New Facilities for Woodbridge Hospital.

Geriatric Psychiatry

NG Li Ling and SENG Kok Han

Development of Services for the Elderly

The first Department of Geriatric Medicine began in 1988 in Tan Tock Seng Hospital with several local geriatricians being trained. In 1991, the training of psychogeriatricians followed and in the Report of the Review Committee on National Health Policies in 1992, improving the health of the elderly and improving mental health care were identified as priority national health programmes for the 1990s (Ministry of Health Singapore, 1992). This report also recommended strengthening psychogeriatric services.

In the original Woodbridge Hospital built in 1928, there were no specific facilities for the mentally ill elderly. Young and old were admitted into general wards and management of the frail elderly in these wards were far from ideal. The Department of Geriatric Psychiatry was formed in the new Woodbridge Hospital and Institute of Mental Health (IMH) in 1993 which consisted of inpatient and specialist outpatient services and satellite clinics at Alexandra and selected polyclinics.

As geriatric services were organised into three regions — East, West and Central — each centred around geriatric medicine departments at Alexandra Hospital, Changi General Hospital and Tan Tock Seng Hospital, psychogeriatric services were also regionalised to complement the existing geriatric services. However, resources were limited and therefore it was essential to actively collaborate with other services and agencies and to have a close association with geriatric medicine departments in order to have a wider impact.

Multidisciplinary mental health professionals from IMH were actively involved in community care networks started by the National Council of Social Service (NCSS) and the Ministry of Health (MOH). The aim of such networks was to provide opportunities for representatives from various health and social agencies to meet, share ideas, improve coordination and access to services. Dynamic partnerships were formed between organisations and innovative services such as psychogeriatric consultancy and on-site support were provided for nursing homes and dementia day care centres. This provided the foundation for the early diagnosis and interventions of psychiatric disorders as well as training of staff in the step-down facilities.

Such collaborations were further extended with the Framework for Integrated Health Services for the Elderly that was implemented by MOH in July 2000 (Ministry of Health Singapore, 2000). Through this framework, community hospitals and nursing homes had access to additional funding for support by geriatricians, psychiatrists and allied health professionals from the restructured hospitals for training and for improving the standards of care. Elderly patients are also seen at the outpatient services run by the psychological medicine departments in restructured hospitals.

Aged Psychiatry Community and Treatment Service (APCATS)

Community-oriented psychogeriatric outreach service was later developed. In 2006, the Aged Psychiatry Community and Treatment Service (APCATS) was set up to provide home assessment and treatment services to elderly people who were frail or had difficulties accessing mental health services in the central region of Singapore. Its role also includes preventing unnecessary admission, minimising the length of inpatient stay and promoting ageing-in-place in the community by supporting caregivers and reducing the burden of care. APCATS came under the National Mental Health Blueprint funding in 2008. With that, the staff strength was increased and Regional Eldercare Agencies Partnership (REAP) was set up in 2008.

REAP aims to promote early detection of depression and dementia in the elderly by partnering with community eldercare agencies and primary care practitioners. It empowers partners to manage the elderly with mental disorders through training, consultation and support. REAP also provides free training for the staff and volunteers of participating agencies who screen their clients for depression and dementia. In 2009, APCATS took over the western region and became the largest service provider, until August 2013 when National University Health System (NUHS) started their community outreach team to cover the western region of Singapore.

Dementia-Friendly Ward and Memory Clinic

In the 2010 departmental retreat, the team embarked on the journey to understand the concept of person-centred care (PCC) and implementing its core objectives in the design and operations of the acute wards. In August 2011, the department engaged Hammondcare consultants from Australia to conduct an environmental design audit and presented their recommendations to make the wards dementia-friendly. The department was awarded a budget of $4.28 million from MOH to renovate the acute wards. These wards were officially opened on 14 February 2014 and named the Sunshine Wing.

The renovation incorporated dementia-friendly design elements and created additional facilities to reduce agitation and aggression in patients by providing a safe and conducive environment for rehabilitation while promoting PCC. Some of the features include improved dormitory layout to provide more privacy and convenience for patients, carefully selected furniture and a colour scheme for calming effect on dementia patients, materials that are safe, new beds and patient care equipment, an occupational therapy room, a reminiscence room, a multisensory, cognitive stimulation room, a fitness gymnasium, an isolation suite, a time-out room, spaces to encourage and facilitate participation and interaction, as well as a therapeutic garden.

Due to the rise of elderly patients with dementia and the increasing need for a memory clinic, IMH Memory Clinic was established on 13 February

2013 to detect early dementia, to recommend various interventions to slow down the progression of dementia, to keep patients in the community for as long as possible and to improve patients' and caregivers' quality of life.

References

Ministry of Health Singapore (1992). Review Committee on National Health Policies: Towards Better Healthcare.

Ministry of Health Singapore (2000). State of Health 2000: The Report of the Director of Medical Services.

Community Psychiatry

LEE Cheng

Mental Health Services in the Community

Community psychiatry has been defined as a community-based mental health service which provides a full range of effective mental health care to a defined population, and which is dedicated to treating and helping people with mental disorders, in proportion to their suffering or distress, in collaboration with other local agencies.

There are three periods in the development of mental health services: rise of the asylum, decline of the asylum and approach to 'balanced care' (Thornicroft and Tansella, 2002).

Mental illnesses were described as early as 1900 BC. During classical times, mental illnesses were believed to be physical in origin. From the Middle Ages to the 18th and 19th centuries, the mentally ill were perceived as spiritually or morally diseased. The emphasis then was on saving souls and not bodies, and treatment was through religious means rather than through medicine. Some were even burned at the stake. Subsequently asylums and large institutions were created, usually remote from their populations, offering mainly custodial containment and the provision of the basic necessities for survival. Patients were typically incarcerated, with many being locked in and also locked up in chains. Not only were the patients segregated, but the mental health professionals were also segregated from the main body of clinical practice.

Mental illnesses were previously considered hopeless and untreatable. The discovery of chlorpromazine by Delay and Deniker in 1952 indicated that drugs could be developed that would have a calming effect on psychotic and agitated patients (Delay and Deniker,1957). By the late 1950s, anti-depressants such as imipramine and anti-anxiety drugs such as meprobamate were also developed. This was the beginning of the de-institutionalisation movement. The movement gradually gained momentum and public support as it focused on the human rights of psychiatric patients, especially with the journalist exposés of abuses and the recognition of the damaging and anti-therapeutic effects of long-stay treatment for psychiatric patients.

Over the past decades, critics have highlighted the ill effects of de-institutionalisation. These include the rampant drug and alcohol use among psychiatric patients in the community. The patients may also be homeless and have untreated physical health problems. There was also a perceived threat to the community by the mentally ill when they relapsed due to poor treatment adherence. Family burden increased when the caregivers were not well supported. 'Trans-institutionalization' occurred when patients with psychiatric illness in the community committed crimes and were incarcerated in prisons.

In the third period, the balanced-care approach, community-based and hospital-based services commonly aim to provide treatment and care that (1) are close to home, including acute hospital care and long-term residential facilities in the community; (2) respond to disabilities as well as to symptoms; (3) are specific to the diagnosis and needs of each individual; (4) are consistent with international conventions on human rights; (5) are related to the priorities of service users themselves; (6) are coordinated between mental health professions and agencies; and (7) are mobile rather than static.

Several critical factors have been identified that have major influences on the success or failure of services provided in the community (Barton, 1966). These include the need for active aftercare and aggressive placement of patients discharged from acute care hospitals, the need for long-term administration of anti-psychotic medications for persons with serious and persistent mental illness, the need for additional acute care hospital beds to treat short-term episodes and the need for more clinicians to work in the community. In general, as mental health systems develop away from an asylum-based model, more services will be community-based; and the new services outside the hospital can only be provided by either using or tapping extra resources (for example, the primary care physicians), or transferring resources from the hospital sites.

Community Psychiatric Services in Singapore

Singapore has developed from a small trading post of the British Empire to a first-world nation in less than 50 years since its independence in 1965. As of 2011, the population stands at 5.18 million (Ministry of Health, 2011). There are 9646 registered doctors, giving a doctor-to-patient ratio of 1:537. Of these doctors, 157 are registered in Psychiatry, with 106 (67.5%) working in the public sector and 51 (32.5%) working in the private sector (Singapore Medical Council, 2011).

In Singapore, the Institute of Mental Health (IMH) (of which Woodbridge Hospital was a part) has been the de facto mental health service provider since 1928. It has about 2100 beds — one third of the beds are for acute care and the remaining two-thirds are generally for chronic care. However, the history of psychiatric care in Singapore dates back much earlier. The first psychiatric hospital in Singapore, 'The Hospital', as it was known then, was completed in 1841 and was located at the corner of Bras Basah Road and Bencoolen Street. Due to the increase in the number of patients, the hospital was shifted to larger premises, Kandang Kerbau Maternity Hospital in 1861 and Sepoy Lines in 1887. In 1967, in order to reach out to the community, two outpatient clinics were opened. The first child guidance clinic was also opened in 1970 (Sengupta *et al.*, 2012; Wei *et al.*, 2005).

IMH has always adopted a balanced-care approach in the provision and delivery of mental health services. The hospital strategic trust is aligned with the 2001 World Health Organisation (WHO) recommendation to provide cost-effective psychiatric care in the community. The Department of Community Psychiatry was formed with the following aims:

1. To provide optimal treatment for chronic psychiatric disorders outside of the hospital. The comprehensive treatment for chronic mental illness includes psychosocial rehabilitation, which aims to minimise disability

and produce the highest possible levels of functioning and well-being for the patients served.

2. To provide early treatment of acute psychiatric disorders. This involves health education and promotion so as to reduce the stigma associated with mental illness, and to encourage early appropriate help-seeking behaviour.

Community Clinics

Currently there are three adult community psychiatric clinics under the purview of the Department of Community Psychiatry. One is located within the campus of IMH and two are satellite clinics located in the east and west of Singapore. They are aptly known as Community Wellness Clinics (CWCs) and serve the local population. They are also located close to the Mass Rapid Transit train stations and both are situated within the premises of a general practice polyclinic. The multidisciplinary staff consists of psychiatrists, medical officers, psychiatric nurse practitioners, psychologists, medical social workers, case managers and occupational therapists, who work together to provide comprehensive assessment and treatment. Psychoeducation sessions are provided for both patients and their family members. On average, there are about 450 outpatient visits per day.

Amongst people identified in a community survey as having a psychiatric disorder, many do not seek medical advice. Whether a person with a psychiatric disorder consults a primary care provider depends on the severity and duration of the disorder, the person's attitude to the disorder, family and friends' attitude, knowledge about the possible help and perception of the doctor's attitude. The WHO World Mental Health Survey Consortium (Demyttenaere *et al.*, 2004) found that although disorder severity was correlated with probability of treatment, 35.5–50.3% of serious cases in developed countries and 76.3–85.4% in less developed countries received no treatment in the preceding 12 months before the interview. The Singapore Mental Health Survey

(Chong *et al.*, 2012) also reported the average time taken to seek help could range from a median of four years (major depressive disorder) up to a median of 13 years (alcohol abuse).

The Department of Community Psychiatry has been working closely with both the general practitioners and polyclinic doctors by providing regular updates and talks on psychiatric disorders. It also facilitates early referrals from the primary care service to the CWCs. We are also embarking on a shared care approach whereby the primary physician can attend to a patient with a psychiatric condition of mild to moderate severity on a regular basis, and where the psychiatrist can review the patient at less frequent intervals. Appropriate training of the primary care doctors is important for the shared care approach. The primary care doctors can also be supported by the allied health staff from IMH or mental health voluntary welfare organisations (VWOs) equipped with allied health staff. Effective coordinated care will require regular communication and feedback between all parties, and working out their respective roles with respect to the patient.

In addition, the Mental Health-General Practitioner (MH-GP) Partnership was introduced by the Ministry of Health in 2005. The programme provides ongoing training for primary physicians to manage patients with stable mental illness, as well as to enhance collaboration between primary physicians and tertiary care. The coordination of care by a case liaison officer ensures smooth transition from the hospital to community-based treatment (Lum *et al.*, 2010).

Community Psychiatric Nursing (CPN) Service

In 1988, the Community Psychiatric Nursing (CPN) service was established to provide care support and follow-up for selected patients in order to prevent relapses and to encourage them to function optimally in the community. During the home visits, the CPNs would assess the patient mental state and functioning level, administer depot anti-psychotic medications when necessary and observe for side effects of the medications.

They also monitor compliance to treatment, deliver continuing psychoeducation and give psychological support to the caregivers. Patients referred include those who have defaulted treatment or who have depended on proxy attenders at outpatient clinics for some time, patients with a history of poor compliance and those whose families had problems looking after in the past. This essential service supports these patients and their families, keeping them well in the community, preventing relapses of their illness and reducing readmissions.

Assertive Community Treatment (ACT)

The Assertive Community Treatment (ACT) programme or assertive outreach model associated with developments in Madison, Wisconsin has been one of the most important approaches in community psychiatry (Marx *et al.*, 1973; Stein and Test, 1980). ACT provides a comprehensive range of treatment, rehabilitation and support services through a multidisciplinary team based in the community. Basic characteristics of ACT programmes include assertive engagement, in vivo delivery of services, a multidisciplinary team approach, staff continuity and responsibility, caseloads with high staff-to-patient ratios and brief but frequent contacts (Scott and Dixon, 1995). The ACT approach has been widely adopted across the world. Evaluations where conducted often concluded that the approach can significantly improve outcome of patients (Mueser *et al.*, 1998). Many have shown ACT to be effective in reducing the number of days spent in psychiatric hospitals in different communities (Hoult *et al.*, 1983; Mulder, 1985; Salkever *et al.*, 1999). Studies have also shown ACT to be cost-effective (Rosenbeck *et al.* 1994; Essock *et al.*, 1998).

IMH adopted the ACT Programme in 2003 and identified the following aims for each patient (Lim *et al.*, 2005):

- To minimise or prevent recurrent relapses of the illness.
- To improve self-care and skills for independent living such as taking transport and handling financial transactions.

- To enhance the quality of life.
- To improve social and/or occupational functioning.
- To lessen the caregiver or family's burden of providing care.

The inclusion criteria of target cases were:

1. Individuals aged 18–65.
2. Moderately severe and persistent mental illness such as schizophrenia, delusional disorder and manic-depressive psychosis.
3. Presence of intractable symptoms and impairments that produce distress and major disability in daily functioning.
4. Individuals who experience significant disability from serious mental illnesses and are not helped by the traditional outpatient management model.
5. Three or more admissions in the last one-year period.

The IMH ACT team provides the treatment monitoring, rehabilitation and support services primarily through visits to the patients at their homes or workplaces. Through case coordination, the team also links the patients with other community resources which can help to meet their needs and goals such as applying through the Community Development Councils (local town councils) for financial assistance or help with job placement or liaising with social welfare agencies to provide free meals for patients in extreme poverty. The IMH ACT programme appears to be effective in reducing the frequency and duration of admissions for patients in Singapore. The employment status of patients also showed improvement over the course of study (Fam *et al.*, 2007).

Mobile Crisis Team (MCT)

The availability of support services to assist patients and their families when they face problems or a crisis can reduce the caregiver's burden and minimise the rejection of patients in society. The IMH Mobile Crisis Team

(MCT) is made up of the 24-hour helpline and the Crisis Intervention Team. The Helpline provides an avenue for them to speak to a qualified counsellor to obtain immediate assistance and appropriate advice. If necessary, a Crisis Intervention Team is dispatched for crisis interventions. These two services were launched by the Department of Community Psychiatry in the beginning of 2004. The IMH MCT consists of two community psychiatric nurses, with assistance from a medical officer or a medical social worker when needed. If necessary, especially in cases of acute relapses of illness when community treatment is not advisable, the MCT also assists in escorting patients for admission to IMH. Depending on the severity of the crisis, the police may be called in to assist in the resolution of the crisis.

In Singapore, we do not have community treatment orders (CTOs) which are a form of compulsory community treatment law that first appeared in the United States, Canada, Australia and New Zealand during

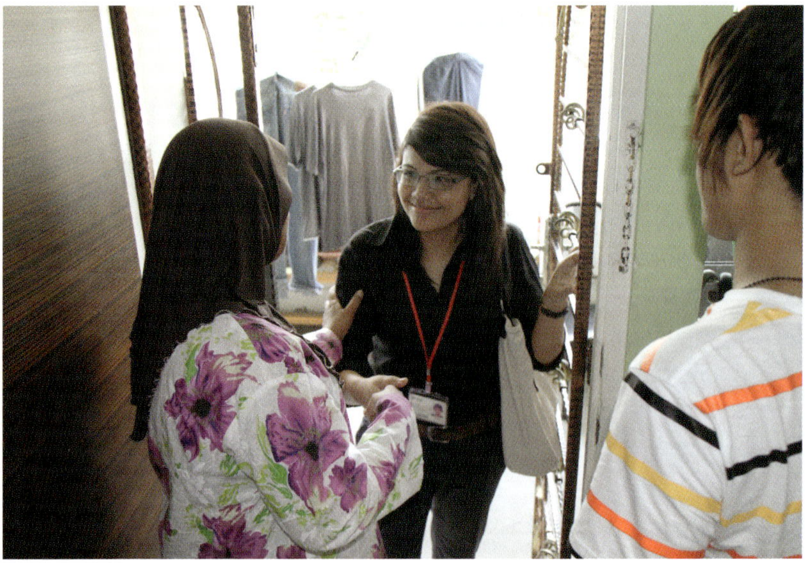

Medical social worker from CMHT visiting patient at home to assess the home environment and financial needs.

the 1980s. They provide a legal framework within which patients with a serious mental disorder are required to accept psychiatric treatment while living in the community, with aims to prevent relapse, hospital readmission and incarceration.

Based on current evidence (Cochrane Database of Systematic Reviews, 2008), CTOs may not be an effective alternative to standard care. It appears that compulsory community treatment results in no significant difference in service use, social functioning or quality of life compared with standard care. There is currently no evidence of cost effectiveness. People receiving compulsory community treatment were, however, less likely to be victims of violent or non-violent crime.

Community Mental Health Team (CMHT)

Currently both the ACT and MCT services are funded by the National Mental Health Blueprint (Ministry of Health, 2010) and renamed Community Mental Health Team (CMHT). The ACT clinical services are decentralised into four sectors, although the whole team meets in the hospital biweekly to maintain team cohesiveness and communication.

CMHT continues to focus on providing psychosocial rehabilitation to patients with multiple readmission episodes (with equivalent long inpatient length of stay) and hence high users of inpatient resources. However, to improve the care services for the many patients in CMHT, patients are categorised into two main groups for a more customised care management. Depending on the history and nature of the patient's psychiatric condition, different care management plans are tailored to treat patients more effectively. The rehabilitation service was thus separated into Assertive Care Management (ACM) and Standard Care Management (SCM) to provide the patients with psychosocial support targeted at their individual needs and required intensity (Department of Community Psychiatry, 2013).

- ACM: For patients who have had three or more admissions in the past year, with more than 30 days hospital stay per admission.

- SCM: For patients who have had less than three admissions in the past year and less than 30 days hospital stay per admission.

ACM patients require more intensive monitoring and they receive home visits every two to four weeks. SCM patients receive home visits at intervals of four to six weeks. In addition to conducting the home visits, the CMHT staff maintains regular contact with their patients via telephone to check on their progress and recovery.

Patients are discharged from CMHT service if they have:

- Successfully demonstrated ability to function in major role areas.
- Enrolled into a psychiatric residential care centre or a nursing home.
- Enrolled in an outreach service provide by another psychiatric community agency.
- Made a self-request — in this instance, the CMHT staff will discuss the case with the referring psychiatrist.

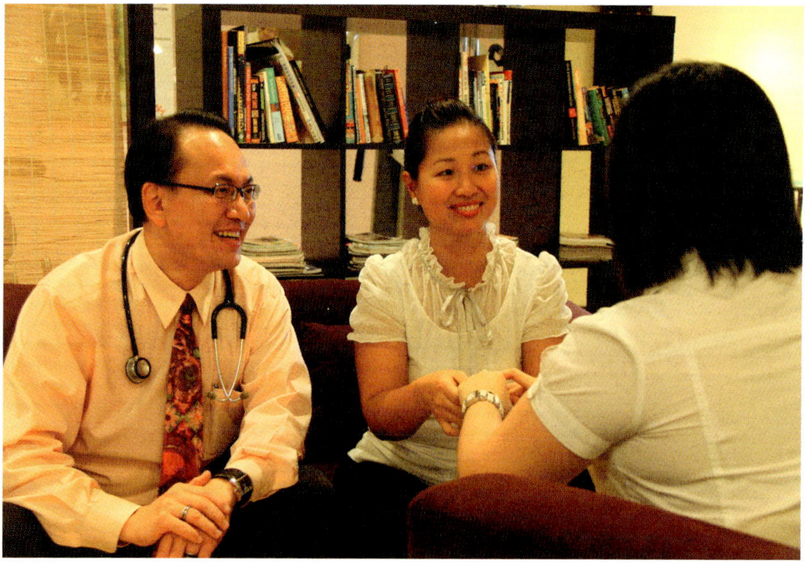

Doctor can conduct mental state evaluation and physical examination during a home visit.

If a patient is deemed not suitable for CMHT service, he/she will be referred to other appropriate community-based support services such as the National Addictions Management Service (NAMS) (see section on Addiction Medicine on page ___) if the primary condition is that of an addiction problem, or the Aged Psychiatry Community Assessment and Treatment Service (APCATS) (see section on Geriatric Services on page ___) if they are older than 65 years old.

Currently CMHT has also extended its psychosocial rehabilitation services to patients who are receiving psychiatric treatment at the different psychiatric departments of general hospitals.

There are many social welfare and religious organisations that reach out generically to the poor, the disabled and the disadvantaged in Singapore. A large number of individuals with mental illness are likely to be disadvantaged by unemployment, social isolation and poverty, and may need to tap the resources of these organisations. There are also mental

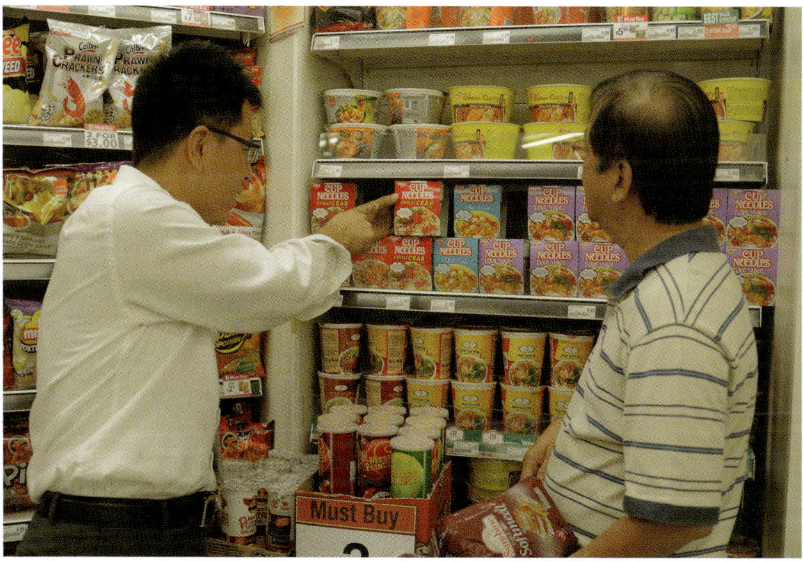

Besides home visits, CMHT staff also bring patients to the neighbourhood supermarket to teach them skills such as grocery shopiing and monetary transaction.

health VWOs (such as Singapore Association for Mental Health and Singapore Anglican Community Services) which are recognised for their services such as residential facilities (supported housing, hostels and long-stay care homes), day facilities (vocational training, activity centres and club houses) and patient support groups. These facilities and services provide opportunities for patients at different stages of the illness to interact. Patients may be more receptive to peers who have had positive experiences with therapeutic modalities and may perceive treatment to be more effective after interacting with their peers.

It is important to build a strong relationship between the providers from the health and social sectors. Traditionally, such a relationship has often been unplanned, piecemeal and episodic. Networking often happens when disagreement occurs between agencies or when an urgent need arises. These have often resulted in the provision of poorly integrated and fragmented services to clients and poor understanding between service providers.

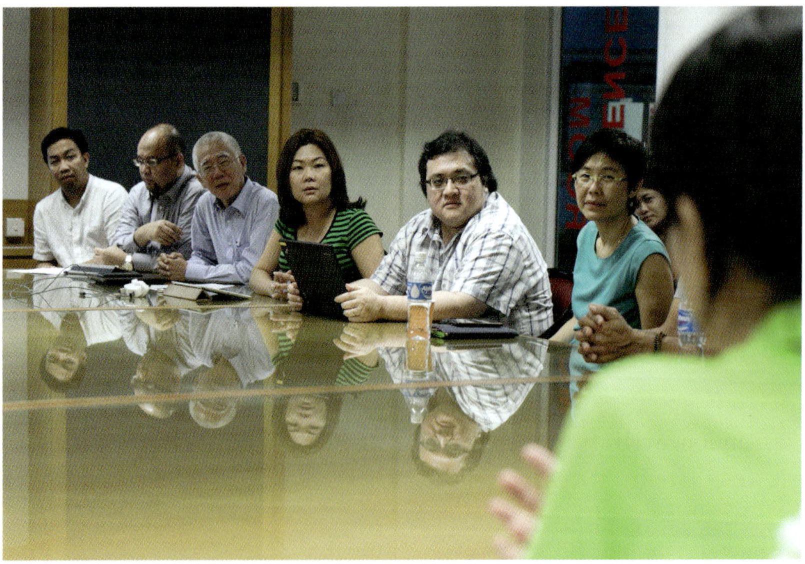

Dr Kelvin Ng *(3rd from right)* from CMHT at a case conference session with other community agencies.

Since its inception, CMHT has met up with social service providers such as Community Development Councils, Family Service Centres, prison service, police, psychosocial rehabilitation service providers and volunteers in the community grassroots organisations. The main goal for this collaborative effort is to provide holistic support to patients and their caregivers. During these networking sessions, CMHT not only shares its objectives and services but also actively addresses any existing service gaps. Additionally, the team offers assistance as requested by these agencies to manage patients in the community through case conferences, telephone consultations and other initiatives.

Mental Health Helpline

The Mental Health Helpline (MHH) is a multidisciplinary team of doctors, helpline counsellors, community psychiatric nurses, case managers and administrators. The key focus of the MHH team is to de-escalate pre-crisis situations, before it turns into a crisis that involves risk to self and others. Being cognisant that distressing situations can occur antime, the 24-hour helpline provides a convenient and immediate access for callers to seek necessary mental health advice and support (including home visits) for their loved ones or clients. As patients and caregivers' needs often go beyond just medical treatment, the team also works closely with community partners, the Singapore Police Force and other social service agencies to ensure continuity of holistic care for the patients.

MHH receives more than 1300 calls per month via the 24-hour helpline and activate more than 20 crisis home visits per month to assess patients' mental state. Approximately 30% of the home visits require admission into IMH so that the patient can receive the required psychiatric intervention. MHH has received compliments from caregivers and partners that were initially at a loss to manage these patients, but managed to do so successfully via collaboration with MHH.

In the community, MHH currently (as at September 2016) has over 140 partners, including family service centres, senior activity centres, town councils, mental health VWOs as well as grassroots organisations and constituencies. Since 2012, it has conducted almost 60 training sessions to all these partners, reaching out to more than 1600 people. In addition, MHH also led case conferences for complex cases involving mental health issues. A total of 402 cases were raised by constituencies and networks at this platform.

Community Psychiatry of the Future

There has been considerable development in community psychiatric services in Singapore and better collaborative efforts between the healthcare sector itself and between the health and social service sectors. We should tap best practices from all over the world but with sufficient modifications to suit our own sociocultural needs. With better collaboration among different providers, we could then provide better post-discharge care for our patients, by delivering efficient outreach and rehabilitation services. A community-based mental health service should be one which provides a full range of effective mental health care to a defined population, and which is dedicated to treating and helping people with mental disorders, in proportion to their suffering or distress, in collaboration with other local agencies.

Adopting a balanced-care approach, community-based and hospital-based services aim to provide treatment and care that (1) are close to home, including acute hospital care and long-term residential facilities in the community; (2) respond to disabilities as well as to symptoms; (3) are able to offer treatment and care specific to the diagnosis and needs of each individual; (4) are consistent with international conventions on human rights; (4) are related to the priorities of service users themselves; (5) are coordinated between mental health professions and agencies; and (6) are mobile rather than static. ACT provides a comprehensive range of treatment, rehabilitation and support services through a multidisciplinary team based in the community.

While tapping best practices from all over the world, there should be sufficient modifications to suit our own sociocultural needs. It is important to build a strong relationship between the providers from the health and social sectors. With better collaboration among different providers, we could then provide better post-discharge care for our patients, by delivering efficient outreach and rehabilitation services.

References

Barton WE (1966). Trends in community mental health programs. *Hosp Community Psychiatry* **17**: 253–258.

Chong SA, Abdin E, Sherbourne C, Vaingankar J, Heng D, Yap M, Subramaniam M (2012). Treatment gap in mental health care: The Singapore perspective. *Epidemiol Psychiatr Sci* **21**: 195–202.

Cochrane Database of Systematic Reviews (2008). Compulsory Community and Involuntary Outpatient Treatment for People with Severe Mental Disorders.

Delay J, Deniker O (1957). Characteristiques psychophysiologiques des medicaments neuroleptiques. In: Garattini J, Ghetti V, eds. *The Psychotropic Drugs*. Elsevier, Amsterdam, pp. 485–501.

Demyttenaere K *et al.* (2004). Prevalence, severity, and unmet need for treatment of mental disorders in the World Health Organization World Mental Health Surveys. *JAMA* **291**: 2581–2590.

Department of Community Psychiatry (2013). Caring for the Community: Community Mental Health Team Programme Report FY2007–11.

Essock SM, Frisman LK, Kontos NJ (1998). Cost-effectiveness of assertive community treatment teams. *Am J Orthopsychiatry* **68**: 179–190.

Fam J, Lee C, Lim BL, Lee KK (2007). Assertive Community Treatment (ACT) in Singapore: A one-year follow-up study. *Ann Acad Med Singapore* **36**: 409–412.

Hoult J, Reynolds I, Charbonneau-Powis M, Weekes P, Briggs J (1983). Psychiatric hospital versus community treatment: The results of a randomized trial. *Aust N Z J Psychiatry* **17**: 160–165.

Lim CG, Koh CW, Lee C, Poon WC (2005). Community psychiatry in Singapore: A pilot Assertive Community Treatment Programme. *Ann Acad Med Singapore* **34**: 100–104.

Lum WMA, Chew J, Lim BL (2010). The successful collaboration between psychiatrists, a mental health institution and general practitioners in primary care. *Singapore Fam Physician* **36**: 19.

Marx AJ, Test MA, Stein LI (1973). Extra-hospital management of severe mental illness: Feasibility and effects of social functioning. *Arch Gen Psychiatry* **29**: 505–511.

Ministry of Health (2010). Healthy Minds, Healthy Communities: National Mental Health Blueprint Singapore 2007–2012. https://www.imh.com.sg/uploadedFiles/Publications/IMH%20National%20Mental%20Health%20Blueprint.pdf

Ministry of Health (2011). Health Facts. Published in Singapore.

Mueser KT, Bond GR, Drake RE, Resnick G (1998). Models of community care for severe mental illness: A review of research on case management. *Schizophr Bull* **24**: 37–74.

Mulder R (1985). *Evaluation of the Harbinger Program, 1982–1985*. Michigan Department of Mental Health, Lansing, MI.

Rosenbeck R, Neale M, Frisman M (1994). Issues in estimating the cost of innovative mental health. *Psychiatr Q* **66**:1–23.

Salkever D, Domino ME, Burns BJ, Santos AB, Deci PA, Dias J, Wagner HR, Faldowski RA, Paolone J (1999). Assertive community treatment for people with severe mental illness: The effect on hospital use and costs. *Health Serv Res* **34**: 577–601.

Scott JE, Dixon LB (1995). Assertive community treatment and case management for schizophrenia. *Schizophr Bull* **2**: 657–668.

Singapore Medical Council (2011). Singapore Medical Council Annual Report 2011.

Sengupta S, Leong JY, Lee C (2012). Community psychiatry in Singapore. In: Chavan BS, Gupta N, Arun P, Sidana A, Jadhav S, eds. *Community Mental Health in India*. Jaypee Brothers Medical Publishers (P) Ltd.

Stein L, Test M (1980). Alternatives to mental hospital treatment. *Arch Gen Psychiatry* **37**: 297–392.

Thornicroft G, Tansella M (2002). Balancing community-based and hospital-based mental health care. *World Psychiatry* **1**: 84–90.

Wei KC, Lee C, Wong KE (2005). Community psychiatry in Singapore: An integration of community mental health services towards better patient care. *Hong Kong J Psychiatry* **15**: 132–137.

Military Psychiatry

SOH Teck Hwee and Christopher CHEOK

'He (the Minister of Defence) has to manage a large conscript army. To do this, he must understand what makes Singaporeans tick and what causes them to switch off. Since there are so many kinds of Singaporeans, this understanding does not come easily ... in the course of my work, I often visit military camps. One of the lasting impressions I get is the image of the National Serviceman on sentry duty — a bespectacled youth of slender proportions, ill at ease in an unaccustomed environment but trying to conceal it. An improbable soldier.'

Dr Goh Keng Swee
Singapore's First Minister for Defence

Psychiatrists in the Military

The words by Dr Goh Keng Swee probably aptly summarises the *raison d'etre* of military psychiatry in the Singapore Armed Forces (SAF). As much as National Service is a part of Singapore society, military psychiatry in the Singapore Armed forces has been an integral part of the local psychiatric community. Since its humble beginnings as a part-time practice by a single psychiatrist in a refurbished storeroom at the then Tanglin Medical Centre, it has grown into an entire multidisciplinary service with its own clinic space and a ward with psychologists and case managers, managing not only clinical work but policies and operational psychiatric issues.

Military psychiatry in the SAF was started by Dr Fong Yen Hoi in 1973. Although it was only a single-doctor section, Dr Fong laid the foundation of what was to become and still is one of the hallmarks of the military psychiatric practice: the complete holistic occupational health approach to psychiatry, focusing not just on clinical well-being but development of policies and shaping of the military environment to ensure that our soldiers are able to perform at their best psychologically in the challenging military environment.

The military environment and the system of conscription intertwined with the changing social fabric of Singapore society present a unique set of stressors for each succeeding generation of soldiers. There is no 'one size fits all' solution, and meeting these demands this has been the challenge for each generation of military psychiatrists.

The Early Years

From 1973 to 1998 the psychiatric section in the Medical Corps grew in strength both in terms of manpower and set-up. It culminated in 1998 with the establishment of the Psychological Care Centre (PCC) providing both clinical services at an outpatient centre in the Military Medicine Institute (MMI) and an inpatient ward in Alexandra Hospital, the Psychological Medicine Inpatient Centre (PMIC), fondly referred to by most doctors and patients as 'the SAF ward'. It was then headed by Dr Ang Yong Guan. By then, the number of military psychiatrists had grown, with many of them being familiar names to the psychiatric fraternity in Singapore. They include Dr Simon Siew, Dr James Lee Tock Eng and Dr Lionel Lim.

The early years of military psychiatry in the SAF focused on basic service and capacity building, and policy guidelines of screening and deployment. The latter years focused on operational demands and enhancement of mental health in the SAF.

Evolving Needs in Operations

The establishment of PCC under Dr Ang Yong Guan with its ability to provide comprehensive psychiatric care marks a maturation of the peacetime clinical services in the SAF. The next cycle of evolution was meeting the evolving demands of the SAF's increasing operational requirements.

There is a psychological cost to all military missions, and the military psychiatrist is called into action following significant incidents or support operations in the SAF. This work was spearheaded by Dr John Wong Chee Meng who underwent a stint at Walter Reed Hospital in the United States where he did work in the area of traumatic stress in the military. Dr Wong and Dr Chew Peng Hoe refined the existing operational doctrine for combat stress based on the principles of proximity and immediacy in treatment. This including drawing up of detailed plans and formalising a training programme and system for handling combat stress in the SAF. Till today, all military medical officers are taught the basics of handling combat stress while military psychiatrists and psychologists undergo training in the Critical Incident Stress Management Model (Everly and Mitchell, 1997) for handling psychological trauma. Dr John Bosco Lee and Dr Christopher Cheok took over from Dr John Wong and continued his work. This was work that spanned several years with continuous refinements based in advances in research as well as the experiences of various SAF psychiatrists in operations. What started as an application of basic principles in battlefield medicine evolved to become a standardised doctrine to be used across all three services in the SAF in 2011 for management of combat stress. Also established was a system for managing traumatic stress with other stakeholders in mental health, which included the SAF Counseling Centre as well as the organisational psychologists from the Defense Psychological Department (formerly known as Applied Behavioural Science Department).

The provision of operational psychological support is the cornerstone of military psychiatry, and SAF psychiatrists have been called upon to serve on numerous occasions. These range from the fields of Indonesia with the deployment of our soldiers in a massive humanitarian mission following the 2004 Asian Tsunami (known as Operations Flying Eagle) to the deserts of Afghanistan where two of our psychiatrists were deployed to a Role 2 hospital while others did psychological screening and debriefing for members of the teams that were deployed in Afghanistan. The SAF deployed soldiers to Afghanistan as part of the International Security Assistance Force to contribute to the stabilisation and reconstruction of Afghanistan. The other notable incidents when SAF psychiatrists have been called to action include the tragic collision of an RSN naval patrol vessel, the *RSS Courageous*, in 2003 as well as the crash of a training jet into a camp in one of our overseas training bases. The nature of the work spans from preventive measures in the form of briefings and screening of deployed personnel to monitoring of psychological health status to management of acute stress disorders and post-traumatic stress disorders.

> *'The team managed different groups of soldiers with a multitude of reactions. At the commander level, they felt personally responsible for their units' loss; immediate superiors felt guilt for sending them to the warehouse where the mishap occurred. Colleagues felt grief and rage in the initial days.'*
>
> LTC (NS) (Dr) Christopher Cheok who lead the psychiatric team following the crash of a foreign jet into a SAF troop training area

It is through this combination of good leadership and incident management that the SAF has been able to mitigate the psychological consequences of such incidents.

Increasing Capacity

The next milestone in PCC came in 2006 with a drive towards further enhancement of psychiatric care in the SAF with the approval of a restructuring of the PCC to increase its capacity. The drivers for this change were the needs to meet increasing clinical demands as well as a progressive move towards mental health promotion and building of resilience. This move towards positive psychology as well as more holistic care aims to equip soldiers with knowledge and skill, becoming more psychologically minded and better prepared to handle challenges so as to reduce occurrence of mental illness. The reorganisation included the establishment of a specific section to look into preventive and operations psychiatry and an increase in number of psychologists providing therapy.

This allowed for dedicated assets to develop the areas of health promotion through formalised education of commanders. Talks and workshops were held at various stages of their careers on the management of soldiers with difficulties coping as well as the understanding of mental illness. There was also the training of recruits themselves. One of the key features was the Building Resilient Thinking in Individuals for Growth and Emotional Wellbeing (BRIDGE) program. It is a PCC-driven tripartite effort with Defence Psychology Department (DPD) and SAF Counselling Center (SCC) to educate soldiers on common faulty thinking errors that negatively impact emotional well-being.

These efforts in primary prevention were complemented by improvements in secondary and tertiary prevention with the introduction of case managers. The case managers function was a link between the units and the psychiatrist and help to shape the workplace environment as well as monitor the progress of the patients at work. The SAF senior leadership led by then Chief of Defence Force Lieutenant General Neo Kian Hon saw a need for greater outreach and coordination of psychiatric care. The Soldier Resilience Hub (SRH) was set up in 2011. This was a joint forum comprising human resource agencies in the SAF as well as clinicians in which the mental health needs of soldiers (as reflected in policies, programmes, campaigns and education) can be addressed holistically. The establishment of the SRH as well as expansion into case management in 2011 marked another major improvement to the practice of military psychiatry in the SAF. This is of particular importance given the nature of military psychiatry. The military environment is a unique one and patients do experience difficulties coping and adjusting. The role of the military psychiatrist is not merely to treat an illness but to ensure that the soldier remains able to serve in the military and to contribute meaningfully. In line with this, there are plans to wind down the inpatient services of the ward and move towards the concept of a day rehabilitation centre. This will allow for the provision of therapy and training of coping skills in a larger group setting more closely mimicking the camp environment.

> *'During my time working at the Psychological Care Center, I had the chance not just to see distressed servicemen in times of need, but I also had the chance to impact their lives during their time in National Service.'*
>
> Maj (NS) (Dr) Jared Ng, former regular SAF psychiatrist on his work at PCC

These changes in the military psychiatric landscape are still ongoing today with a continual buildup of the capacity of PCC. They would not have been possible without the relentless efforts of various military psychiatrists spanning the tours of several heads starting with Dr Christopher Cheok to Dr Wong Sheau Hwa to Dr Adrian Loh. Credit must also go to the long-serving clinical psychologist Ms Dorothy Teo and the PCC clinic manager Ms Cecilia Tan for driving the psychological portions as well as the daily administration of PCC along with teams of full-time National Service (NSF) medics. These NSF medics often display a maturity beyond their years as they assist in the delivery of healthcare.

The increase in capacity demanded an equal increase in the number of military psychiatrists. The SAF has also leveraged upon the national system for the training of its doctors, including postgraduate training via various hospital rotations. In 2001, the Advanced Specialty Training Programme was revised and PCC, which was previously an accredited training centre, was not audited. In 2003, PCC began its journey to become an accredited postgraduate training centre for AST once again. This was to allow the time which advanced trainees spent in PCC to be recognised towards their certification for advanced specialty training. The then chairman of the Specialist Training Committee, Prof Kua Ee Heok, was consulted and a training roadmap was drafted and subsequently endorsed by Headquarters Medical Corps and implemented. This was again changed in tandem with the changes towards a seamless training programme in psychiatry training. PCC become an accredited training centre for AST again in 2010 under the then Head of PCC Senior Lieutenant Colonel (Dr) Wong Sheau Hwa. A new challenge arose in 2012 with the move towards residency. Head of PCC Dr Robin Goh undertook another review and once again PCC was recognised and accredited by ACGME from 2013.

From the Tanglin Barracks in the 1980s to the establishment of outpatient clinics at MMI in 1998, the physical structure housing military psychiatry has its own colourful history. The familiar façade of the current PMIC in Alexandria Hospital was only established in 2004. In 1997, the SAF ward was established at the old Ward 9 of Alexandria Hospital. It actually shifted to Nee Soon Camp for a period of time in 2003 due the SARS outbreak and it shifted back to a newly renovated SAF ward which is its current premises. The ward and the clinic have always been separate and this poses logistical challenges. There are plans to relocate once again, along with a move by the Headquarters Medical Corps (HQMC), so that all the various SAF specialist healthcare facilities (currently at Kent Ridge) are with the Medical Classification Centre (currently at the Defence Technology Tower at Depot Road) altogether at the brand new medical complex at Gombak. This will allow for merging of the ward with the clinic. The proposed new move also increases the area for the ward to eventually become a day centre focusing on outpatient rehabilitation of patients with space for conducting group therapy and plans for setting up of physical simulations of military environment to slowly acclimatise patients back to work.

Part of the National Mental Health System

Military psychiatry does not stand alone. It is an integral part of the national mental health landscape. It is not possible to speak of military psychiatry and not mention its links with the rest of Singapore psychiatry. There is no clearer evidence of this than our greatest resource, the people that make up PCC. Just as National Service is the rite of passage for all male Singapore citizens, serving at PCC as part of their posting as

NSF medical officers or operationally ready NS men has been an integral part of many male psychiatrists' clinical careers. PCC alumni include Dr George Fernandez, Dr Leslie Lim, Dr Alex Su, Dr Marcus Tan, Dr Tan Hao Yang, Dr Seng Kok Han, Dr Chan Herng Nieng and Dr Soo Shunqiang.

> *'It is a privilege to be able to assist people with mental health issues in the SAF. It is an honour to be part of the PCC team which is at the forefront of doing this critical work.'*
>
> Dr Chan Herng Nieng, consultant NS man psychiatrist at PCC

This collaboration continues as SAF psychiatrists continue to work together with their civilian counterparts to co-manage patients. This collaboration extends beyond individual patient care to research projects. The SAF works with numerous partners to conduct research into areas that pertain to the mental health of our servicemen. This is of particular importance given the epidemiology of certain mental illnesses, such as psychosis, having an early age of onset. Research projects include Longitudinal Youth-at-Risk Study (LYRIKS), Early Psychosis Intervention Program (EPIP) at Institute of Mental Health (IMH), epidemiology of pre-enlistees and a project to identify biomarkers for depression with IMH and Khoo Teck Puat Hospital. Such collaborations aid in improving the screening processes, deployment and management of the mainly young NSF population.

Dr Fong Yen Hoi said about being a pioneer, 'We had to set up the protocols and policy not knowing if they would work. But we refined them through the years.' And refine them we did. While military psychiatry has taken huge strides through the years, it is timing to reflect that these were refinements upon the works of those that tread before us.

The core business and fundamental principles have not changed. The military psychiatrist in the SAF is there to help the soldier cope better mentally within the military context.

Reference

Everly GS, Mitchell JT (1997). *Critical Incident Stress Management (CISM): A New Era and Standard of Care in Crisis Intervention*. Chevron Publishing, Ellicott City, MD.

Forensic Psychiatry

Jerome GOH, Kenneth KOH, Stephen PHANG and ONG Say How

Introduction

Forensic Psychiatry in the Institute of Mental Health (IMH) has its roots in general psychiatry and traditionally follows an 'integrated model', where forensic assessments were performed by doctors in general psychiatric departments, but more concentrated in one of these departments. Doctors would balance their ward rounds and clinics commitments and forensic assessments.

With the move to the current Buangkok Green Medical Park premises in 1993, one block was designated 'Forensic'. Although the ward layout is similar to other blocks, the Forensic block possesses infrastructure that meets the requirements of a 'medium secure' unit, with external fencing, security screening, surveillance and monitoring systems as well as reinforced steel gates. There are also security staff deployed in certain forensic wards where there is a need for higher security.

The bulk of forensic work in IMH has traditionally been concentrated in two areas: forensic assessments for the State Courts, and treatment of mentally disordered offenders. Being the national centre for psychiatry also means that IMH doctors are often involved in policy and programme discussions with the Police, the Singapore Prison Service (SPS), the Ministry of Home Affairs (MHA) and the Ministry of Social and Family Development (MSF), and interface with the legal profession over laws that concern the mentally ill.

The Courts may remand individuals who are arrested for offences for psychiatric evaluations if they are suspected to be mentally unwell or unfit to plead, and hundreds of such assessments are done each year in IMH. All homicide cases also require a forensic psychiatric evaluation, where diminished responsibility is a potential defence. There are also forensic evaluations done in outpatient settings, who are either referred by the police or defence counsels. Individuals involved in criminal proceedings are sometimes referred to IMH during the pre-sentencing phase, for assessment of risks and to explore treatment options.

IMH also has inpatient wards for the treatment of mentally disordered offenders who are detained under the Criminal Procedure Code, as they have been found to be of unsound mind or unfit to plead by the Courts. These inpatient wards are known as Visitors' Board (VB) wards, and they also treat individuals who are detained under our Mental Health Act. Risk assessments, a multidisciplinary team and psychiatric treatment and rehabilitation are important features of these VB wards, and regular reviews by the Board of Visitors on their progress or need for continuing their detention are informed through progress reports from doctors, nurses, medical social workers and occupational therapists.

Forensic Subspecialisation

There is growing recognition for the need for further specialisation in Forensic Psychiatry. This is reflected by a rapidly growing body of knowledge in Forensic Psychiatry, and higher expectations and scrutiny of forensic work, as well as the need to adopt and incorporate best practices in forensic evaluation and treatment.

Adult Psychiatry Services in IMH

The Adult Psychiatry Department 2 adopted a forensic nomenclature in January 2010, and was renamed the Department of General and Forensic Psychiatry, and a 'parallel model' was thus adopted. The bulk of capital cases have since been done by specialists in this department, and cases remanded by the Courts in IMH are assessed by both specialists as well as specialists in training.

Forensic evaluation work

Forensic evaluation work is a critical part of our work, and recent focus has been on adopting the best practices of forensic mental health assessments, given the role the Forensic department plays. There is a continued appreciation of the importance of psychiatric opinions in sentencing considerations, especially in capital cases. In the current context, ongoing risk assessments have become an integral part of the forensic practice of psychiatry, with assessing psychiatrists being expected to not only perform risk assessments, but also recommend, and in some cases, even arrange for the care of offenders deemed to pose a significant risk, either to themselves, or others.

Having staff predominantly doing forensic work has predictably accelerated forensic skills acquisition, building up relevant experience and forensic service development. The advent of the new generation of formally trained forensic psychiatrists dates back to the late 1990s, when the first specialists were sent to such world renowned centres as the Institute of Psychiatry in London, UK, as well the Victorian Institute of Forensic Mental Health, Melbourne, Australia. Prior to this era, general psychiatrists performed forensic evaluations, as alluded to above. Training has also, of course, been targeted at clinical and allied health staff engaged in specific areas of forensic work.

Work with the Singapore Prison Service (SPS)

Discussion with SPS on the provision of psychiatric services led to the establishment of the Psychiatric Housing Unit (PHU) for male mentally disordered offenders in April 2011. With the support of IMH's Psychiatric Rehabilitation Service, the Illness Self-Management and Recovery (ISMR) model was adopted for use in a correctional population in the PHU. Under this model, Nurses and Occupational Therapists perform a crucial role in the inmates' rehabilitation, by teaching skills such as illness and medication management, and the importance of structured activities in community reintegration upon their release. The PHU is located in one of the housing units within Changi Prison where clinical and allied health staff are stationed, so that offenders with mental disorders can be managed centrally and more effectively. It complements the current 'in-reach' model that SPS already offers, where prisons psychiatrists would review and treat offenders with mental disorders who are housed in the broader prison population. Since its creation, up to 600 inmates have benefited from placement in the PHU, substantially higher than the numbers managed in forensic inpatient 'treatment' wards in the same period. A recent notable development is the setting of a PHU for female inmates in Changi Women's Prison in November 2013, also run by IMH's Forensic Psychiatry department.

Reintegration of ex-offenders with mental illness into the community

In the third quarter of 2011, the Forensic Psychiatry Community Service (FPCS) began operations. With pilot funding by the Ministry of Health (MOH), it focuses on the continuity of psychiatric care in the community of offenders upon their release from incarceration. Mental health staff would review inmates in prisons referred by the mainstream parts of SPS or the PHU, to assess their clinical risks and needs. This is to facilitate the exploration of appropriate interventions in advance, rather than at the point of release or only on presentation to mental health services outside of the penal environment. The FPCS thus serves as a crucial 'bridge' for continuity of care and access to services for released inmates to facilitate reintegration into the community. Most of these cases continue to receive outpatient follow-up at IMH and, in a few cases, the FPCS has facilitated admissions to IMH to stabilise their mental health conditions. The FPCS complements the work done by the PHU. It is envisaged that both will help to reduce the 'revolving door' phenomenon that some mental health sufferers find themselves in, caught in a cycle of mental unwellness and re-offending.

Community-based sentencing option — the Mandatory Treatment Order programme

The third major initiative started in 2011 was the Mandatory Treatment Order (MTO) programme. At its inception and even now, the MTO is unique and innovative in its approach among diversion schemes worldwide. It is a community-based sentencing option, and allows the Courts to order an offender to undergo compulsory psychiatric treatment in-lieu of imprisonment for a maximum period of two years. Its objectives are three-fold: to provide an effective and targeted approach to rehabilitating mentally ill offenders, for better utilisation of resources which would otherwise be allocated to incarceration, and giving a 'second chance' for mentally ill persons charged with relatively minor offences. Among the various community-based sentences, the MTO has become the most utilised and 'over-subscribed' programme.

Recent developments

The revision of Singapore's drug trafficking laws in 2012, where diminished responsibility can be a potential defence, has led to the involvement of IMH's psychiatrists in forensic evaluations for arrested drug 'couriers', thus expanding the scope of forensic assessment work in the department.

Yet another more recent initiative in forensic evaluation work is the forensic department's collaboration with the Criminal Legal Aid Scheme (CLAS) in doing forensic evaluations for those involved in criminal proceedings and represented by pro bono lawyers. The forensic department also worked with the Attorney General Chambers (AGC) and MSF in exploring a diversionary scheme for offenders who commit minor offences.

The expanding forensic programmes development in recent years requires IMH to work even more closely with criminal justice agencies, to achieve a shared goal of reducing re-offending. Co-morbidities, such as substance misuse and personality disorders, are common in mentally disordered offenders, and these individuals also have multiple and complex risks and needs.

The Forensic Psychiatry department has worked with the Courts on improving coordination and usefulness of forensic psychiatric evaluations to the Courts, and to understand their needs better. The department also hosted visits to forensic wards for the judiciary, AGC's legal officers, defence counsels, prisons staff and the police.

To drive programme development, the Forensic Psychiatry department has also focused on trainings and skills acquisition for forensic staff, and benefitted from a network built up over the years. The department has invited overseas experts to teach staff on risk assessments (2010 and 2015), forensic community psychiatry (2012), high secure forensic services (2012), psychiatric rehabilitation (2011) and offender treatment programme (Reasoning and Rehabilitation 2, 2013). Staff are also sent on postings to forensic services in other countries like the UK, Australia and Canada to learn about provision of forensic services to their mentally ill populations.

The Forensic Psychiatry Department has also benefitted from training jointly organised with criminal justice agencies in areas such as Courtroom Skills and the criminal justice framework. In return, it has organised training on mental health issues for correctional officers, encompassing the sharing of best practices. Recent years have also seen the Forensic Psychiatry Department's clinicians involved in teaching medical students and law students.

Being the only forensic service and the centre of expertise for forensic psychiatry in Singapore, the Department of Forensic Psychiatry continues to be involved in consultancy work, on the revision of legislation affecting the mentally ill, such as Mental Capacity Act, Mental Health (Care and Treatment Act), Criminal Procedure Code, Criminal Law reform work and improving mental health services for correctional population, as well as direct consultations by such agencies as AGC in respect of freighted cases, with potentially prominent medicolegal/social implications. In these instances, the department's specialists have appeared in court to professionally assist the judicial process, akin to psychiatric 'amicus curiae'.

With the nationwide adoption of the Residency programme, the forensic department is privileged to be recognised as a key psychiatric subspecialty, and all psychiatric residents pass through the department to pick up skills in forensic report writing, risk assessment and management.

Child and Adolescent Forensic Psychiatry Services in IMH

Introduction

Juvenile delinquency and anti-social behaviour is a significant problem that adversely affects not only the individual and his immediate family, but also imposes a serious and significant social, psychological, emotional and economic burden on his community and society. If left unchecked, there is a high risk of the juvenile delinquent or anti-social youth becoming an anti-social adult and embarking on a criminal career. Often, it has been found that delinquent and anti-social children and youth have mental health problems that perpetuate and aggravate the problem.

Recent scientific studies using well-standardised procedures have shown that as many as 65% of youths in the juvenile justice system have diagnosable disorders (Garland *et al.*, 2001; Teplin *et al.*, 2002; Wasserman *et al.*, 2002). However, many juveniles with mental health difficulties come into the justice system without having been either identified or treated in their communities. In one study of juvenile detainees, only 40% of those with a diagnosed substance use disorder and only 34% of those with anxiety, mood, or disruptive behaviour disorders had received earlier services (Novins *et al.*, 1999).

Fortunately, such negative outcomes are not inevitable. There is increasing recognition of the importance of identifying and responding to the mental health needs of these children and youth. With early screening and identification of mental health conditions in the juvenile delinquents or children at risk and the provision of appropriate treatment and intervention, such a negative trajectory can be averted.

Child abuse, in its various forms, not only causes child mortality, but also leads to significant physical, psychological and social–emotional morbidity. Child abuse can cause immediate or short-term damage to the individual as well as affect his or her development and future functioning as a competent and well-adjusted individual. Adverse psychosocial outcomes associated with child abuse include the development of anti-social and aggressive behaviour, criminality, depression, borderline personality disorder and low self-esteem, amongst a whole host of various mental disorders. Abused children also have an increased risk of growing up to be dysfunctional parents who batter or neglect their offspring — the so-called intergenerational transmission of abuse and neglect. Such tragic outcomes are avoidable with early identification and appropriate intervention.

In the past, the Department of Child and Adolescent Psychiatry did not have a dedicated forensic assessment and treatment service for children and adolescents presenting with abuse-related trauma issues or forensic issues. Such patients were usually only seen by the psychiatrist for an assessment. However, there was no standardised assessment format. Treatment was provided by the psychiatrist on an ad-hoc basis, without much input from allied health professionals such as the medical social worker or the psychologist. In addition, the psychologists assigned to provide treatment to this patient population were not specifically trained in child and adolescent forensic issues. In such situations, the psychologist used generic treatment methods often applied in general child psychology.

Previously, juvenile offenders incarcerated in the corrective homes run by the then Ministry of Community, Youth and Sports (MCYS), were brought handcuffed to the clinic if they needed a psychiatric assessment or therapy. We realised that this practice had the potential of undermining the youth's fragile self-esteem. Additionally, the presence of the police escort during the assessment or treatment sessions also posed a hindrance to the development of a positive therapeutic relationship between the patient or his or her doctor or therapist. Furthermore, we noticed that often the person who brought the juvenile to the clinic was usually not directly involved in the care of the patient. Thus we were unable to get useful information about the juvenile's condition in the corrective home or have a meaningful discussion about how the corrective home staff could positively work with the patient in various areas of need or concern. To address these issues, we felt that it was best if clinical services could be provided on-site at the corrective homes to better support the assessment and management of these troubled children and adolescents.

Establishment of the Forensic Rehabilitation, Intervention, Evaluation and Network Development Services (FRIENDS)

With MOH's special Reinvestment funding, the Forensic Rehabilitation, Intervention, Evaluation and Network Development Services (FRIENDS) was established in the Department of Child and Adolescent Psychiatry in 2010 to provide a comprehensive, integrated, multi-systemic and multidisciplinary assessment, treatment and intervention service to juvenile offenders and abuse victims with mental health issues.

In addition to child psychiatrists, the FRIENDS team is staffed by a group of psychologists and social workers who have been specifically trained in child and adolescent forensic issues and assessment and treatment methods. Besides prescribing medication for any underlying or co-morbid psychiatric conditions such as attention deficit disorder with hyperactivity or depression, a range of specialised psychological therapies are offered to the child or adolescent who presents with either abuse-related issues or at-risk or offending behaviours. The individual psychotherapies for abuse victims include cognitive–behaviour therapy, trauma-focused cognitive–behaviour therapy, trauma-informed therapy, eye movement desensitising reprocessing therapy and creative expressive therapies like play and sand therapy. Individual psychotherapy for juvenile offenders includes supportive therapy and cognitive therapy that address the offending behaviour and the underlying contributory or co-morbid factors.

A holistic management involving the multiple ecosystems in which the child or youth lives is needed to attenuate risk factors for child abuse or juvenile anti-social behaviours. The child's or youth's family, school and community are roped in to support the therapeutic process and promote positive parenting and family functioning.

Besides providing direct care to the child abuse victim and the juvenile delinquent, the FRIENDS team also provides advice, consultation and training to other professionals dealing with troubled children and youth. By providing these professionals with information on child abuse, childhood trauma, juvenile delinquency and other mental health issues, it is believed that they will be better equipped to help troubled children and youth under their care.

In addition to providing help to abused and at-risk juveniles, the child psychiatrist in the FRIENDS team also conducts custody and access assessments when children are caught in complex and acrimonious child custody and access proceedings. To improve the process, a standardised assessment framework has been put in place following the establishment of the FRIENDS team.

Besides providing direct clinical services, training and consultation to helping professionals, the FRIENDS team also liaises and collaborates with agencies such as the Police, MSF, AGC and the Courts to enhance our common understanding of the juvenile offender or abuse victim so that this particular vulnerable population can be better helped.

Finally, the FRIENDS team also runs a helpline to provide support and advice to pre-appointed contact persons in the various collaborating agencies. The forensic team helps to provide preliminary assessment and advice when collaborating agencies encounter suspected or complicated cases that might need psychiatric input. The forensic team also facilitates case conferences or multi-agency meetings to share information about the particular juveniles, if needed, or to help fine-tune the work processes and services that will best help the vulnerable child victim or the troubled juvenile offender population.

Conclusions and Future Plans

Forensic psychiatry is in essence a subspecialty of psychiatry in which medical, neuroscience, mental health expertise and clinical experience are applied to court cases in order to form an objective opinion in legal litigation. Forensic psychiatrists are retained as experts in a variety of criminal (as well as civil) cases. Generally, their assistance is most critical in high-stakes cases, those in which either life or liberty are in jeopardy. The provision of expert testimony in the courts of law is, of course, the most visible aspect of the forensic psychiatrist's work. An expert states the facts and assumptions on which he bases his opinions, and present evidence to the court which is independent and uninfluenced by the exigencies of litigation, or any other group. In other words, the expert opinion is objective, unbiased and pertains only to matters within the professional expertise of the expert.

A competent forensic psychiatrist is a highly experienced clinician, familiar with legal issues, who can weigh psychiatric evidence and present logical and compelling explanations for their opinions based on the evidence available in the case and the background of scientific knowledge pertaining to mental disorders and human motivation. When an expert gives an opinion on an issue, and that opinion is not challenged, the court will normally accept the opinion if it is based on a sound foundation and is not otherwise objectionable. Of course, it is manifestly clear that an expert opinion is not the mere guesswork, surmise or speculation of the expert: it is his judgement on a matter of professional fact; it differs from ordinary evidence on matters of fact in that it is not based on the use of untutored senses or on the observation of the average man, but on specialised training, uncommon experiences and recondite theoretical information.

Forensic psychiatry is a relatively nascent field in Singapore and forensic development in IMH has seen major changes in recent years, with the setting up of the PHU, forensic community service and the MTO programmes. In addition, other changes in recent years are a combination of forensic specialisation, focus on training and building a network of communication and collaboration with criminal justice agencies, with the shared goal of reducing recidivism and breaking the 'revolving door' phenomenon of treatment disengagement, mental unwellness and re-offending. The new services help to ensure greater access to services and continuity of care for mentally disorders offenders, who often have multiple co-morbidities and complex risks and needs.

Forensic evaluation remains a core part of forensic work in Singapore, and recent focus has been on adopting best practices of forensic mental health assessments and communication with criminal justice agencies on relevance and utility of forensic reports, and promoting an understanding of forensic psychiatry work to them in return.

References

Chee KT (2017). Chapter 7 Law and Psychiatry. *Psychiatry in Singapore: A Guide (pp. 121).*

Garland AF *et al.* (2001). Prevalence of psychiatric disorders in youths across five sectors of care. *J Am Acad Child Adolesc Psychiatr* **40**(4): 409–418.

Goh J, Tomita TM (2014). Forensic psychiatry. In: Sim K, Sengupta S, Fung D, Chee KT, eds. *Essential Guide to Psychiatry*. Pearson, Singapore, pp. 339–352.

Heilbrun K, Grisso T, Goldstein A (2008). *Foundations of Forensic Mental Health Assessments*. Oxford University Press.

Ng BY (2016). *Till the Break of Day: A History of Mental Health Services in Singapore, 1841–1993 (2nd Edition)*. NUS Press.

Novins D.K. *et al.* (1999). Utilization of alcohol, drug, and mental health treatment services among American Indian adolescent detainees. *J Am Acad Child Adolesc Psychiatr* **38**: 1102–1108.

Simon RI, Gold LH (2010). *Textbook of Forensic Psychiatry (2nd Edition)*. American Psychiatric Publishing.

Teplin LA *et al.* (2002). Psychiatric disorders in youth in juvenile detention. *Arch Gen Psychiatr* **59**: 1133–1143.

Wasserman GA *et al.* (2002). The Voice DISC–IV with incarcerated male youth: Prevalence of disorder. *J Am Acad Child Adolesc Psychiatr* **41**: 314–321.

Suicide in Singapore

CHIA Boon Hock

Introduction

For a practising psychiatrist, the management of a suicidal patient can be challenging. Fortunately, for most psychiatrists, only a handful of their patients will commit suicide. When it occurs, however, the psychological trauma can be tremendous. Even after 45 years of practice, the news that one of my patients has committed suicide still leaves me with an unhappy and uneasy feeling.

The origins of suicide are often complex, influenced by a variety of personal, social, psychological and medical factors which may or may not culminate eventually in the act of suicide. These factors vary between different cultures and societies, and between individuals and countries.

Although it is estimated that 60% of all suicides occurs in Asia, the amount of the research focused on suicide in Asia is insignificant compared to that in the West. As such, much of our early understanding and management of suicide were based on Western models. However, with more Asian-based studies now available, we are able to better understand unique characteristics of suicidal behaviour in China, Taiwan, Hong Kong, Japan, Korea, India, Pakistan and Singapore. An online search of the literature suggests that there are about 50 Singapore-based publications related to suicide with the first being published in 1954 (Murphy, 1954). These publications cover various aspects of suicide: demography, trends, risk association, methods, letter, media guidelines, assessment and prevention.

Recently, a colleague asked me whether I was ever emotionally affected by the study of such a morbid subject. I told him I was not. Rather, I feel I have learned a lot about life from my studies. In particular, I have learnt about the importance of having good health and peace of mind. To achieve these, one could aspire to a simple life with a healthy sense of one's self-worth, a well-developed family and social support network, and a general acceptance of the tribulations and stressors of life. I hope you will understand why I have come to this conclusion after you finish reading this chapter.

My understanding and management of potentially suicidal patients have changed through the decades, ever since my early forays into the subject in the 1970s. In the beginning, I was simply interested in determining the rate of suicide in Singapore and the factors associated with it. However, over the years, I have become more interested in prevention of suicide. In particular, I feel it is important that we, as mental healthcare professionals, are able to assess and manage patients' suicide risk, so that we are able to 'bring them off the edge' when risk is acute, and to 'keep them off the edge' in the longer term (Chia and Chia, 2012). Medication can help but in those who are more unwell and resistant to treatment, careful follow-up to ensure appropriate use and compliance to treatment is necessary. However, medication itself is not enough, and mental healthcare workers must try to understand and address all underlying social, psychological and physical problems which has caused the individual to consider suicide in the first place.

Here I will summarise some points that Singaporean psychiatrists may find useful in their management of a potentially suicidal patient. Much of this information is based on my 50 years of practice, the findings from published literature and on my study of 1717 cases of suicides occurring in the years 2000–2004.

Suicide Rates

Suicide rates can be difficult to ascertain and are often underestimated. They are calculated from number of deaths documented as being due to suicide in each country's death registry, and are often reported as suicides per 100,000 population per annum. Much, therefore, depends on whether such suicides are identified and reported accurately. In some countries, social, cultural and religious factors may influence whether a death is attributed to suicide. In Islamic countries, like Malaysia, suicide by a family member can bring tremendous shame on the family (Maniam, 1995). In Pakistan, there are punitive laws against attempted suicide which result in marked under-diagnosis and under-reporting of both attempted suicide and suicide (Khan, 1998). In Taiwan, suicide may be underestimated by more than 30% because some suicides are 'hidden' among deaths certified as due to other causes (Chang, 2010). It is important to know these facts, as without accurate data, it is difficult to carry out any meaningful research on suicide in these countries.

In Singapore, we are fortunate that there is a well-standardised process where each suspicious death is carefully investigated to determine the cause of death. This includes a police-led investigation of the place of death, interviews of eye witnesses and close relatives, and acquisitions of affidavits from close relatives and friends detailing the deceased's personality, social situations and behaviour prior to death. Medical reports are obtained from all doctors caring for the victims. These, together with post-mortem and toxicology findings, are presented to a coroner's court held three to six months after the death (Chia and Chia, 2010). A verdict of suicide will only be returned by the Coroner where it is shown beyond reasonable doubt that death has occurred as a result of a deliberate act by the deceased and that in so doing, the deceased intends that the consequence would be his own death (Coroner, 2008).

However, in some cases, the cause of death may be difficult to determine. This occurs when the death was unwitnessed, when discovery of death is delayed and the body is severely decomposed, or when death may have conceivably been accidental. In these cases, the Coroner may return an open verdict. In a review of open cases in 1978, there was sufficient doubt that up to 57% of these cases might have been 'undeclared suicides', which suggested that the official suicide rate in Singapore could be under-reported by some 13% (Chia, 1978).

Singapore's Suicide Rate

Compared to suicide rates reported in other Asian countries, Singapore's suicide rate has remained at approximately 8–16:100,000 over the last five decades. It is similar to that in China, India and Hong Kong, higher than that in the Philippines (2:100,000); and much lower than that in Sri-Lanka, South Korea and Japan (35–45:100,000) (Table 1).

Table 1: Suicide rate: an Asian perspective (2011).

Country	Year	Male	Female	Sex-ratio
Sri Lanka	91	44.5	17	2.7:1
S Korea	09	40	22	1.8:1
Japan	09	36	13	2.7:1
Hong Kong	09	19	10.5	18:1
China	99	13	15	0.9:1
India	09	13	8	1.7:1
Singapore	06	13	7.5	1.7:1
Thailand	02	12	4	3.2:1
Phillipines	93	2.5	1.5	1.5:1

Ref: WHO suicide rates by country, year and sex.
http://www.who.int/mental_health/prevention/suicide_rates/en/.

The long-term review of suicide rates in Singapore shows that rates have remained quite stable over the last five decades with peaks occurring during pre-war/war periods, and during times of financial depression and recession (Figure 1). There are roughly 350–400 suicides per year, which means one person will commit suicide every day. Differences in the rate of suicide in ethnicity, age and gender do exist (Chia and Chia, 2010).

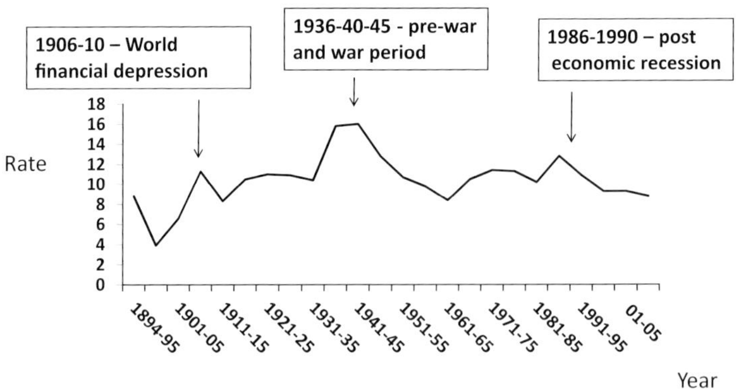

Figure 1: Trend of suicide rate.

Ethnic Differences

Among the three main races in Singapore, the Chinese and Indian suicide rates are very similar, while the Malay rates are strikingly low (Table 2). Obviously, cultural differences in attitudes, values and religious beliefs exist; and perhaps, the Malays who are generally quite tolerant, humble and unassuming people, preferring a simpler and slower-paced life, may be less prone to committing suicide. There are also strong cultural and religious taboos against suicide in Islam, and the restrictions against alcohol and drug use, and a greater acceptance of 'God's will' may also be contributing factors. Required to fast from dawn to dusk for a full month may also build a greater fortitude and a better ability to withstand adversity. In contrast, religion appears to have less influence on the Chinese and Indian psyche and suicide is more acceptable and even encouraged in some social contexts (Chia *et al.*, 2010).

Table 2: Trend of suicide rate by race.

	Rate		
	Chinese	Indian	Malay
Tan and Ting (1955–64)	12	12	2
Chia (1970–76)	13	15	2
Tsoi and Kok (1980)	14	14	2
Peng and Choo (1986)	15	21	2
Ng and Lau (1991–00)	14	16	3
Chia (2000–04)	14	13	3

Elderly Suicide Rates

Suicide rates tend to increase with age in many countries including Singapore (Figure 2). There are exceptions in countries such as India and Thailand where the higher status of the older individual within families is thought to lessen risk. In Singapore, it can also be noted that the Indian

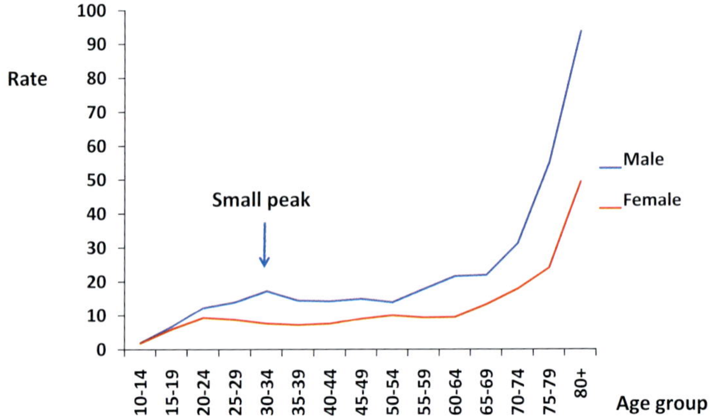

Figure 2: Suicide rates in different age-groups.

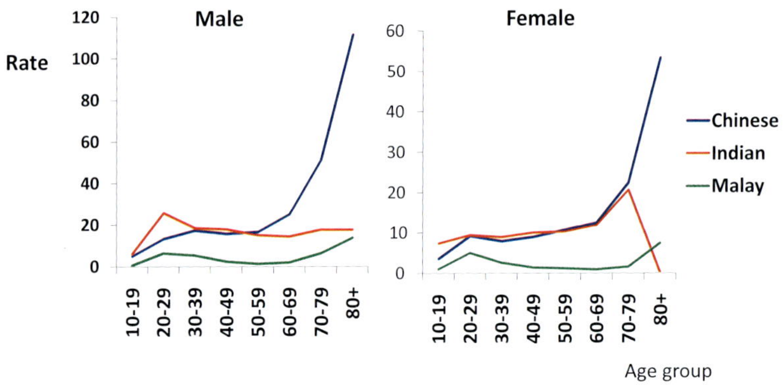

Figure 3: Suicide rate by race, sex and age (2000–04).

male and female suicide rates both flatten with age, rather than increase steeply as it does in the older Chinese population (Figure 3). The Malay suicide curves for both genders are much lower.

Recently, however, there has been some reduction in elderly suicide rates possibly as the new elderly are now more likely to be locally born with better social support and in better economic and physical health (Chia *et al.*, 2010). However, rates in the elderly Chinese male population remain unacceptably high.

Gender Differences

In many studies based in the West, the male: female suicide ratio is about 4:1; males are much more likely to commit suicide than females. In Singapore, as in South Korea, Hong Kong, India and the Philippines, the male: female ratio of suicide is 1.7:1, while in China, it is close to 1 (Table 1). The higher female propensity to suicide in East Asian subjects has been attributed to lower status, lower self-esteem, lower level of education, lower degree of society and familial support, and increased subjugation of females in these societies. When faced with overwhelming odds, these women may feel there is no option but suicide.

In Singapore the low male: female suicide ratio is mainly secondary to a lower-than-average male and higher-than-average female suicide rate. This ratio, however, tends to increase with age (Chia *et al.*, 2010). It is difficult to attribute our higher female rates to disadvantage and subjugation as our young Singaporean women enjoy good education and employment prospects. Rather, it is possible that with an equalisation of gender roles, they are now subject to the same social expectations as their male counterparts, but with continued pressure to fulfil their traditional roles.

Protective Factors

Marriage in Singapore appears to be protective. Suicide rates are highest in divorced individuals, followed by the widowed and singles (Table 3). However, if we look more closely at the age-breakdown, we find that marriage is not as protective for young males and old females (Figure 4), and in both Singapore and Hong Kong, suicide rates for elderly married

Table 3: Suicide rate by marital status (Singapore years 2000–04.

	Rate	
	Male	**Female**
Single	22	11
Married	14	10
Divorced	42	22
Widowed	25	12

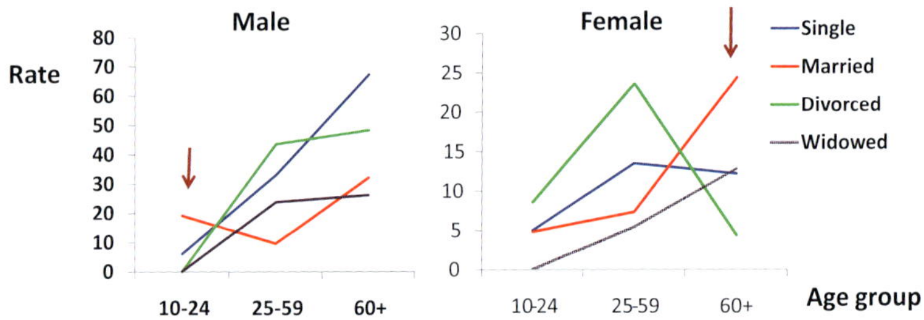

Figure 4: Suicide rate and marital status (2000–04).

women are higher than for those who are widowed, single or divorced (Yip, 1998). Detailed analysis of data suggests that in older married women, depression and an unwillingness to be a burden to their families are strong risk associations.

Risk Factors

The risk factors associated with suicide in Singapore can broadly be categorised into four domains: recent life event (65%), mental illness (62%), physical illness (35%) and mental-related factors (34%) (Figure 5a). The impact of these factors can vary through life with recent life events being more important in the young, with mental illness peaking in adulthood, and with physical illness becoming more prevalent

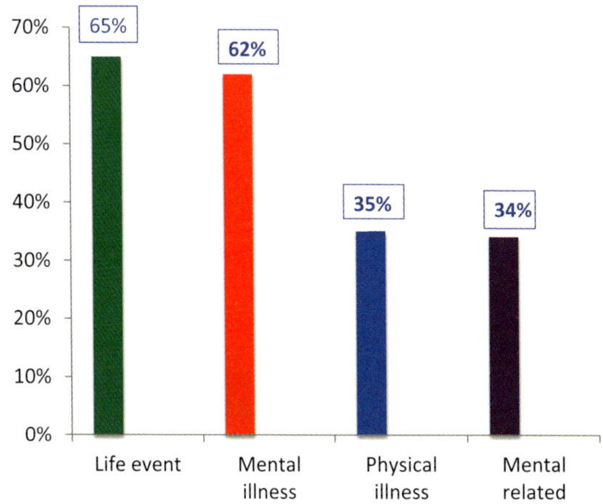

Figure 5a: The importance of the various risk Factors found associated with suicide in Singapore

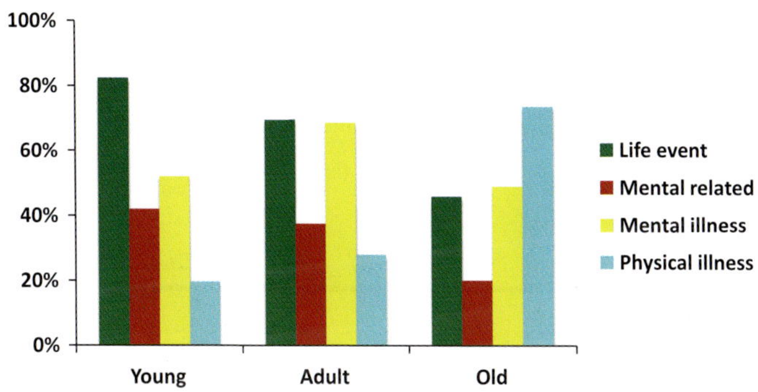

Figure 5b: Risk factor versus age (2000–04).

in the old. Mental-related factors are important in young and adult suicides (Figure 5b).

Life Events

Recent life events that may have contributed to suicide can be ascertained from affidavits of family and close friends, and from suicide notes. From these, several common themes emerge. Relationship issues (girl-boy and parent-child), academic stress (exams) and national service are common themes in young persons (aged < 24 years) (Loh *et al.*, 2012). However, in working adults, marital, financial (employment) and legal problems become more important. Bereavement, financial problems (debt), feeling lonely and unwanted, and the 'fear of being a burden' are problems in the elderly (aged > 60 years) (Table 4).

Table 4: Life events found associated with suicide in the different age groups (2000–04).

Young (10–24y)	Adult (26–59y)	Old (60+)
Relationship	Relationship (36%)	Relationship
Love (30%)	Marital (16%)	Bereaved (9%)
Family (26%)		
Social	Job (18%)	Finance (11%)
Study (19%)	Finance (28%)	
National Service (2%)	Unemployment	Social
Loneliness (2%)	Failed business	Being a burden (13%)
Unwanted (4%)	Gambling debt	Loneliness (5%)
		Being old (7%)
	Legal (13%)	Unwanted (3%)

In Singapore, like many Asian countries, unemployment is a major risk factor in suicide. The suicide rates for the unemployed for both genders in Singapore are 18 to 22 times higher than those of the employed (Table 5). There is little social security support in Singapore, and while charity organisations cater to the very poor and very sick, the able-bodied unemployed may find it necessary to rely on their savings or on the generosity of family and friends. The social stigma, coupled with the stress of trying to find a job quickly while supporting a household, can be enormous (Chia and Chia, 2008).

Table 5: Unemployment and suicide (2000–04).

	Rate	
Occupation	**Male**	**Female**
Employed	8	5
Unemployed	142 (18x)	107 (22x)
Economically inactive	23 (retired)	9 (homemaker)

Data suggest that many of the unemployed suicides in Singapore also suffer from major mental illness (e.g. depression) while a high percentage of economically inactive suicides (too old to work or retired) are associated with severe physical illness.

Mental-related factors

Persons at greater risk include those who are proud, secretive and lonely, those with low self-esteem and a tendency to worry unnecessarily and those with poor problem-solving skills (Chia and Chia, 2010). These people may find it difficult to relate to others, share their problems and seek solutions. This effect is compounded if they also have less developed family and social support systems.

People with addiction problems are also disadvantaged. These include those with substance abuse, alcohol abuse, gambling problems and sexual issues. In Singapore, alcohol abuse is more prevalent amongst the Indian suicide victims (13%), while substance abuse (13%) and sexual deviance are more common amongst Malay suicide victims and gambling problems are more common amongst the Chinese (5%) (Figure 6).

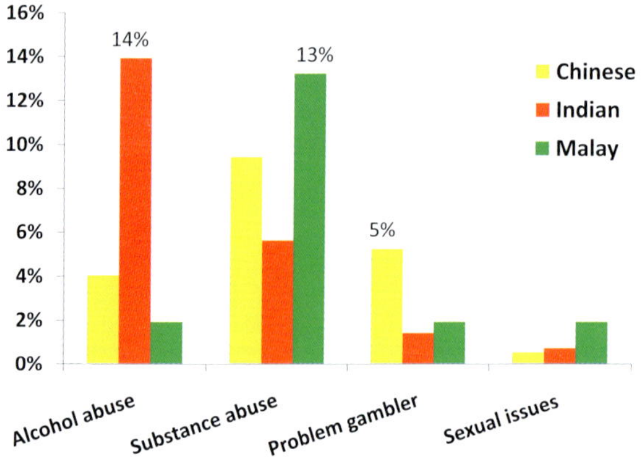

Figure 6: Mental-related factors versus different races (2000–04).

Mental illness

Mental illness in Singapore is associated with 62% of all suicides (Table 6). This means that in 38%, no mental illness is identified, a finding which is consistent with that in a review article involving six studies where it was found that 37.1% of suicide had no Axis 1 and sub-threshold/mild mental conditions (Milner *et al.*, 2013). Suicides, in general, are less likely to be attributed to a mental illness in Asian countries (such as China and India) than in Europe, North America or Canada. This may be due to how different cultures conceptualise and diagnose mental diseases. In Chinese traditional medicine, mental illness is not an illness but a symptom resulting from a depletion and disharmony of flow of 'vital life energy' originating from the various vital organs in the body.

Table 6: Mental illness and suicide (Singapore 2000–04).

	Percentage (n = 1717)
Minor mental illness	35%
Major mental illness	27%
No mental illness	38%

Where mental illness exists, it can be divided into 'minor' or 'major'. Minor mental illness most associated with suicide includes minor depression, generalised anxiety, obsessive-compulsive disorder, panic-phobia and anorexia nervosa (Table 7), while major mental illness includes psychoses (mainly schizophrenia), and affective (unipolar and bipolar) and organic psychoses (mainly early dementia) (Table 8).

Table 7: Minor Mental Illness and suicide (Singapore 2000–04).

Minor mi	Suicide (n = 1717)
Minor depressive	29%
Generalized anxiety	5%
OCD	0.6%
Panic-phobia	0.3%
Conduct disorder	0.3%
Somatic	0.1%
Anorexia nervosa	0.1%
Total	35%

Table 8: Major Mental Illness and suicide (Singapore 2000–04).

Major mi	Suicide (n = 1717)
Schizophrenia	15%
Psychosis	4%
Paranoid	2%
Tourette's syndrome	0.2%
Dementia	0.5%
Depression-bipolar	2%
Depression-unipolar	4%
Unknown	0.6%
Total	27%

Physical illness

Physical illness is associated with 35% of suicides. In Singapore, as in many countries, suicide associated with physical illness, not unexpectedly, increases with age with physical illness, being present in 75% of all elderly suicides in Singapore. Physical illnesses associated with suicide include cancer, and cardiorespiratory, cerebrovascular, gastrointestinal, renal-urinary, orthopaedic/rheumatic and eye diseases. Those with chronic illnesses, which result in physical pain, disability and suffering (such as breathlessness, nausea and vomiting) despite treatment, are at greatest risk. A study from Denmark recently concluded that physical illness constitutes a significant risk factor for suicide independent of psychiatric and socioeconomic factors (Qin *et al.*, 2013).

Good pain management and palliative care, especially as our population ages, is very important, and the recent government's focus on better palliative services and building of hospices is both timely and encouraging.

Identifying Suicidality

Help seeking behaviours

In Singapore, 72% of people who committed suicide had contact with medical or mental health providers prior to their suicides (Table 9). Fourteen percent had contact with general practitioners (GPs) or the polyclinic, 23% had admission to a general hospital, and 30% had a previous admission to a

Table 9: Percent of suicide which had been treated for mental or physical condition (Singapore 2000–04).

	Suicide (n = 1717)	
Mental health care provider	30%	
Medical health care provider	21%	
Both	21%	72%
No contact	28%	

mental hospital (Table 10). Of those who had contact with mental health care providers, 67% had contact with them within one month of the suicides (Table 11).

Table 10: Types of treatment received by suicide victim prior to suicide. (Singapore, 2000–04).

	Suicide (n = 1717)
GP/polyclinic	14%
Admission to mental hospital	30%
Private psychiatrist	6%
Psychiatric OPD	2%
Other psychiatric treatment	0.9%
Admission to general hospital	23%
Specialist centre	9%
Other medical treatment	0.6%

Table 11: Last contact with mental health care provider

	Sucide (n = 880)	
1 day	7%	
<1 week	16%	
<1 month	44%	67%
<1 year	28%	
>1 year	5%	
Known	93%	
Unknown	7%	

Despite this, post-mortem toxicology was found to be often negative for therapeutic agents, suggesting that patients were either not adequately treated or poorly compliant to treatment (Table 12). This suggests that it

Table 12: Types of mental illness and toxicology findings for drug level at autopsy. Singapore 2000–04.w

	Anti-anxiety	Anti-depressive	Anti-psychotic	Anti-convulsant	Lithium
Schizophrenia (n = 248)	37%	8.5%	26.5%	0.8%	—
Major depression (n = 61)	39%	39.5%	11.5%	1.5%	—
Manic depression (n = 30)	37%	16.5%	16.5%	6.5%	3.5%
Minor depression (n = 495)	34.5%	18.5%	4.5%	2%	—
Anxiety (n = 65)	97%	—	—	1.5%	—

may not be the 'lack of care' but inadequate 'level of care' that is to be blamed. The reasons for these are varied:

- The patient, family member, or medical and mental health care providers may have underestimated the severity of the patient's illness.
- The medical or mental health provider may not have been adequately trained in suicide assessment and prevention.
- An inadequate dosage or inappropriate medication (e.g. anti-depressant or anti-psychotic agent) may have been prescribed.
- There may have been a reluctance to use more effective new drugs because of cost.
- There may have been an inadequate emphasis on compliance, a failure to hospitalise the high-risk patient or a lack of proper follow-up care.
- There may have been a failure to educate and involve the patient's family and friends in the patient's care and management.

Communicating and attempting suicide

Although many suicide victims (54%) (Table 13) provided some warning of their intent to commit suicide, their relatives or friends often did not

Table 13: Types of warning provided pre-suicide. Singapore 2000–04.

Warning	Total (n = 1717)
Verbal warning	45%
Pre-suicidal planning	11%
Behavior change	6%
Total	54%

take them seriously, and so they tragically lost the opportunity to provide the individual with the help and services he/she needs.

Notable exceptions include those with a major mental illness (such as schizophrenia) who are less likely to express their suffering or to leave behind suicide notes. My belief is that this is not so much that they are not suffering as much as other suicide victims but that they are mentally so preoccupied with their abnormal mental symptoms or are so disturbed in their thinking that they would find it difficult to express themselves (verbally or in writing). They are, however, more likely to have a past history of suicide attempts (Table 14).

Table 14: Warning given, past suicide attempt, letter left behind and expressed suffering in those with and without mental illness. Singapore 2000–04.

	Warning given	Past suicide attempt	Letter left behind	Expressed suffering
Major mental illness (n = 460)	53%	36%	14%	69%
Minor mental (n = 601)	63%	25%	37%	99%
No mental illness (n = 656)	46%	11%	23%	61%

Indeed, about 23% of all suicide victims in Singapore would have had previously attempted suicide. So, having attempted suicide before places a person at higher risk. That said, elderly victims are less likely to have a history of a past suicide attempt (Table 15) possibly because they are often more serious in their intent such that their first attempt is more likely to be their last.

Table 15: Types of warning provided pre-suicide by age Singapore 2000–04.

	Young	Adult	Old
Verbal warning and planning	55%	52%	58%
Past suicide attempt	23%	26%	17%
Suicide note	49%	27%	11%
Grand total	81%	72%	68%

Suicide letters

In Singapore, 25% of all suicide victims and 50% of young suicide victims leave behind suicide notes. By contrast, older individuals and those who have a mental illness are less likely to do so (Chia *et al*,. 2008). These letters provide an insight into the emotional state of individuals just prior to death; and both positive emotions (a sense of care and concern for those they left behind) and a wide range of negative emotions (e.g. despondency, emptiness, self-blame, guilt/shame, hopelessness and anger) are expressed. In many cases, the individuals contemplating suicide felt they had little choice but to kill themselves, although they might be reluctant to do so.

Such letters may express the mental pain a person is enduring:

- *'I am living in agony. The last few years have been hell.'*
- *'Shedding tears on my pillow until dawn just like raindrops falling on the doorsteps. The tree wants to be at rest but the breeze will not cease blowing. The evening breeze cannot blow away my suffering.'*
- *'It is difficult to describe my suffering. I cannot sleep at night. Past few years, I have unspeakable misery.'*

Or the physical pain they can no longer tolerate:

- *'Words cannot describe the chest and abdominal pain I am suffering.'*
- *'The pain of urinating is unbearable.'*
- *'I am in pain every day and there is not a single day I feel well. I can no longer take it.'*

And their reluctance to leave their loved ones behind:

- *'Father is reluctant to leave all of you. I have failed so badly that I have no choice. I have no regret. Life is a dream. I am leaving happily.'*
- *'I feel bad that I have to leave like this. Can I continue to live on? I do not want to die so young.'*

And, finally, the lack of alternative but to die:

- *'With great pain, I made this decision to part. Parting is inevitable in life. All these gave me courage to end it all. It is better to go through pain once than to suffer emotionally for a long time.'*

Often the decision to commit suicide is not a simple one, but has occurred after much thought and consideration. This suggests that if in this process, the individual is helped with support and a provision of alternatives, and then suicide may have been averted.

Methods of Suicide

The choice of a suicide method depends on availability, accessibility and cultural acceptability. In urban Singapore, where more than 80% of the population live in high-rise buildings, it is not surprising that most would choose to jump from them (72%). It is a lethal, easily accessible means of death, which requires very little planning. In a recent review of suicide methods, 90% of young Singaporean suicide victims (Chia *et al.*, 2011) and

73% of the elderly suicide committed suicide by jumping. Also, most of those suffering from major mental illness jumped from high-rise flats. Most flat residents jump from their own flat/building (67%), with the most common sites being the common corridor (50%), kitchen (30%), bedroom (16%) and living room (5%), and the most common floor being the 10th–12th floors (30%).

Interestingly, the proportion who jump in Singapore is much higher than that in Hong Kong (59%) where much of the population also live in high-rise flats (Figure 7). Possible reasons could be that the flats in Hong Kong are much smaller and closer together with little common space, whereas many of the older flats in Singapore have long open corridors and large well-ventilated kitchen spaces for residents to hang their laundry, thus affording victims with more private areas from which to jump.

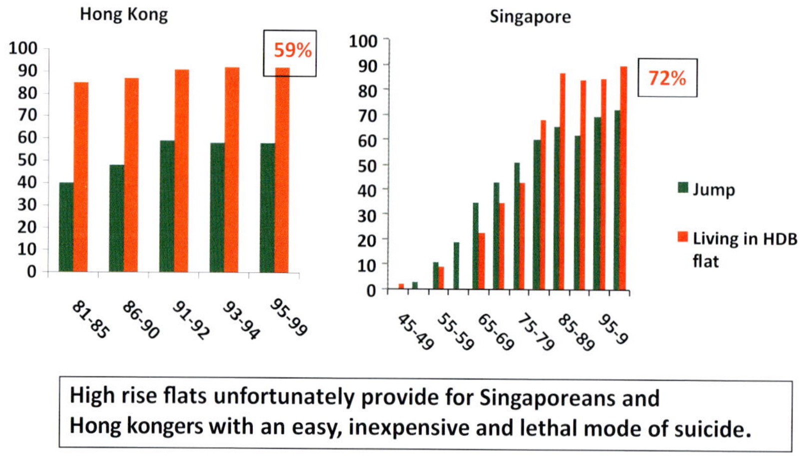

Figure 7: Jumping as a method of suicide and percentage of the population living in high-rise flats in Hong Kong and Singapore.

Other methods of suicide include older methods such as hanging and drowning, and newer methods such as using domestic gas and overdose of prescribed medication (Table 16). Charcoal burning which is now commonly used in Hong Kong and Taiwan (Liu *et al.*, 2007) has, fortunately, not taken root in Singapore (0.3%). Other methods like shooting oneself with a gun which is common in more gun-liberal

Table 16: Methods of suicide used (2000–04).

	Old method		New method
Hanging	17%	Jumping	73%
Poison	2%	Gas	2%
Drowning	1%	Drug	2%
Burning	1%	Charcoal burning	0.4%
Knife	0.4%	Plastic bag	0.3%
Gun	0.3%	MRT train	0.2%
		Other	0.2%
		Multiple	2%

countries, or pesticide poisoning which is common in rural areas, are also not common in Singapore.

The Role of the Media

The media can do their part by addressing the factors (social, psychological, mental and physical), which may predispose one to suicide. They should, however, avoid sensationalising one particular suicide or providing details of a suicide act so as to avoid triggering copycat suicides

Suicides are rarely reported in Singapore newspapers, with only 0.6% of total suicides reported in our two English newspapers, *The Straits Times* and *The New Paper*, from 2000 to 2004. Unfortunately, some reports such as the MRT train suicides and Bedok reservoir drowning suicides may have led to several copycat suicides. The press should also not reinforce suicide myths.

Those suicides which newspapers find most newsworthy include murder-suicides and the methods of suicide (e.g. MRT train and Bedok reservoir drowning) (50–70% of cases were reported) while suicides associated with physical and mental illnesses are rarely mentioned (fewer than 0.3% of cases were reported).

There are World Health Organisation (WHO) media guidelines which detail how suicides and their risk associations can be responsibly reported

(Pirkis *et al.*, 2006). Indeed, the media can help by highlighting the risk associations of suicide, and how these can be managed so as to prevent suicides. The media should also avoid focusing on any one single suicide or provide details of a suicide method which may teach people how to commit suicide or make it socially acceptable.

Conclusion

Although the suicide rates of many Asian countries are rising, the suicide rates in Singapore have remained quite stable (Chia *et al.*, 2010). There have even been falls in suicide rates in the elderly, in middle-aged males and in young females (Chia *et al.*, 2010). I feel that this is because our unemployment rates and the percentages of alcohol and illegal substance abuses in the population are relatively low and, most importantly, because there is relatively easy access to good health care. However, we cannot be complacent, and there is room for improvement, especially in treating those who are mentally or physically ill. With proper interdisciplinary cooperation, planning, education and action, we could conceivably lower our suicide rates by a further 10% over the next decade.

Since suicides are multifactorial, any successful suicide prevention programme must be directed at all these related factors (Chia and Chia, 2012). On an individual level, we should begin in our families and schools to help raise well-balanced children with good communication and coping skills, strong family and social support, and realistic long-term ambitions and expectations.

In addressing lifestyle risk factors, there needs to be adequate community awareness of the dangers (i.e. academic and relationship problems in the young, financial and addiction problems in adulthood, and bereavement and loneliness in old age), and proper training of teachers, counsellors, social workers, police and healthcare workers (nurses) so that they can adequately identify those at risk, and link them with existing social or mental-health programmes.

As our population ages, physical illness will become increasingly important, and there is a need for physicians to be more holistic in their care. In the pursuit of a cure, physicians may neglect the impact of chronic pain, particularly in those who are terminally ill. Careful attention to minimising the amount of pain and suffering patients need to endure may help the patient decide to go on living despite a poor medical prognosis.

Much more needs to be done for the mentally ill. We know that those with more severe illness and who are more resistant to treatment are at greater risk (Thong *et al.*, 2008). However, therapeutic drugs are often not detected in the blood during autopsy, suggesting that many suicide victims had not been taking their medication. A greater emphasis may need to be placed on ensuring that patients receive adequate treatment and follow-up. However, simply treating the mental illness (e.g. depression or anxiety) does not eliminate risk as suicide is multifactorial; and other risk-associations need to be explored and managed appropriately.

As healthcare professionals we need to be vigilant and to know how to assess for suicide risk in our patients. Knowing the demographics and risk associations helps, but physicians, nurses, counsellors and psychiatrists also need to consider the possibility that their clients may be contemplating suicide, and not forget or be afraid to ask that one question — 'Do you have any intention of killing yourself?' A person contemplating suicide will often have thought about and made plans for their suicide. One may fear that asking this question may trigger suicidal ideations, but I find that the person not thinking of committing suicide will simply dismiss the suggestion. Those contemplating suicide, however, will often be relieved that someone has finally broached the subject, that someone finally understands how they feel, and he/she may in fact open up more, allowing you to work better with them in finding solutions for their various problems. Without asking that one question, we would not have done a proper suicide assessment (Shea, 2002).

References

Chang SS, Sterne JA, Lu TH, Gunnell D (2010). 'Hidden' suicide amongst deaths certified as undetermined intent, accident by pesticide poisoning and accident by suffocation in Taiwan. *Soc Psychiatry Psychiatr Epidemiol* **45**: 143–152.

Chia BH (1978). Suicide in Singapore. MD thesis. University of Singapore.

Chia BH, Chia A (2008). Singapore. In: Yip SF, ed. *Suicide in Asia: Causes and Prevention*. Hong Kong University Press, Hong Kong, pp. 101–120.

Chia BH, Chia A (2010). Suicide in Singapore. *Singapore Fam Physician* **36**: 26–29.

Chia BH, Chia A (2012). Prevention of suicide in Singapore. *Ann Acad Med Singapore* **41**: 375–376.

Chia BH, Chia A, Ng WY, Tai BC (2011). Suicide methods in Singapore (2000–2004): Types and associations. *Suicide Life Threat Behav* **41**: 574–583.

Chia BH, Chia A, Tai BC (2008). Suicide letters in Singapore. *Arch Suicide Res* **12**:74– 81.

Chia BH, Chia A, Yee NW, Choo TB (2010). Suicide trends in Singapore: 1955–2004. *Arch Suicide Res* **14**: 276–283.

Coroner's practice in medical cases (2008). Academy publishing. Monograph series.

Khan MM (1998). Suicide and attempted suicide in Pakistan. Crisis **19** (4): 172–6.

Liu KY *et al.* (2007). Charcoal burning suicides in Hong Kong and urban Taiwan: An illustration of the impact of a novel suicide method on overall regional rates. *J Epidemiol Community Health* **61**: 248–253.

Loh C, Tai BC, Ng WY, Chia A, Chia BH (2012). Suicide in young Singaporeans aged 10–24 years between 2000 and 2004. *Arch Suicide Res* **16**: 174–182.

Maniam T (1995). Suicide and undetermined violent deaths in Malayasia, 1966–1990: Evidence for the misclassification of suicide statistics. *Asia Pac J Public Health* **8**: 181–185.

Milner A, Sveticic J, De Leo D (2013). Suicide in the absence of mental disorder? A review of psychological autopsy studies across countries. *Int J Soc Psychiatry* **59**: 545–554.

Murphy HBM (1954). The mental health of Singapore: Part 1 — Suicide. *Med J Malaya* **1:** 1–45.

Ng DW, Lau G (2003). Suicide trends in Singapore: Two decades down the road. *Med Sci Law* **43**: 141–147.

Peng KL, Choo AS (1992). Suicide in Singapore, 1986. *Aust N Z J Psychiatry* **26**: 599–608.

Pirkis J, Blood RW, Beautrais A, Burgess P, Skehans J (2006). Media guidelines on the reporting of suicide. *Crisis* **27**: 82–7.

Qin P, Webb R, Kapur N, Sorensen HT (2013). Hospitalization for physical illness and risk of subsequent suicide: a population study. *J Intern Med* **273**: 48–58.

Shea SC (2002). *The Practical Art of Suicide Assessment: A Guide for Mental Health Professional and Substance Abuse Counsellors*. John Wiley and Sons, Inc, New Jersey.

Thong JY, Su AH, Chan YH, Chia BH (2008). Suicide in psychiatric patients: Case-control study in Singapore. *Aust N Z J Psychiatry* **42**: 509–519.

Ting SK, Tan KK (1969). Post-mortem survey of suicides in Singapore. *Singapore Med J* **10**: 248–259.

Tsoi WF, Kok LP (1981). Suicidal behavior in Singapore for the year 1980. *Singapore Med J* **23**: 299–305.

Yip PS (1998). Age, sex, marital status and suicide: An empirical study of east and west. *Psychol Rep* **82**: 311–322.

Psychotherapy Movement

GWEE Kok Peng

Introduction

Psychologist Hans J. Eysenck (1999) defined psychotherapy in its broadest sense as 'the use of psychological theories and methods in the treatment of psychiatric disorders'. It is the branch of psychiatry concerned with the use of psychological methods of treatment as opposed to physical ones such as medications and electroconvulsive therapy.

The first form of psychotherapy, psychoanalysis, was developed by Sigmund Freud at the turn of the last century. It was about half a century later, in the 1950's, that the first modern antipsychotic and antidepressant drugs were developed. In that span of 50 or so years between the introduction of the first psychotherapy and the first pharmacotherapy in psychiatry, various psychological treatments (in rough chronological order — psychoanalytic psychotherapies, group therapies, family therapies, cognitive and behavioural therapies) had been developed and employed in the practice of psychiatry universally.

In Singapore, the timeline of the introduction of psychiatric treatments seems to have reversed this order, with electro convulsive therapy and psychotropic medications being introduced decades before the psychotherapies, and the most 'physical' of the psychotherapies — behaviour therapy — before the other therapies. The very first universally practised psychotherapy, psychoanalytic psychotherapy — which could be considered the most 'psychological' of the psychotherapies as it deals with the unconscious psychogenic roots of psychiatric disorders — was established locally around the turn of this century, about a hundred years after it was developed by Freud. The overarching direction in Singapore over the decades has been from a primarily biological to a more holistic bio-psycho-social approach, in keeping with the increasing psychological sophistication that accompanies the development of a nation.

Universal Historical Development

Psychoanalytic psychotherapy

Universally, Psychoanalysis and its derivative, Psychodynamic Psychotherapy, was the first specific school of psychotherapy. Sigmund Freud originated it at the turn of the last century in Vienna, Austria, initially applying it to patients with conversion hysteria, who presented with physical symptoms that turned out to have psychological rather than organic origins. Psychoanalysis was subsequently developed over the century primarily in Europe and America by the likes of Melanie Klein, Anna Freud, D.W. Winnicott, Heinz Kohut, Wilfred Bion, and John Bowlby into various sub-schools of theory and practice, addressing the unconscious psychological roots of psychiatric disorders ranging from hysteria (conversion and dissociative), depression, anxiety, phobias, obsessions and later personality disorders and even some cases of psychosis.

Group therapy

The founders of group psychotherapy in the United States were Joseph H. Pratt, Trigant Burrow and Paul Schilder (Barlow *et al.*, 2000; Barlow *et al.*, 2005). In the early 1900's, Pratt recognised that apart from cost-effectiveness, therapy done in groups benefited from certain therapeutic factors that stem from being part of a group, observing that his patients became concerned about and influenced one another. Years later, group therapy became a widely used approach, especially in the United Kingdom, by the likes of Wilfred Bion and S.H. Foulkes, partly to address the many needs of military troops returning from World War II. By the mid-1950's, it was applied across a wide range of populations and settings.

Family and couple therapy

The roots of family therapy were established in the early 1900's with the emergence of the child guidance movement (1909) and marriage counselling (1920's) although the formal development of family therapy dates to the 1940's and early 1950's (Broderick and Schrader, 1991; Sholevar, 2003). By the mid-1960's, a number of distinct schools of family therapy had emerged.

Cognitive and behaviour therapy

Thorndike first wrote about 'modifying behaviour' in 1911 and Wolpe (1958) described behaviour modification in the 1940's and 1950's. Skinner's group in the United States focused on contingency management such as the token economy and behavioural activation, using the principles of operant conditioning, to improve the functioning of people who were diagnosed with chronic schizophrenia (Lindsley *et al.,* 1953).

In the 1950's and 1960's, others began to consider the role of cognition in psychiatric disorders. In the 1960's, Aaron Beck, developed his approach called Cognitive Therapy. Initially, cognitive and behavioural approaches conflicted, with the former looking at mental causes and the latter simply assessing stimuli and behavioural responses. However, in the 1970's behavioural modification and cognitive therapy techniques were merged to form Cognitive Behavioural Therapy.

Physical/biological treatments

In contrast, antipsychotic and antidepressant medications were only introduced in the 1950's.

The Development of Therapies in Singapore

Pre 1960's — From custodial care to physical treatments

In Singapore, before the 1940's, custodial care, rather than treatment, and asylums, rather than mental hospitals, were the order of the day. The first credible treatments introduced were biological, rather than psychological, ones. Electroconvulsive Therapy was introduced in the late 1940's, soon after it gained widespread use universally. Likewise, anti-psychotic drugs started being used in the mid-1950's and antidepressants and anxiolytics in the late 1950's, soon after their introduction in other parts of the world.

The 1970's — Introduction of the first psychological treatment — behaviour therapy

In the early 1970's, psychiatrist Dr Chee Kuan Tsee and clinical psychologist Mr Long Foo Yee (personal communication) — who trained under Isaac Marks and H.J. Eysenck in the United Kingdom — started Behaviour Therapy in Woodridge Hospital for a range of problems such as phobias, obsessive- compulsive disorder, sexual dysfunction and disorders of sexual preference. Mr Long also introduced Token Economy in the rehabilitation of chronic inpatients, mostly with schizophrenia, in 1972 (Long *et al.*, 1973).

The 1980's — Families and groups

Child psychiatrist Dr Goh Choo Woon started the practice of Family Therapy in the Child and Adolescent Department of Woodbridge Hospital after training at the Tavistock Institute in London in the early 1980's (Tan, 2003). Also in the 1980's, Ms Seng Boon Kheng (personal communication) introduced Family Therapy for adult patients and their families through the Medical Social Work department of the hospital.

The practice of family therapy was also emerging in the community, with Anthony Yeo and Juliana Toh of Counselling and Care Centre receiving their training in the United States and the United Kingdom, respectively in the mid 1980's. Subsequently, they introduced 'live' supervision and the use of the one-way mirror, and set up the first introductory course in family therapy in 1989 (Sim, 2012).

At about the same time, Dr G.S. Devan (1992) trained in Group Therapy during his residency in the United Kingdom in the early 1980's;

and subsequently ran groups from 1984 to 1989 while working in Woodbridge Hospital. Psychiatrists Dr G.S. Devan and Dr Pauline Sim Li Ping, clinical psychologist Lyn Chua and occupational therapist Kamaldin Ibrahim helped to further develop Group Psychotherapy in the late 1980's and early 1990's, reinforced by training at the Menninger clinic and the Institute of Psychiatry in London. The Occupational Therapy Department, under Mr Kamaldin Ibrahim, ran Projective Groups using art, drama and games.

The 1990's — From groups to individuals

1990 saw the first Cognitive Behaviour Therapy clinic being opened at the Tampines Psychiatric Clinic — a satellite clinic of Woodbridge Hospital — by Dr Leslie Lim Eng Choon, after he trained from 1987 to 1988 at the St George's Medical School in the United Kingdom (Ng, 2001). With the help of the author and clinical psychologists, Elizabeth Pang, Teresa Foong, Shirley Tan, Vivienne Ng, Clare Yeo, Yap Ann Keong, Matthew Woo and Khoo Sue Anne, Cognitive Behaviour Therapy services were further developed in the 1990's, initially for depressive disorders, then extending to an increasing number of psychiatric problems including generalized anxiety disorder, panic disorder, obsessive compulsive disorder, somatoform disorders and eating disorders.

In 1998, the Royal College of Psychiatrists sent Professor Jan Scott, an expert in Cognitive Behaviour Therapy from Cognitive Therapy Centre, Newcastle, United Kingdom, to Singapore to be an external examiner for the Masters of Medicine examinations in Psychiatry (Ang, 2001). In the same year, the Ministry of Health, Singapore (MOH) invited Dr Christopher Dare from the Institute of Psychiatry, London, to be a visiting expert to help train mental health professionals in psychotherapy, mainly from a psychoanalytic perspective. These visitors gave feedback to MOH on psychotherapy training as part of the strategy to upgrade mental health services in developing Singapore. A local working committee was formed — comprising six psychiatrists and a clinical psychologist, including Professor Kua Ee Heok, Professor Ko Soo Meng, Dr Anthony

Ang Wee Kiat and psychologist Lyn Chua — which started the Graduate Diploma in Psychotherapy run by the National University of Singapore School of Postgraduate Studies starting in July 1999. The diploma course comprised of an initial three-month theoretical module followed by a nine-month practicum in either psychoanalytic or cognitive-behavioural therapy that involved clinical supervision, case conferences, lectures, reading seminars and written assignments.

The New Millennium — Back to the Beginning

At about the same time as the local training programme was kicking off, the Institute of Mental Health and Woodbridge Hospital sent its first psychiatrist (the author) to train in individual psychoanalytic psychotherapy at the Institute of Psychiatry, London, United Kingdom and New York University Medical School, United States, from 2000 to 2001. The new century (and millennium) heralded a return to the very first psychotherapy developed a century earlier.

Subsequently, two more psychiatrists were sent for training in psychoanalytic psychotherapy. Dr George Joseph Fernandez spent a year in the Halliwick Psychotherapy Department in St Anne's Hospital, North London, United Kingdom, under the tutelage of Professor Anthony Bateman, specialising in treating personality disorders (especially borderline personality disorder), a group of particularly complex and difficult conditions which had previously been regarded as "untreatable" in Singapore. The following year, Dr Samuel Cheng Eng Teck trained with Dr Jeremy Holmes at the University of Exeter in Devon, United Kingdom. Subsequently, Dr Habeebul Rahman went to the United Kingdom to complete his psychiatric training which he had started in Singapore, and while training in the United Kingdom, he gained further experience in psychoanalytic psychotherapy, as well as cognitive behaviour therapy, before returning to Singapore. The author then added further training in psychoanalytic psychotherapy in the United Kingdom, comprising a Masters of Science in Theoretical Psychoanalytic Studies from University College London under Professors Peter Fonagy and Mary

Target; further clinical experience and supervision from Halliwick Unit, St Anne's hospital; and further personal training analysis during a one-year unpaid leave from 2006 to 2007. With that, a psychoanalytic psychotherapy service was established in the Institute of Mental Health and Woodbridge Hospital.

Over the rest of the decade, the Institute of Mental Health continued to beef up its Psychotherapy Service so that the service, under the directorship of the author, now straddles several hospital departments in an integrated effort to meet the psychological and psychiatric needs of rapidly developing Singapore. Interpersonal needs and problems are addressed by family and couple therapists, led by Ms Chan Lay Lin, followed by Ms Goh Min Hui, primarily from the medical social work department. Employing a systemic approach, the focus is on the relational context, addressing patterns of interaction and meaning, and aiming to facilitate personal and interpersonal resources within a system as a whole. Intrapersonal problems are mostly handled by a team of clinical psychologists led by Clare Yeo Kwang Ngee, followed by Ong Lue Ping. They primarily employ a cognitive behavioural approach, addressing patterns of thinking and beliefs within individuals that contribute to a wide range of problems including panic attacks, anxiety disorders, depressive disorders, obsessive compulsive disorders, post-traumatic stress disorders and eating disorders. Intrapsychic problems are dealt with by the psychoanalytic psychotherapy service, headed by the author. The focus is on conflicts arising from early experiences that are being re-enacted in adult life, producing mental health problems; and the aim is to resolve these conflicts and problems through the vehicle of the relationship with the therapist, giving new opportunities for emotional assimilation and insight. Personality disorders, depressive disorders, disorders of sexual preference, eating disorders, shoplifting, anxiety states, bereavement and adjustment disorders are some of the problems addressed through this approach.

An Art Psychotherapist, Kirsty McTaggart joined the psychotherapy service towards the end of the decade, reinforcing the psychoanalytic mode of treatment for patients who work better through the medium of art.

Two Occupational Therapists, Ho Soo Fung and Wan Sau Peng, completed their training in Art Therapy with the LASALLE School of Fine Arts and joined Kirsty in offering this form of therapy. Likewise, a Play Therapist in the Child and Adolescent Department, Anne Marie Lo Castro, provides play as a modality for children to communicate feelings and experiences which they are unable to articulate. Play and Art Therapy address child developmental and other psychopathologies such as child abuse; divorce and family relationship problems; selective mutism; sibling rivalry; trauma, stress and anxiety issues; conduct disorder; grief and childhood mood disorders, death and dying; health psychology issues; self-esteem and self-confidence issues; resilience, coping and adjustment management.

On a smaller scale and to varying degrees, similar integrated psychotherapy services were also developed in the psychiatric departments of the various general hospitals, as well as in private practice. Dr Samuel Cheng moved to Changi General Hospital and worked with psychologists such as Christopher Choo, Velda Chen and Constance Png to run a psychotherapy service while Dr Habeebul Rahman migrated to Tan Tock Seng Hospital. Dr Leslie Lim, who started the first Cognitive Behaviour Therapy clinic in Tampines Polyclinic/Institute of Mental Health, moved to Singapore General Hospital, working with Psychologists Evelyn Boon, Kevin Roy Beck, Vivien Yap Lian Hiang and Evangeline Tan Sue Lin. Several of the clinical psychologists who helped run the cognitive behaviour therapy service in the 1990's have moved to other hospitals and private practice. Psychiatrist Dr Lim Yun Chin, who started out in the Institute of Mental Health addiction medicine services, started the Raffles Counselling Centre with Raffles Medical Centre and Dr Ang Yong Guan, previously Chief Medical Officer in the Singapore Armed Forces, practices psychotherapy in private practice.

The 2010's and Beyond — Facing the Future

With integrated, comprehensive psychotherapy services being established, the natural progression is the training and development of future therapists.

The newly established psychotherapy service in the Institute of Mental Health started by organising two national psychotherapy conferences: the first in 2001; the second in 2003. A range of psychotherapies and therapeutic issues was discussed at these conferences — including Interpersonal Therapy; Psychoanalytic Therapy; Hypnotherapy; Dream Analysis; and Cognitive Behaviour Therapy for bipolar disorder, for anxiety in adults and children, and for addictions.

The clinicians, psychologists and other therapists from the service also joined hands with those who had moved to other restructured and private centres to teach a yearly postgraduate theory course in psychoanalytic psychotherapy and cognitive-behaviour therapy organised by the National University of Singapore School of Post-Graduate Studies. This course is/was open to both medical and non-medical professionals and has received avid interest from professionals of widely divergent circles including teachers, religious leaders, engineers, human resource managers, artists, counsellors, mental health and other health professionals.

Within the mental health profession, psychotherapy is also increasingly being included as an integral part of training, helping to further the move away from a purely biological to a more comprehensive and holistic bio-psycho-social approach. Psychotherapy is taught as part of the psychiatry curriculum to medical students from the Duke NUS (National University of Singapore) medical school as well as the NUS Yong Loo Lin School of Medicine.

In addition, the MOH, after discussions with the Specialists Accreditation Board (SAB), recommended the introduction of the medical residency programmes with the aim of enhancing quality of care by improving the structure of formative graduate training. The Ministry worked closely with the United States Accreditation of Graduate Medical Education (ACGME-I) in carrying out this transformation. Psychiatry was one of the seven specialties of the first phase (Phase I) that began in July 2010. With this change, a major difference from previous training of psychiatrists in Singapore is the requirement of competencies in three psychotherapies, namely psychoanalytic, cognitive behaviour and supportive; and exposure to family therapy. The result will be that all future psychiatrists will have knowledge and skills in the main psychotherapies.

The first batch of psychiatry residents under this scheme started their residency in 2010 and completed their first year of psychotherapy training in their third year — 2013. It seems that the development of the cognitive-behaviour therapy and psychoanalytic psychotherapy services and the psychotherapy training of mental health professionals that took place in the 1980's, 1990's and 2000's had been well-timed to prepare us for this challenge of producing future generations of psychotherapeutically-competent, holistic psychiatrists.

At the same time, it has also enabled us to start training other mental health professionals locally, as opposed to requiring overseas stints. In the Institute of Mental Health, a system of privileging and supervision was put in place in the last five years to recognise and support various levels of depth and specialisation of psychotherapeutic work that help the wide spectrum of patients with widely varying needs; and to try to ensure that training therapists of every level have adequate supervision to deliver safe and effective care.

Since 2012, candidates with the Master of Art, Art Therapy Programme, LASALLE College of the Arts, Singapore have had clinical internships with the Psychotherapy Service, Institute of Mental Health.

Giving Back

In addition to training our own therapists, local psychotherapists have also presented and published observations from local and regional perspectives that affect and refine the way we practise these therapies that had their origins primarily in the Western world. As early as 1992, Dr G.S. Devan (1992), based on the groups that he ran from 1984 to 1989, presented his observations about how Asian culture and values affect processes in group therapy. More recently, Dr Patricia Michelle Eng Hui Yap and Tan Boon Huat (Yap and Tan, 2011) published their findings about work with families of Asian origin in the *Journal of Family Therapy*. This latter was based on a qualitative study employing interviews with four Singaporean Chinese family members from two families. Interestingly, both presentations, made about 20 years apart, had a common observation about the high value that Asian patients placed on harmony — in families and in the social network. Dr Devan observed that, unlike in the West, where full individuation and separation was valued; in the East, the attachment to parents are valued throughout life, described as healthy mutuality, mature interdependence or mature dependence.

Some other publications about psychotherapy in Singapore, or written by Singaporeans, singly or in collaboration with overseas authors include the following:

Foo KH, Merrick PL, Kazantzis N (2006). Counselling/psychotherapy with Chinese Singaporean clients. *Asian J Couns*, **13**: 271–293.

Groot JD, Cobham V, Leong J, McDermott B (2008). Individual versus group family-focused cognitive-behaviour therapy for childhood anxiety: Pilot randomized controlled trial. *Aust N Z J Psychiatry* **41**: 990–997.

Jennings L, D'Rozario V, Goh M, Sovereign A, Brogger M, Skovholt T (2008). Psychotherapy expertise in Singapore: A qualitative investigation. *Psychother Res* **18**: 508–522.

Lee BO (2002). Chinese indigenous psychotherapies in Singapore. *Couns Psychother Res* **2**: 2–10.

Ng KS (1998). *Counseling Asian Families from a Systems Perspective* (The Family Psychology and Counseling Series).

Ng KS (2003). *Global Perspectives in Family Therapy: Development, Practice, Trends*.

Ooi YP, Lam CM, Sung M, Tan WTS, Goh TJ, Fung DSS, Pathy P, Ang RP, Chua A (2008). Effects of cognitive-behavioural therapy on anxiety for children with high-functioning autistic spectrum disorders. *Singapore Med J* **49**: 215–220.

Ooi YP, Raja M, Sung SC, Fung DSS, Koh JBK (2012). Application of a web-based cognitive-behavioural therapy programme for the treatment of selective mutism in Singapore: A case series study. *Singapore Med J* **53**: 446–450.

Sim K, Gwee KP, Bateman A (2005). Case formulation in psychotherapy: Revitalising its usefulness as a clinical tool. *Acad Psychiatry* **29**: 289–292.

Sung M, Ooi YP, Goh TJ, Pathy P, Fung DSS, Ang RP, Chua A, Lam CM (2011). Effects of cognitive-behavioral therapy on anxiety in children with autism spectrum disorders: A randomized controlled trial. *Child Psychiatry Hum Dev* **42**: 634–649.

References

Ang A, 2001. Psychotherapy training in Singapore. *Psychiatr Bull* **25**: 112–113.

Barlow SH, Burlingame GM, Fuhriman A (2000). Therapeutic application of groups: From Pratt's 'thought control classes' to modern group psychotherapy. *Group Dyn* **4**: 115–134.

Barlow SH, Burlingame GM, Fuhriman A (2005). The history of group practice: A century of knowledge. In: Wheelan SA, ed. *The Handbook of Group Research and Practice*. SAGE Publications, Thousand Oaks, CA, pp. 39–64.

Beck AT, Rush AJ, Shaw BF, Emery G (1979). *Cognitive Therapy of Depression*. The Guilford Press, New York, p. 11.

Broderick CB, Schrader SS (1991). The history of professional marriage and family therapy. In: Gurman AS, Kniskern DP, eds. *Handbook of Family Therapy, Vol. 2*. Brunner/Mazel, New York.

Brown D (1983). Dr SH Foulkes (1898–1976). *Int J Psycho Anal* **64**: 109.

Devan GS (1992). Group Psychotherapy in Singapore: Modifying UK/USA Experience in Singapore Context. Presented at the College of Medicine Building, Singapore.

Ellis A (1975). *A New Guide to Rational Living*. Prentice Hall.

Eysenck H (1999). In: Gregory RL, ed. *Oxford Companion to the Mind* (2004). Oxford University Press, Oxford, pp. 92–93.

Lindsley O, Skinner BF, Solomon HC (1953). *Studies in Behavior Therapy (Status Report I)*. Metropolitan State Hospital, Walthama, MA.

Long FY, Phua EC, Tan KH (1973). Token economy programme in Singapore (report of a trial). *Nurs J Singapore* **13**: 103–109.

Ng BY (2001). *Till the Break of Day: A History of Mental Health Services in Singapore, 1841–1993*. Singapore University Press, Singapore.

Rioch MJ (1970). The work of Wilfred Bion on groups. *Psychiatry* **33**: 56–66.

Sholevar GP (2003). Family theory and therapy. In: Sholevar GP, Schwoeri LD, eds. *Textbook of Family and Couples Therapy: Clinical Applications.* American Psychiatric Publishing Inc, Washington, DC.

Sim T (2012). The growing pains of family therapy in Singapore. *J Fam Ther* **34**: 204–224.

Tan A (2003). The emergence of family therapy in postmodern Singapore. In: Ng KS, ed. Global Perspectives in Family Therapy: Development, Practice, and Trends. Brunner-Routledge, New York, pp. 39–55.

Thorndike EL (1911). Provisional laws of acquired behavior or learning. In: *Animal Intelligence.* The McMillian Company, New York.

Wolpe J (1958). *Psychotherapy by Reciprocal Inhibition.* Stanford University Press, Redwood City, CA.

Wolpe J (1982). *The Practice of Behavior Therapy*, 3rd ed. Pergamon Press, New York.

Yap, PMEH, Tan BH (2011). Families' experience of harmony and disharmony in systemic psychotherapy and its effects on family life. *J Fam Ther* **33**: 302–331.

Yates AJ (1970). *Behavior Therapy.* John Wiley & Sons, New York.

The Development of Psychiatric Nursing

Samantha ONG

The Pioneering Years

Almost a century has gone by and psychiatric nursing services have made major contributions to Woodbridge Hospital/Institute of Mental Health. When the hospital was established in 1928, care of the mentally ill was borne by the medical pioneers and a handful of expatriate nurses. Custodial care was the practice at that time.

The next decade brought about significant development in the history of psychiatric nursing service. With the introduction of modern standards of administration and treatment, there was an increasing demand for adequate and competent nurses, both male and female. The evolution of psychiatric nursing started in 1954, where it established formal training of psychiatric nurses through the School of Psychiatric Nursing. Nursing training was granted reciprocal recognition by the General Nursing Council of England and Wales in 1958.

This led to the development of better care and treatment for mentally ill patients. Graduating from basic care, psychiatric nursing took on an earnest pursuance of professional progress and trends in modern psychiatric care. Psychiatric nurses took on a new role of education and prevention.

The seventies saw landmark changes in the Nursing leadership at the Institute of Mental Health (IMH). Before 1975, the female and male wards were managed by different categories of Nursing Administrators. It was only in 1975 that the whole Nursing Department was integrated. Leading the new team was IMH first Principal Nursing Officer (PNO), Mrs M Thurairajah.

The eighties were revolutionary as we saw the birth of Community Psychiatric Nursing (CPN) to provide care and support for selected

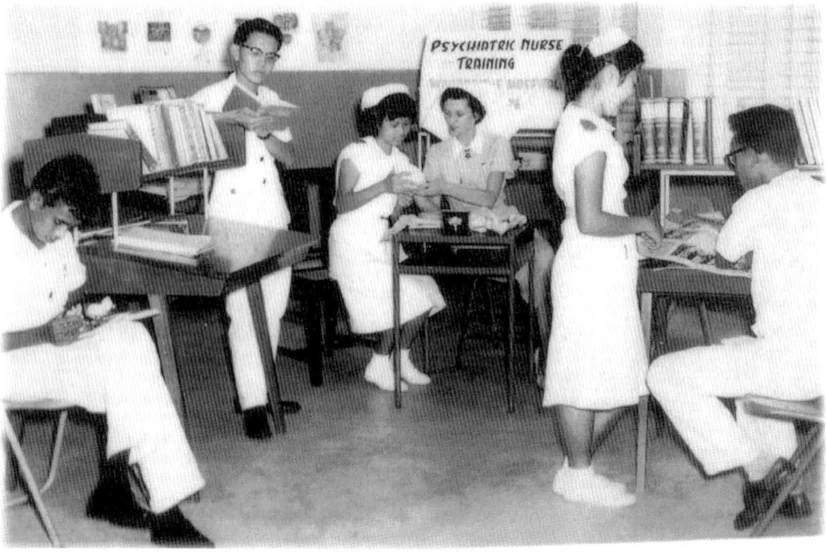

School of Nursing, 1954.

patients discharged from Woodbridge Hospital. The aim was to enhance our client's optimal functioning in the community and minimise and prevent relapses/re-admission.

On 1 October 1982, the Psychiatric Nurse Practitioner (PNP) service was introduced at IMH. This was in line with the overall upgrading of nursing skills and clinical career pathway as charted by the National Healthcare Group (NHG). Ten nurses were selected for two-week training. The PNP scheme ceased operations in 2004 with the introduction of the Advance Practiced Nurse (APN).

Beginning of a New Era

The nineties saw a beginning of a new era of Nursing at IMH. In May 1993, led by PNO Mdm Lucy Cheng Gueh Eng, the nurses moved into the new campus with the patients. It was an exciting year for IMH as 100 nurses from other government hospital joined us.

One of our primary concerns is the quality of care we deliver to the patients and the competency of the nurses in the process of care delivery. Hence, training and development of our nurses continued to play a pivotal role in Nursing. In 1991, the Nursing Training department was set up to provide learning and professional growth and development for nurses and the ancillary support staff. The Nursing Training oversees the overall management of the training and development functions of the Nursing Department, which includes among others:

- Policies and procedures related to nursing training;
- Nursing scholarships, locally and abroad;
- Training courses, seminars and conferences, including overseas and local attachment;
- Practical attachments for mental health training for nursing students and overseas nursing trainees; and
- Clinical teaching and practical attachment for basic, post-basic, degree and master nurses.

From 1994 to 1995, with the establishment of the School of Health Science at Nanyang Polytechnic, the Advanced Diploma courses were initiated for post graduate trained nurses. Our hospital continued to provide psychiatric nursing training for the nursing student. Assistance was also given to students from the Basic Diploma and Advanced Diploma courses from the Nanyang Polytechnic during their attachment to the hospital. The first batch of seven nurses graduated with a Bachelor of Health Science (Nursing) in November 1996. The first group of 49 National Certificate of Nursing students from the Institute of Technical Education (ITE) had their attachment in our hospital for four weeks of psychiatric elective postings.

Many new in-house nursing training were developed and implemented in the years. These in-house programmes aimed to provide new or higher nursing skills and raise the level of nursing practices for our nurses. Nurses from the clinical areas conducted training/education programmes for nursing colleagues at hospital and block level. In 1993, the Control and

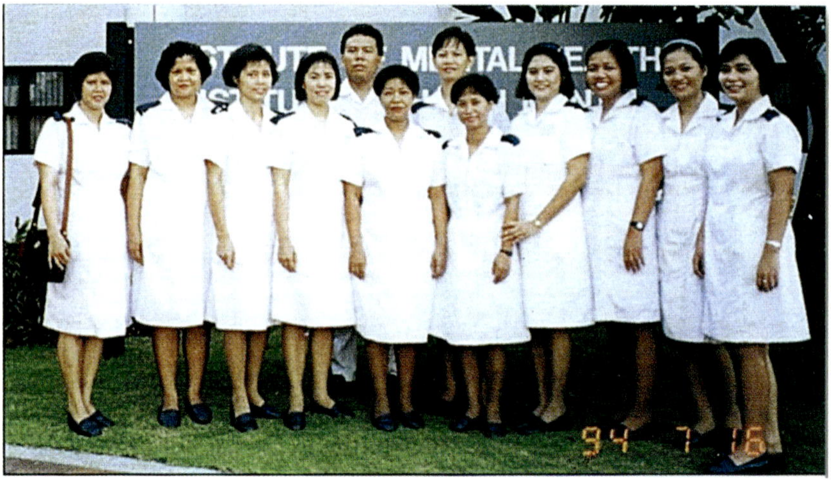

Pioneer group of Filipino nurses, 1994.

Restraint Technique programme was started to train nurses in handling aggressive and violent patients in a safe manner.

A milestone in the development of psychiatric nursing was the appointment of the first Nurse Therapist on 1 July 1993. Nurse therapists were trained psychiatric nurses who primarily looked into the psycho-educational aspects of rehabilitation.

In 1994, IMH opened its door to foreign Nurses from Myanmar and the Philippines. Nursing care was improved with the establishment of Psychiatric Nursing Standards and Patient-Centred Nursing System, which were used to measure the standard of care delivered. Another major initiative was the Re-Categorisation of Patients in the Long-Stay Wards. This was to ensure that the rehabilitation programmes could be planned to meet the needs and abilities of patients with the same level of functioning. In 1995, the Patient Education Programme (PEP) was implemented at IMH. The Programme aimed to help the individuals or group of patients to comply with treatment, reduce relapses and re-admission and to prevent or alleviate their deterioration in mental and social functioning. Three full-time Nurse Therapists conducted the PEP for both inpatients and

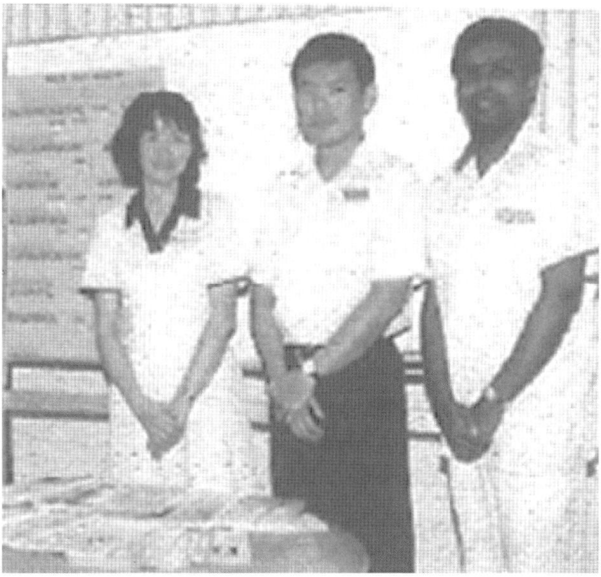

Patient educators (from left to right): N.O. Jane, N.O. Peter and S.N. Arumugum.

outpatients. The Programme was structured into five modules to meet the needs of the patient including *Understanding Mental Illness, Psychotropic Medication and You, Coping with Stress, Coping with Emotion, Family Values and Relationship*. The PEP ceased in 2003.

In 1996, a Nursing Documentation Committee was formed to revise the psychiatric nursing care plan with the aim of improving the quality of documentation. A new documentation format was developed based on the McGill's Nursing Model and implemented on 1 October 1997. A guidebook titled *A Guide to Mental Health Nursing Documentation* was also produced by the Committee to help the nurses in their care plans.

In connection with the MOH Nursing Research and Nursing Ethics Committees, two sub-committees were formed in 1997: the Nursing Research Sub-Group Committee and Nursing Ethics Sub-Group Committee, which dealt with ethical concerns on hospital admissions.

In 1998, at the PS21 WITs (Public Service for the 21st Century Work Improvement Teams) Convention, IMH was awarded the Distinguished

Departmental Effort Award for showing continuous commitment to WITs for the four consecutive years through active participation in WITs Conventions and awards attained in these Conventions.

In 1998, the Nursing Ethics Workgroup was formed. Some of the issues reviewed by the team included informed consent, physical restraint and nurse–patient relationships. Nursing articles on ethical issues were distributed to the wards to keep staff current and updated. The Nursing Ethics Workgroup was relinquished with the development of IMH Research Ethics Committee.

In all, the nineties were enriching as nursing took on a holistic approach together with the multidisciplinary team. At the new hospital, psychiatric nursing also became much modern evolutionary due to the

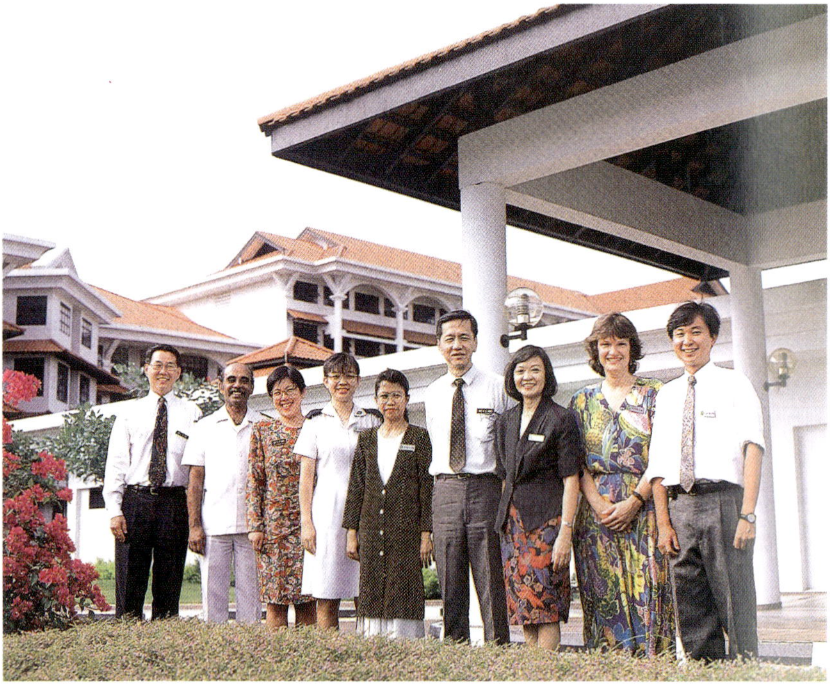

Multidisciplinary team for better patient care.

high-rise living. Structured activities and group therapy session became intensified. Changes were inevitable and it rejuvenated the nurses to spur towards better patients' care and community involvement.

Psychiatric Nursing in the New Millennium

The year 2000 marked the beginning of a new chapter of the nursing service at IMH. The hospital underwent restructuring on 1 October. The Department of Nursing Administration, led by Mdm Mary Yeo Kim Luang, took on the challenge to manage and prepare the nursing service in the new millennium.

The nursing service was guided by a new vision for nursing:

- Providing quality nursing care through fostering a safe and supportive environment conducive to the promotion of mental health and the rehabilitation of individuals into the community; and
- Upholding professional nursing standards through continuing education and evidence-based clinical practice to meet the changing needs in mental health education and promotion.

The beginning of the hospital's restructuring status was indeed exciting. There were vast changes in the hospital: environmentally, clinically and administratively. The Department of Nursing Administration continued its relentless effort to improve nursing standards and in training and development of nurses to provide safe quality care to meet the changing needs of the patients, families and the community in the new millennium. Mary and her team put in tremendous effort to revise the nursing organisation chart and develop 36 job descriptions of the various nursing grades.

In the new millennium, there was a strong emphasis on service quality and staff development as the hospital prepared for the People's Developer Standard certification, the Joint Commission International (JCI) certification and Quality Environmental Health Standards (QEHS) and other standards/accreditations.

In 2001, in preparation for the new standards, the Nursing Policies and Procedures Committee charted new nursing policies, procedures and guidelines to incorporate the maintenance. The changes include:

- Guidelines on the maintenance of Data and Document Control for ISO 9000;
- Revision of the Procedure on Triaging;
- Revision of Guidelines on Outing for Long-Stay Patients;
- Development of the Psychiatric Crisis Intervention procedure; and
- Revision of Infection Control systems and procedures.

The year 2003 was a tragic period when the nation was hit by SARS (severe acute respiratory syndrome). It was a wake-up call for the healthcare sector as we realised that we were not well prepared to face the pandemic outbreak. However, it showed how courageous and resilient our nurses were in the wake of such calamity. From then on, our infection control nurses played a pivotal role in the Infectious Disease Outbreak Taskforce. Our hospital also set up a new medical and isolation ward, which saw brought a team of nurses to IMH with competency in treating general medical conditions and infectious diseases.

The year 2005 was a golden period for IMH when it became the first psychiatric hospital in Asia to be accredited with JCI. It was an exciting journey whereby the nursing team, led by Director of Nursing, Ms Pauline Tan, played a pivotal role to ensure that processes and patient safety areas were of the highest standards. In addition to receiving the accreditation, IMH was cited by the JCI surveyors for exemplary performance in the Competency Assessment Process for Nursing. JCI helped IMH to improve patient care. There was an environment of continuous improvement so that the best care is ensured for our patients. The accreditation helped to demonstrate commitment to quality care. It benchmarked our standards against other similar organisations. With this accreditation, patients can be assured that the quality of patient care and clinical quality are kept at a standard that is consistent with other renowned hospitals. It promotes a safe environment for patients and staff. With our focus on patient safety and clinical quality, any lapse in these will immediately be detected and remedied. IMH went on to receive JCI re-accreditation in 2008, 2011 and 2014.

Patient Safety and Quality Improvement

In 2001, in pursuit to provide continuous quality improvement in the nursing service in the hospital, the Nursing Quality Improvement Committee (NQIC) was formalised. It provided a framework for coordinated quality improvement programmes. In addition, five quality improvement committees were set up to monitor areas that are problem prone and high risk. The NQIC identified the aspects of care that needed improvement and implemented changes to nursing documentation, administration of medication, care of patient on restraint and prevention of falls. Till today, the spirit of quality improvement is deeply embedded in the nursing culture as our nurses continue to participate actively in quality improvement projects and receiving numerous awards and accolades at various quality conventions.

In 2008, in conjunction with NHG lean initiatives, IMH embarked on the Kaizen journey. This focuses on pursuing seamless and cost-effective mental health services to our patients and builds a continuous improvement culture. To date, nursing has produced many improvement initiatives, 6S and lean projects to improve care processes and quality of patient care.

In 2009, in an effort to create greater awareness on healthcare safety issues at IMH, nursing organized the Patient Safety Carnival. Since then, the Patient Safety Carnival has been an annual event at IMH. The carnival offers a fun and interactive way of learning safety tips, with exhibition, live demonstrations, delightful games and quizzes. The carnival shows how innovative and creative our nurses are in their quest for safety awareness. Each year it attracts more than 500 staff from the different disciplines to participate in the activities.

Advanced Practice Nursing

The year 2004 was an important milestone for nursing profession in Singapore as it saw the birth of the Advanced Practice Nursing in Singapore. To prepare our nurses for this new role, six senior nursing staff were selected to undergo an 18-month Master of Nursing (Psychiatric) programme at the Yong Yoo Lin School of Medicine at the National University of Singapore (NUS).

Since then, IMH has built a pool of Advanced Practice Nurses (APNs) in Mental Health. Currently, IMH has 18 SNB certified APNs, and 6 APN Interns. The role and responsibilities of the APNs include:

- Conduct advanced triaging at the Emergency Department;
- Manage long stay patients with medical problems;
- Conduct chronic disease management at the annual review clinic;
- Review patients at B and satellite clinics;
- Conduct psycho-education at clinics; and
- Clerk new cases for Associate Consultants and above.

The APNs work closely with the Chairman of the Medical Board and his team of doctors in acute, long-stay, psycho-geriatric, child and adolescent unit and outpatient clinics. The APNs support the nurses to identify cases for daily multidisciplinary ward review, flag complex cases for case presentation by the wards nurses and develop nursing strategies for collaborative multidisciplinary management and treatment. This initiative now becomes the impetus to transform nursing practice from one that is task-driven to one that engages critical enquiry and analytical clinical decision-making in the patient care management process.

Since 2005, APNs had clinic sessions daily to off-load the doctors from having to see voluminous 'common-pool' patients. Aside from achieving our global effort to right site care and provide for an appropriate care model for mental health practice, this strategic move also marks the onset of autonomous mental health nursing practice and is indicative of the cluster's support in advancing the nursing profession for Singapore. In 2007, the APNs resume their outpatient clinic from seeing common-pool patients to team consults. At the team consult, the respective consultants will refer their respective unit cases to the APNs for follow-ups and continuous care. They see remission cases and also recent readmissions as well. In 2008, the APNs clerked new cases at outpatient clinic to reduce waiting time for patients.

The APNs have piloted a project to improve the management of patients with medical co-morbidities in the long stay wards. This project involved a resident physician, who will review patients in the long stay wards together with the APNs. With continual assessment and reviews of patients with medical co-morbidities, the APNs hope to improve patients' outcomes by reducing the number unnecessary transfers to the acute hospital.

Mental Health Nursing Education

Training and development of our nurses remains a key focus of Nursing Department in the new millennium. To date, IMH has sponsored three nurses to pursue their PhD:

- Dr Xie Huiting, a PhD Nurse Researcher, graduated in 2012 with a PhD from the renowned Case Western Reserve University in Ohio, USA; and
- Ms Li Ziqiang, a final-year PhD candidate at NUS, who is working on examining the effectiveness of peer-led self-management program on empowerment, perceived recovery, medication adherence, social support and reducing symptom severity in people with schizophrenia.

In addition, IMH has 18 Advanced Practice Nurses equipped with a Master of Nursing. To add to its growing army of highly qualified nurses, IMH has also sponsored two nurses in the field of Information Technology to lead the nursing informatics scene at IMH. These nurses will graduate with Master in Knowledge Management and will plan and develop IT enhancement programmes to support nursing practices across all levels.

Centre for Mental Health Education

IMH envisages being a tertiary centre of excellence and global leader in mental health care in Asia by 2020. IMH's forte in mental health treatment and nursing care delivery has distinguished us from other general hospitals. This makes strengthening nursing human capital an important goal for IMH to deliver valuable services to our customers, retain our valued employees and attract new talent. In view of these, it is imperative to improve our current capability and capacity catered for continual professional development of our nurses and harness technology to support various innovative pedagogies that will help us in achieving our vision. As such, IMH has established the new Centre for Mental Health Education (CMHE) within its premises. The new facility becomes an integral part of the whole IMH Learning Hub. This centre comprises the following:

- Joanna Briggs Institute (JBI; an IMH Research and Evidence-Based Affiliated Centre of Mental Health) and library;
- A control and restraint cum basic cardiac life support (BCLS) training room;
- A nursing skills laboratory;
- Three seminar rooms;
- A SMART classroom;
- A nursing training department; and
- An e-learning courseware development laboratory.

The main focus of CMHE is to develop and hone the innate capabilities of our nurses, keep in tandem with changes, and preserve our competitiveness in the ever-changing local, regional and global healthcare markets and trends. The centre was officially opened on 30 July 2010.

JBI — IMH Affiliate Centre for Mental Health Care

A major initiative in 2010 was the application to be a Centre for Evidence-Based Practices with the JBI, Australia. The Institute is a recognised global leader in evidence-based health care, collaborating internationally with 60 centres and groups across the world to promote and support the transfer and utilisation of research evidence into practice that improves healthcare outcomes. The Centre is physically located within the new CMHE, where there are resources available for nurses to engage in evidence-based and research-related activities.

American Nurses Credentialing Centre Accreditation with Distinction

In June 2012, the IMH Nursing Education Department was awarded the American Nurses Credentialing Centre's (ANCC) Accreditation with Distinction. It is the highest accolade from ANCC. IMH is the only mental health institution outside the US to receive this recognition. Established in 1974, the Accreditation Program of the American Nurses Credentialing Centre recognises healthcare organisations worldwide that offer highest quality continuing nursing education activities for nurses. Accredited organisations use evidenced-based ANCC criteria to plan, implement and evaluate such continuing nursing education activities.

With this accreditation, IMH's Nursing Education Department is now certified to provide continuing nursing education activities to upgrade the clinical skills of nurses who work in mental health settings and to improve their care delivery.

The Department currently offers three continuing nursing education activities that are accredited by ANCC, namely: Nursing Management of Acute Psychiatric Patients, Nursing Management of Elderly Patients with Mental Illness, and Management of Disturbed, Aggressive and Violent Patients with Mental Illness. Three new continuing nursing education activities are in the pipeline: Basic Mental Health Course, Management of

Chronic Medical Conditions for Nurses and Nursing Management of Patients with Mental Illness and Intellectual Disability.

The Department is developing more of these continuing nursing education activities to beef up the standard of mental health care. These continuing nursing education activities will be open to nurses in Singapore, the region and around the world.

National Resuscitation Council Accreditation

One of the most significant continuous improvement initiatives that the Nursing team achieved in 2012 is the National Resuscitation Council (NRC) Accreditation of IMH Life Support Training Centre (CMHE) earlier in May. The accreditation brings IMH a step closer to being a tertiary centre of excellence by establishing the institution's status as an accredited AED (automated external defibrillator) training centre certified to roll out internal Basic Cardiac Life Support (BCLS) and AED training programme founded upon proficient facility and equipment as well as a pool of certified internal trainers.

Since the commencement of a series of tailored training which caters to various levels of staff in Jun, a total of 352 medical, nursing, ancillary and allied health professionals have been trained in AED via 17 training sessions, each consisting of 16 participants. With increasingly more staff trained in Life Saver, BCLS, community AED and AED, the benchmark of patient safety has been significantly raised because all trained professionals are empowered to deliver resuscitation during code-blue situations where time is of essence. The Nursing team is targeting to complete the intermediate training for all medical, nursing, ancillary and allied health staff within two years before the next NRC audit occurs in 2015.

Management of Aggression and Violence Training

In January 2013, IMH became the only hospital in Singapore who is accredited by the Management of Aggression and Violence (MOVA) Training Academy, UK, to be certified trainers for the MOVA course. A total of 15 nurses attended the train-the-trainer programme conducted by Mr Anthony Rowe, Director of Training and Senior Tutor of the MOVA Training Academy.

Nursing Research and Evidence Based

The beginning of the new millennium was a challenging, demanding and fruitful year for the Research Workgroup. It has seen an increase in the number of nurses showing active interest in research, the formation of five research sub-workgroups and the publication of the nursing research paper entitled 'Incident of Falls in a State Psychiatric Hospital' in the *Psychosocial Nursing Journal and Mental Health Service* in September 2000.

Being Singapore's only tertiary institute for psychiatric care, IMH continues to emphasise on research to advance patient care. In 2007, a new mentorship scheme for nurses, the Research Residency Programme for nurses was established to encourage selected nurses to be engaged in research. Under the mentorship of clinicians, the programme aims to establish a pool of nurses with the capability to conduct research, mentor, coach other nurses who are also interested in research.

The research journey continued to flourish with the introduction of evidence-based practice in 2008. In 2009, five Clinical Practice Guidelines were developed to guide nursing practice in IMH after an intensive workshop with Dr Marita Titler, a guru of evidence-based practice.

The members of the Nursing Research Workgroup continued to encourage more nurses to come forward to be involved in nursing research. Talks and seminars were organised to create awareness of the important of research among nurses. For the first time, a Mental Health Research Award was given to Nursing during the 6th IMH Annual Scientific Meeting, which was held on 6 October 2011 in IMH. It was opened to all the other hospital in both clusters. The research paper entitled 'Seepage and Other Local Complications: A Comparative Study of Three Intra-Muscular Injection Techniques' won the award.

Since then, more nurses have been seen taking up research projects which led to the establishment of JBI, an internationally recognised leader in evidence-based practice centre in IMH in 2010. The team at JBI–IMH is made up of ward based Staff Nurses (SNs), Senior Staff Nurses (SSNs) and APNs who have expressed interest in, and are competent to conduct research and translate evidence into clinical practice. To date the centre has produced three systematic reviews all conducted by nurses.

Further headway in projects by nurses saw the start of the Nursing Journal Club. Led and managed by a group of APNs, this platform is used to promote evidence-based practice among IMH nurses. Thirty nurses meet every two months to appraise research articles and discuss about the applicability of the research evidence into clinical practice. Nurses are coached and mentored to understand that research evidence is important but not all research findings can be translated into clinical practice. For well-researched evidence deemed useful for translation into clinical practice, the nurses work on strategies to adopt them.

This momentum was further fuelled with the set-up of an Evidence-Based Utilization Workgroup under the JBI International Evidence-Based Utilisation Network. This workgroup aims to advance mental health evidence-based practices and research in the region and translate these to enhance practice, improve patient outcomes and promote mental health. The Evidence-Based Utilisation Workgroup works together with clinical domain areas at the NQIC to ensure that clinical standards are met and quality checks are in place to maintain optimal patient safety.

The gradual increment in the number of nurses participating in nursing research and evidence-based activities has seen IMH clinching a total of three Gold and one Bronze awards at the Singapore Health and Biomedical Conference for the past three consecutive years.

Name	Achievement	Year
APN — Intern Mao Rui	Singapore Nursing Award (Gold)	2012
SSN Rajni Parasurum	Singapore Nursing Award (Gold)	2011
APN Zhou Zhenyu	Singapore Nursing Award (Gold)	2010
SSN Li Ziqiang	SHBC Best Poster Award (Nursing Gold Award)	2011

Seeing the potential in research and benefits to the nursing profession, the JBI–IMH Centre team has collaborated with the National University Health System (NUHS) and NHG Health Services and Outcomes Research (HSOR) to host the inaugural JBI Singapore Colloquium in 2014. The event attracted approximately more than 300 delegates from 52 JBI centres located worldwide. This colloquium will provide a platform for networking and knowledge-sharing with renowned experts from various healthcare fields. It also features a mental health track that allows various research and evidence-based projects to be presented at an international level.

Dr Xie Huiting is IMH first nurse (2013) to complete her PhD in Nursing Research from NHG after four years, following the successful completion of her PhD studies. As Singapore's first Nurse Researcher, Dr Xie will harness her expertise in leading nursing research and evidence-based practices, as well as mentoring aspiring nurse researchers in IMH to consider a dual career in integrating clinical and research activities.

Community Psychiatric Nursing Services

In 2000, the Community Psychiatric Nursing Services (CPNS) was reviewed to reflect a more focused and effective service. The referral system were revised. The CPNS would no longer carry out crisis intervention but could now source and identify suitable cases for referral. A pilot project on family psycho-education was carried out jointly by the CPNS and Patient Educators. The project included 20 patients and their families from April to July. Objectives of the project were to encourage more family involvement in the management of the patients, training on case management.

In 2009, the community mental Health Team implemented the Illness Self-Management and Recovery (ISMR) programme. The programme was developed to help patients who were discharge and referred to Community Psychiatric Nurses (CPNs). The program uses behavioural tailoring and social skills training to help patient cope with their mental illness. All CPNs would be trained in the programme. The programme is currently being conducted in groups at the satellite clinics by our trained CPNs.

The Commcare@IMH Project started in 2008 and was completed in 2009. The project aimed to improve the management of patient's information particularly in community nursing. CPNs now have access to patients' information from the various IT systems at IMH. Patients' clinical assessments are also captured directly into the IT system. The programme has been incorporated into the hospital wide IT initiative on nursing cocumentation aka 'E-Notes'.

Nursing Projects

Trendcare project

One of the major nursing IT projects was the TrendCare, a joint project between MOH and two healthcare clusters funded by the Ministry of Finance (MOF) through the Reinvestment Fund. Trendcare is a patient acuity system, with the objective of matching the nurse staffing to identified patient needs. It utilises inpatient acuity measurement to improve staffing situation and patient care quality thus helping to manage nursing manpower more effectively through findings from Trendcare project. TrendCare was implemented in IMH wards in stages starting in May 07 and completed successfully in November 2007. Inter-rater reliability test was conducted for all staff Nurses from October to December. This is to ensure accuracy of categorisation.

Everglow Nurses project

In 2008, as part of keeping older employees in the workforce, the Everglow Nurses' Programme was launched to offer retired nurses creative job options and an opportunity to remain in the workforce under a flexi-hour scheme. The programme is a novel approach to allowing retired nurses to continue in roles of training, promoting patient safety and maintaining clinical standards of care, while contributing their expertise gathered through the years of service.

Ergonomically designed equipment

In 2009, nursing secured funds worth S$228,000 from the Workforce Development Agency (WDA) to purchase ergonomically-designed equipment to reduce the burden of our senior nursing staff. The equipment made the jobs of our nurses less manual, menial and strenuous thus promoting a friendlier work environment. The equipment purchased included:

- Electronic sphygmomanometer;
- Arjo basic shower chair;
- Arjo basic shower trolley;
- Blood collection trolley;
- Fully motorised patient trolley;
- Magnifying glass; and
- Pat slides.

In our effort to continually upgrade and train our nursing leaders on the ground with the necessary skills and knowledge to meet future challenges, nursing developed the Nurse Clinician Course for 60 Nurse Clinicians (NCs) and SSNs at IMH. The course had a funding of S$98,000 by the WDA. The 178-hour in-house course was specially tailored for the psychiatric setting and consisted of 10 modules. It was also accredited by the Singapore Nursing Board. The modules taught included Clinical Problem Solving, Decision Making Skills, Advanced Clinical Skills, Clinical Supervisory Skills, Risk Management and Patient Safety. All 60 nurses completed the course in 2009.

Awards

Over the past 20 years, our Nurses have achieved outstanding recognition for their exemplary efforts. IMH had produced Nursing Presidents' Award winners and Tan Chin Tuan Award winners, both prestigious awards for nurses.

- Presidents' Award
  - Mdm Chua Siew Hong (2000)
  - Dr Pauline Tan (2006)
  - Mdm Yang Chek Salikin (2008)
  - Ms Poh Chee Lien (2012)
  - Mr Raveen Dev (2016)

- Tan Chin Tuan Award
  - Mdm Zubaidah Bte Mohd Saad (2006)
  - Mdm Hardev Kaur (2007)
  - Mdm Soonthrammal d/o Nalappan (2009)
  - Mdm Lee Poh Gim (2010)
  - Mr Mohd Aliff Bin Adran (2014)
  - Mdm Qiu Baoyi (2014)
  - Mr S Mogana (2015)
  - Mdm Wong Chi Shi (2016)
  - Mdm Sim Kian Kian (2016)

Conclusion

Psychiatric nurses play an integral role in the treatment of people with mental illness, in inpatient and outpatient settings, community, academic, research, private, public and government institutions. The profession of psychiatric nursing is continually evolving. In the past, nurses were involved mainly in providing institutional care, patient education and therapy. Now they play important roles in research and evidence-based nursing, nursing informatics, advanced practice nursing, quality and patient safety and management. What remains unchanged, however, is that psychiatric nurses have a deep desire to provide high-quality care for people living with mental illness, and that they are steadfast in the belief that their care makes a difference.

Acknowledgement

We would like to thank Ms. Pauline Tan for her inputs on this chapter.

Reference

Ong S, Dev R (2014). Psychiatric nursing. In: Sim K, Sengupta S, Fung D, Chee KT, eds. *Essential Guide to Psychiatry*. Pearson, Singapore, pp. 547–558.

Psychiatric Social Work in Singapore

Lilian MARK and Siti Sohanah Binte KASMANI

'Over 60 years, as Singapore moved from third world to first, medical social service has progressed in response to changing needs and has become more sophisticated, from dealing with merely financial welfare issues to providing counselling and dealing with first-world health challenges such as chronic diseases, obesity, mental health problems, addictions, discharge care arrangements and end-of-life issues.'

Khaw Boon Wan, Former Minister of Health

How the Past Shaped the Future

Social work evolved as a profession in Singapore in later 19th century. Medical social workers (MSWs) were known as 'almoners' then and the first Almoner's Department was established in Singapore in January 1949 by Miss M. Eastaugh.

Psychiatric Social Work is a branch of medical social work which specializes in programmes and services for patients with mental illness and their families which is often based within a psychiatric hospital setting. In Singapore, it began taking shape in the fifties. The first psychiatric social worker in Singapore, Mrs A.V. Francis was appointed in December 1955. The same year also saw Psychiatric Social Work instituted in parallel with Psychiatric Occupational Therapy and Psychological services which set off the beginnings of the Multidisciplinary Team (MDT) concept in psychiatric care in Woodbridge Hospital (WH).

In 1962, WH had one psychiatric social worker and two students receiving training in psychiatric social work at the University of Singapore. This team expanded through the seventies and eighties to six social workers, two clerical assistants and an investigator. Three decades later by 1993, there were 18 social workers with 12 support staff (Seng, 1994).

Over the next three decades till the eighties, psychiatric social workers' scope and role evolved in tandem with Singapore's economic and social development. Social issues had evolved from poverty, hygiene-related problems to those related to rapid industrialization.

While in the **fifties**, social workers were primarily concerned and focused on providing **practical assistance** to meet the basics of food, shelter and the physical health of patients, the **sixties** saw the consolidation of its role and functions with the provision of **casework services** to help patients cope with the multiple social problems they faced. There were more family related issues and there was also the need to develop services to meet specific needs such as rehabilitation of offenders and drug addicts and those with disabilities. Their role included getting a comprehensive social history for psychiatrists, acted as a liaison for the patients with the community and aided with discharge of patients back to their own homes.

In the **seventies**, psychiatric social workers became heavily involved in **rehabilitative work** at View Road Hospital (VRH) which offered residential stay as well as employment for patients who could not return to their own homes. During this period, the Employment Scheme was initiated for female patients in domestic and social skills enable them to become domestic servants. This was subsequently introduced to male patients as well. With industrialization in the country, farming and animal husbandry, factory work assembly and packing, cleaning services and security work were also available and found suitable for patients who have been discharged.

The **eighties** saw social workers taking an **expanded role** in another aspect of **rehabilitation** when WH set up more day centres in the community. Social workers became involved and occupied with preparing patients and their families for day release and sheltered employment. By the late eighties, with the further evolution of the MDT concept, social workers took on a more integral position in the MDT and carried out programme specific roles including multi-skill intervention approaches. In programme such as the Alcoholism programme, social workers went beyond the traditional role of financial and social assistance and function as an educator, individual therapist, group facilitator and family counselor in treatment process alongside the MDT members.

A New Era

The relocation and downsizing of WH to the current site at Buangkok Green 1993, heralded a new era which saw more intervention-based approaches initiated whilst securing an increase in the staff ratio.

Systemic perspectives began to influence social work services and approaches in the nineties. A wider perspective was adopted with the view that financial problems when surfaced, in reality represent problems of a wider unique and deeper set of issues and difficulties. In response, the department started sending MSWs for short-term skills attachments in mental health areas such as psychiatric rehabilitation, eating disorders, family psycho education, vocational counseling, group work, forensic social work and family therapy. These training and on-site attachments further equipped social workers with skills to manage complex familial problems that involved multiple interacting factors that span across mental health symptoms, physical illnesses and psychological, emotional and social difficulties.

The **late nineties** saw MSWs venturing outside the hospital to do more **outreach work into the community**. MSWs provided social work and assessment services to day care centres at Sunlove and New Horizon Day Centres. This role continued and later expanded to include MSWs directly giving mental health education and training or through Social Service Training Institute.

Enhancing **patient reintegration into the community** became an added focus of that era. In addition to casework and care planning, the department continued its close involvement in vocational rehabilitation in WH as well as VRH which remained open till 2003. Thereafter the inpatient psychiatric rehabilitation known as the "Stepping Stones" programme took over this function with a more consolidated, structured and holistic package. Patients who were assessed as needing further rehabilitation enroute to eventual reintegration into the community, were referred and supported by MSWs to step down to psychiatric rehabilitation residential care facilities namely Bukit Gombak Group Home, Hougang Care Centre and Simei Care Centre.

An interesting development in this era was MSWs' work with a sizeable number of migrant patients from neighbouring countries some of whom needed psychiatric treatment. MSWs were heavily involved in arranging for repatriation to their countries of origin.

At the **turn of the century, psychiatric social work faced a few serious challenges**. The manpower resource management of MSWs underwent another extensive revamp. Until the nineties, MSWs were employed predominantly in the Civil Service. When WH was converted to a restructured hospital in 2001 and renamed the Institute of Mental Health, several MSWs sought transfers out of WH as they preferred to remain in the Civil Service scheme. As a result, this era saw an increase in new and younger entrants to the department. This transition presented a new strain on existing build-up of demands on psychiatric social workers.

The changing needs of society demanded a greater array of skills and greater adaptability of MSWs. There were expectations for MSWs to expand their role in the community, in tandem with the hospital's focus towards community psychiatry. While social workers were required to work with diverse social problems in the community, they were also expected to hone competencies in specific areas of specialization. The department thus began sending MSWs overseas for longer term training as the post-graduate Master's level. Some training areas included community mental health, forensic social work, vocational counseling, family therapy and geriatric social work.

Meanwhile work circumstances remained challenging, given an increasing lack of social services in the community to support rehabilitation and the issues of stigmatization which impacted patients as much as the workers. Coupled with low remuneration and high caseload, it was not surprising that despite the earlier increase in headcount, there remained difficulties retaining MSWs. This was compounded by a vibrant job market in the booming new economy which limited the recruitment of existing professionals in the field and new graduates.

Nevertheless MSWs were steadfast in their involvement in IMH's efforts to expedite discharge of acute patients and the development of care of acute and long stay patients to establishments that were made available by the Ministry of Health (MOH) and Ministry of Community Development, Youth and Sport (MCYS). These places included Pelangi Village, Tai Pei Home, Sunlove Home and some nursing homes.

The above issues pre-empted a renewal of focus as per call by the Minister of Health, Mr Khaw Boon Wan who challenged the MSW fraternity that as our population ages further, and their expectations change, the medical social services must continue to evolve and stay responsive to their needs (Khaw, 2009).

A Renewed Focus — Towards Advanced Practice in Psychiatric Social Work

Manpower and competency development

The National Mental Health Blueprint (NMHB) in 2007 presented another opportunity to further the manpower enhancement efforts. The department was given additional manpower over a five-year period to address persistent issues relating to heavy workload and a high turnover of social workers due to burnout. Additional staff was also required for new outreach programmes initiated at the hospital level as part of the move towards community psychiatry. While these measures helped to partially stem the fast turnover of younger staff, it surfaced a new challenge — difficulties in hiring.

As a more immediate measure, remuneration of social workers was addressed with MOH's support and new entrants saw a significant increase in their entry salary. Efforts were also made to attract mid-career staff through post graduate diploma training at NUS and UniSIM. The longstanding internship programme with the universities was enhanced to further interest graduates in the area of mental health. In IMH, counselling was established as a basic core competency in addition to social work training at the degree level. Advanced practice areas for the more experienced workers were also established in the areas of family therapy, forensics work, psychogeriatric social work, addictions, intellectually disabled and psychiatric rehabilitation.

Intensifying destigmatisation through public education

The changing profile and evolving role of the family in the country has heightened the emphasis on preventive care and for the MDT to be pay heed to the family functioning of patients. Domestic violence was on the increase alongside social changes. Social workers networked systematically with specialist agencies and also became resource persons on committees overseeing family violence cases, such as with the Elder Protection Team, Promoting Alternatives to Violence (PAVE). Such participation in the national-level framework was seen as helpful to service partners as well as IMH in view of the complexities of these cases which required a multi-agency, multidisciplinary approach.

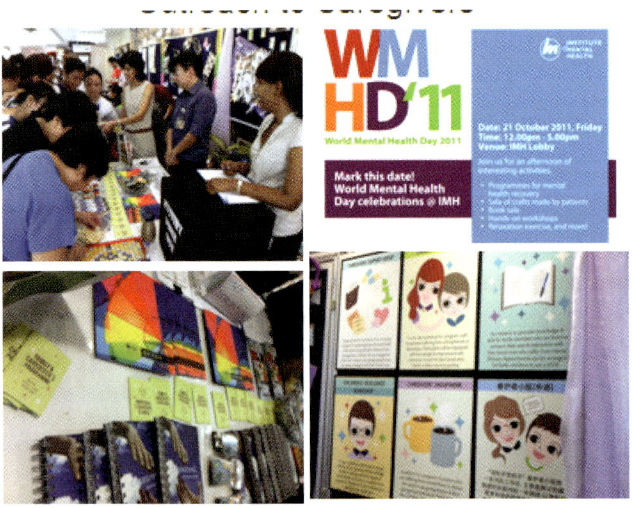
WM
HD'11
World Mental Health Day 2011
Mark this date!
World Mental Health
Day celebrations @ IMH
Date: 21 October 2011, Friday
Time: 12.00pm - 5.00pm
Venue: IMH Lobby

Outreach to caregivers.

Family psychoeducation (FPE) continued to be a key focus of the department to educate the family on the physical and psychosocial needs of its members and the ways they could access internal and external resources. FPE was delivered through individual sessions using materials adapted from Support and Family Education Programme (SAFE): Mental Health Facts for families (Sherman, 2003). In addition, full-day workshops were also held on weekends to provide working caregivers access to a team of multidisciplinary professionals who would gather to interact with them to teach and to lend support to their struggles. Structured group work programmes were initiated for identified groups to support and affirm their caregiving experiences, seek reconciliation in the challenging situations they are in and work towards greater self-care.

A team of social workers also advocated for the needs of children who had parents with mental illnesses. These children, often in the mainstream, were often acknowledged as 'silent victims' who were at risk of the negative impact of mental illnesses. The programme 'I am a Resilient Kid' was started in collaboration with Covenant Family Service Centre (FSC).

Direct services and responsiveness in meeting evolving society needs

- *Changing landscape in financial assistance and resources* — With the introduction of the means testing framework in Singapore to guide government disbursement of subsidies and services, MSWs became key stakeholders as gatekeepers or advocates for the needy population to access treatment and services. To complement this role, MSWs were also challenged to be creative, astute and well informed of resources within IMH and in the community. For example, in addition to practical welfare assistances, new funds were created to meet specific needs in the home improvement, employment and caregivers programmes.
- *Expansion of roles* — The various initiatives in the NMHB gave rise to opportunities for MSWs to expand their roles in preventive services. Some of these services included the roles of the social workers in the outreach services at the young, adult and elderly age groups, including

Response, Early Intervention and Assessment in Community Mental Health (REACH), Adult Community Mental Health Team (CMHT) and Aged Psychiatry Community Assessment and Treatment Service (APCATS), respectively. Besides outreach, this paved the way for specialisation as well.

- *Advocacy* — MSWs, being well placed to sense needs of patients on the ground, would serve as strong advocates for patients as well as their caregivers. In this respect, efforts were made by various representations at workgroups and networks set up with community partners as well as government agencies. Examples of the department's participation in committees include family violence management workgroups with the Ministry of Social and Family Development (MSF) and network meetings with Community Development Councils (CDCs), the Agency for Integrated Care (AIC), the National Council of Social Service (NCSS) and MOH.
- *Employment* — The MSW Department partnered the Occupational Therapy Department to start the Job Club in 2009 with the aim of establishing a structured approach to provide job matching, training and support for patients on the recovering path.

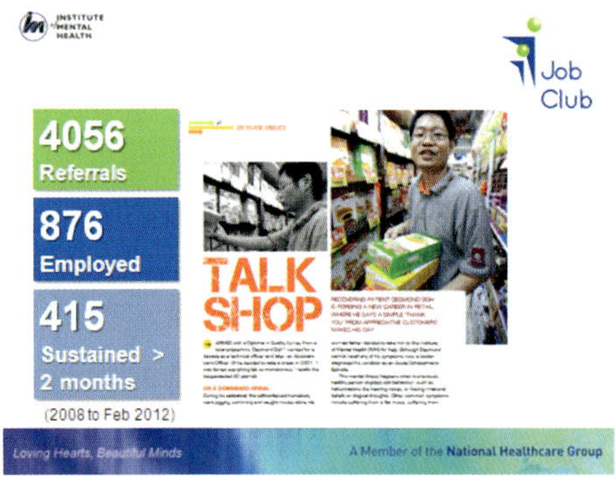
Job Club
4056 Referrals
876 Employed
415 Sustained > 2 months
(2008 to Feb 2012)
TALK SHOP
Loving Hearts, Beautiful Minds
A Member of the National Healthcare Group

'There is little point in rehabilitating patients only to release them back to the same environment that triggered the illness in the first place. While the core work in casework and counselling remains, we now also collaborate with the government and voluntary agencies to advocate services that are lacking and to close service gaps that hinder patients' efforts to return to live in the community.' (Heartening Minds IMH 80th Anniversary, 2008)

- *Care and Discharge Coordination* — A Care Coordination Team was also set up to organise placements to stepdown care facilities in the community. The team would work very closely with service partners through joint or pre-assessments of patients, training, workgroups and sharing of resources involving care coordination units with rehab and nursing homes to better match clients' needs and to increase referrals from IMH to care centres.

- *Crisis Intervention and Training* — The role of MSWs as CARE officers remain steadfast during times of disasters or crises at the national level. IMH MSWs also took on the role of trainers in these areas.

Conclusion

"Mr Khaw Boon Wan, then Minister for Health, challenged the MSW fraternity that 'as our population ages further, and their expectations change, the medical social service must continue to evolve to stay responsive to their needs' (Khaw, 2009).

Psychiatric social work in Singapore has achieved a solid base in the last 70 years and has responded to the changing needs of each era alongside overall changes in psychiatric care. Going forward, more needs to be done cross sector collaborations in health, social and community care."

References

Bentelspacher, CE, Seng BK (1994). A description and analysis of Woodbridge Hospital's employment scheme for ex-mental patients. *Social Dimension* (Issue 1).

Khaw BW (2009). Speech "Medical social workers are key to holistic care for patients" at the launch of the book *Tapestry of care — Voices of Medical Social Workers* on life's joys and pains through the eyes of medical social workers.

Loving Hearts, Beautiful Minds, Woodbridge Hospital Celebrating 75 years, Institute of Mental Health, 2003 (Armour Publishing Pte Ltd).

Mark L, Chan LL (2014). Social work interventions and services. In: Sim K, Sengupta S, Fung D, Chee KT, eds. *Essential Guide to Psychiatry*. Pearson, Singapore, pp. 503–513.

Sherman MD (2003). The Support and Family Education (SAFE) program: mental health facts for families. *Psychiatr Serv* **54**(1): 35–37.

The Growth and Development of the Psychological Services in IMH

Clare YEO, Carolyn KEE, Kala MEHROTRA, GOH Tze Jui, ONG Lue Ping, Jolly CHUA, Nikki LIM, ONG Li Min, GWEE Kenji, HUANG Wanping, Chermain WONG, Siva PENCHALIAH, Haanusia Prithivi RAJ, Matthew WOO, Ann-Marie LO CASTRO, Shannon PEH, Jade JANG, WONG Chin Meng, Clare KWAN and KOK Yun Fern

Early Years

The psychological services in Singapore originated in 1956 when Australian psychologist V. W. Wilson initiated the development of psychological services within the Woodbridge Hospital (Long, 1987). From a handful of psychologists conducting mainly intellectual assessments, the psychological service grew in manpower and scope as psychologists began to provide personality testing and behaviour therapy, thus expanding their contribution to the clinical management of patients. Over the years, the work done by psychologists became increasingly recognised and requested by social and governmental organisations and in 1984, the Department of Psychology was officially established as a centralised psychological service for the Civil Service with Mr Long Foo Yee as its head. The psychologists were active in meeting requests by various government offices and agencies for psychological studies, assessment and input. Psychological input and evaluation was provided for political candidates, President's and Overseas Merit Scholarship candidates and even hostage negotiation situations (Wikipedia, 2016).

'Apart from the continual efforts of the Department of Psychology towards clinical excellence, the department also prided itself on its longstanding collaboration with the Public Service Commission (PSC) which plays an active role in the grooming of existing and future leaders of Singapore and awards the prestigious PSC scholarship to post-"A"-level students with excellent academic calibre and leadership qualities. Utilising their strength in conducting interviews during their clinical work, the psychologists from the department conduct psychological interviews during the annual PSC Scholarship Selection Exercise to assist in the selection of eligible candidates. Tapping on their clinical skills, they also corroborate the psychological interview findings with other essential sources of information such as personality tests. All in all, the psychologists are honoured and privileged to be able to contribute their expertise towards the mammoth task of selecting the potential leaders of Singapore.'

Ms Eunice Seah
Psychologist who coordinated PSC Scholarship interviews at IMH
Psychological Assessment Service

1993–2000

In 1993, the Woodbridge Hospital was renamed the Institute of Mental Health (IMH) and relocated to its new premises at Buangkok Green. Under the strong support of the Institute's first appointed CEO, Ms Luisa Lee, the Department of Psychology further expanded its scope of service to include neuropsychological testing, cognitive–behavioural therapy, individual and group psychotherapy, as well as the provision of mental health education, smoking cessation and stress management workshops for the community. The psychologists were also active in providing talks, lectures and training for students and professional staff. At the Child Guidance Clinic, under the leadership of Mr David Oon, Senior Psychologist, social skills groups, ADHD (attention-deficit/hyperactivity disorder) behavioural management workshops for parents and anxiety management groups were offered to patients and their parents. The

Department of Psychology at IMH played a pivotal role as a centre of deployment and supervision for psychologists from the various ministries and agencies who converged regularly for professional growth and development. Newly recruited psychologists for the Civil Service were given training within the hospital and subsequently deployed to various psychology service units set up at the Ministry of Community Development, Youth and Sports (MCYS, now Ministry of Social and Family Development, MSF), Singapore Prison Service (SPS), Singapore Police Force (SPF), School Health Services, Tan Tock Seng Hospital (TTSH) and Singapore General Hospital (SGH).

In July 1994, following the Hotel New World disaster, the Ministry of Home Affairs (MHA), together with the Ministry of Health (MOH) and other government agencies, established the National Emergency Behaviour Management System (NEBMS) with Mr Long Foo Yee as the Chief Emergency Behaviour Officer and Mr Oh Teik Guan as Deputy to develop a system of psychological support for victims of critical incidents (Long, 2001). The first Emergency Behaviour Officer course was conducted in February 1994 with 30 participants from various ministries attending. The NEBMS was activated during the North–South Highway accident in 1996, the Silkair Flight MI 185 crash in 1997, the SQ006 air disaster in 2000 and the Asian tsunami in 2004.

In 2000, IMH was restructured and public hospitals and health services were corporatised. The Psychological Service as a centralised scheme of service for the Civil Service was discontinued, and individual ministries and agencies proceeded to expand and develop their services within their respective domains. The Department of Psychology continued to champion the growth and development of psychological services in Singapore through the provision of training, supervision and placement opportunities for psychologists from the various ministries and agencies.

2000–Present

With the turn of the century came an era of rapid growth and expansion of the psychological services in IMH. Headed by Dr Lyn Chua and subsequently by Adjunct Assistant Professor Clare Yeo from 2004, the department of psychology initiated and developed new clinics, services and interest groups to address the mounting psychological needs of the population as well as to meet the increasing call for research and publication in the area of clinical psychology and mental health.

Clinical Units and Services

2004 — Neuro-Behavioural Clinic (ADHD Services) at the Child Guidance Clinic

Formerly established as the Children's One-Stop Psycho-Educational Service (COPES) in April 2004 with the assistance of the Medical Capability Development Fund (MCDF), COPES was renamed as the Neuro-Behavioural Clinic (NBC) ADHD services in 2011. NBC (ADHD services) offers specialised multidisciplinary assessment and therapy for children and youth with ADHD and mental health co-morbidities. Educational and Clinical Psychologists provide individual behavioural therapy, social skills training and academic intervention, working collaboratively with parents and caregivers and conducting parent education and workshops to empower them to support their children's needs. The team has also partnered with the Society for the Promotion of ADHD Research and Knowledge (SPARK) in 2012 to conduct a series of parent workshops.

Psychologists have been involved in various research projects and presented at several international conferences. A study on the 'Prevalence of behavioural and emotional problems in children at-risk for learning difficulties' headed by Educational Psychologist Ms Kala Mehrotra was presented as a poster at the European Congress of Psychiatry in 2011, while another poster on 'A hyperactive avatar's quest to save the dolphin: A cognitive-based online gaming program' was put up at the 57th Annual Meeting of the American Academy of Child and Adolescent Psychiatry in 2010.

As part of the team's continuous efforts in learning and building internal capacity, staff at the ADHD clinic have been actively pursuing training to upgrade their skills. Educational Psychologists Ms Suhana Manzur and Ms Elizabeth Tan, together with a specialist teacher Ms Sally Ang, went to the Duke University Medical Centre in the US from January to March 2012 to learn about the Duke ADHD Programme so as to inform and guide the delivery of services at the ADHD clinic.

The team is currently looking into the possibility of manualising some of its core psychosocial programmes and studying its efficacy with the aim of providing evidence-based treatment for its patients.

2005 — Neuro-Behavioural Clinic (Autism Services) at the Child Guidance Clinic

In 2005, the NBC (Autism Services) was the first specialty clinic in Singapore providing holistic and multidisciplinary management of autism spectrum disorder (ASD). It started under the Medical Capability Development Fund (MCDF) and provides diagnostic and psychological assessments of ASD as well as intervention for children between 6 and 19 years old. The service compliments and bridges the gap in service provision in restructured hospitals in Singapore, and has a strong working alliance with schools and community agencies to develop services to cater to the needs of children with ASD and their caregivers beyond the age of 19 and across the lifespan.

In 2008, psychologist Ms Sheila Tan and team went to North Carolina in the US to observe the TEACCH programme, an established ASD-oriented facility, and returned to share important observations to implement improvements to the clinic resources. The psychologists in the team also attend regular courses to update their skills such as Solution-Focused Therapy and the Stop-Think-Do programme. Of note, all the psychologists were trained in administering the Autism diagnostic tests such as the Autism Diagnostic Interview (ADI) and Autism Diagnostic Observation Schedule (ADOS).

In 2011, an inpatient service for children with ASD was initiated at Sunrise Wing, led by Educational Psychologist Ms Kheng Joo Lian. Psychologists in the team conduct regular parent training workshops as well as seminars and training programmes for fellow professionals to equip the community with skills in working with individuals with ASD and raise awareness of ASD.

Psychologists from NBC (Autism Services) have also been actively engaged in research programmes and studies and are strong advocates for evidence-based practices in the field of ASD. In 2005, Ms Goh Tze Jui developed a manualised Cognitive–Behavioural Therapy program for children with ASD and the team headed by Dr Sung Min was awarded a National Medical Research Council (NMRC) grant to study the efficacy of the programme in a randomised controlled trial. Since then, Ms Goh, together with Dr Sung, has led the research efforts of the NBC (Autism Services) team in several studies and secured various grants. Recent projects include a collaboration with Duke-NUS in 2010 titled 'A striatal synaptic dysfunction hypothesis for repetitive behaviours as evaluated by the resequencing of candidate genes', a NAO robot project titled 'Robot-facilitated therapy for children with Autism Spectrum Disorders' under the NTU-NHG (National Healthcare Group) Innovation Seed Grant 2011 and a study titled 'Effectiveness of a multi-professional training module focusing on Autism Spectrum Disorders' under an NHG Homer grant in 2012.

The team presented at the 20th World International Association for Child and Adolescent Psychiatry and Allied Professionals (IACAPAP) Congress 2012. Ms Jade Jang participated in the Donald J. Cohen Fellowship, as part of the conference program, while Ms Goh Tze Jui presented a poster on 'Factors that influence access to services for individuals with Autism Spectrum Disorders'. Ms Goh has also presented at the Asian Conference of Psychology and at the 19th European Congress of Psychiatry in 2011. Together with other team members, she was invited to conduct a pre-conference workshop at the 16th Malaysian Conference on Psychological Medicine during the same year. The team has been publishing extensively on the results of the studies in various international peer-reviewed journals and was awarded the NHG Excellence in Action (Team) award in 2013 for their work and contribution to the field.

2007 — REACH (Response, Early Intervention, Assessment for Community Mental Health)

REACH (Response, Early intervention, Assessment for Community mental Health) is a community-based mental health service in Singapore. The first three REACH teams (REACH North, REACH South and REACH East) were set up by IMH under the National Mental Health Blueprint (NMHB) in 2007 to support schools, community agencies and family doctors help children and adolescents with emotional, behavioural or neurodevelopmental problems. Besides conducting mental health assessments and providing early intervention for students in schools or homes, the multidisciplinary REACH teams also provide helpline advice and training to community partners on child and adolescent mental health. Clinical and educational psychologists in the REACH team conduct cognitive assessment and psychological therapy. In order to increase mental health resources and awareness within the community, they have set up a website (www.roc-n-ash.com) to provide information on childhood anxiety and developed a computer game (CASTLE-AC) to teach upper primary school children anxiety management skills. The REACH psychologists have also conducted research to determine the efficacy of this computer program.

2008 — Research Unit at the Child Guidance Clinic

The Research Unit at the Child Guidance Clinic (CGC) was established in 2008. It comprised a multidisciplinary team of child psychiatrists, allied health specialists and research staff, all of whom have to go through the pre-requisite Proper Conduct Research Training or the Singapore Guideline for Good Clinical Practice (SGGCP) to equip them with the appropriate knowledge to conduct research ethically and with scientific standards. Since the inception of the unit, there has been a gradual increase in the number of psychologists contributing to research, offering expertise to a number of research studies within the Department of Child and Adolescent

Psychiatry (DCAP). In recent years, some have chosen to take the lead as the Principal Investigator of research studies.

In particular, Dr Sharon Sung, a Senior Clinical Psychologist with DCAP, is involved in several clinical research projects including the following studies: a) examining patterns of mood and anxiety disorders in parents of clinically referred youth for which she is the Principal Investigator; b) developing a virtual-reality exposure therapy for children with selective mutism; c) evaluating patients with panic disorder in the emergency ward (a pilot study); and d) developing a mobile application for cognitive–behaviour therapy that patients can use to perform self-guided treatment. Dr Sung's passion in research paid off when she was awarded the Allied Health Bronze Award at the Singapore Health and Biomedical Congress (SHBC) 2012 for her poster on 'Depressive symptoms in Singaporean primary care patients: Do they differ based on age, gender or ethnicity?'

Moving forward, the team hopes to engage more psychologists to take the lead as Principal Investigators and attract a new generation of clinician-scientists who are keen to take research in the clinic to a whole new level. By keeping abreast of the most modern and systematic intervention approaches for managing children with behavioural problems and fostering research collaborations with other major institutions, it is believed that this would not only establish the research unit as an institution where research and clinical work goes hand in hand, but would also constantly challenge the way we think about current clinical practice.

2009 — Mood and Anxiety Clinic at the Child Guidance Clinic

The Mood and Anxiety Clinic (MAC) was established in 2009 as an initiative to develop teams that provided specialised services to address specific areas of need in the community as well as target specific mental health conditions. Under the leadership of Ms Ong Li Min, Principal Clinical Psychologist, the multidisciplinary team comprising psychiatrists, psychologists and social workers provides assessment and intervention services for a range of mood, anxiety and related disorders.

Since MAC was formed, a formal system of triage as well as a database for cases referred to MAC psychologists was established. This ensured right-siting of care and enabled MAC to better understand the profile of patients requiring our services. Existing psychological services were further improved, an example being the standardisation of intellectual assessment report formats as well as psychologists personally providing feedback of test results to parents of patients. Furthermore, the creation of a position for an inpatient child and adolescent psychologist increased access to psychological services for inpatients. MAC psychologists attended various training courses for continuous professional development and to keep abreast of developments in a variety of therapy modalities such as Child Centred Play Therapy, Advanced Therapeutic Play Skills, Creative and Expressive Therapy, Dialectical Behaviour Therapy (DBT), Acceptance and Commitment Therapy (ACT) and client-directed outcome informed approaches to psychotherapy, amongst others. Interest groups among psychologists have been set up in the areas of DBT, ACT and Child Centred Play Therapy. A number of psychologists from the team have received Health Manpower Development Plan (HMDP) awards to pursue postgraduate studies in Clinical Psychology. In 2013, MAC helped to coordinate the visit for a HMDP Visiting Expert from Canada, Dr Mary Nixon. Insights were gained from Dr Nixon's sharings on non-suicidal self-injurious behaviour in young persons.

Several milestones in the area of research were reached. In April 2012, two MAC psychologists, Assistant Professor Dr Sharon Sung and Ms Clare Kwan presented at a symposium on 'Recent advances in the assessment and treatment of children with selective mutism' at the 32nd Annual Conference of the Anxiety Disorders Association of America held in Arlington, Virginia. Currently, a study examining family factors in mood and anxiety disorders, and another study exploring the use of a virtual reality exposure task for selective mutism are underway. Two abstracts were accepted for the 4th Asian Cognitive Behaviour Therapy Conference in Tokyo in August 2013. Ms Clare Kwan presented a poster on 'A novel attempt at adapting Dialectical Behavioural Therapy for

Adolescents (DBT-A) in outpatient group treatment at a Singapore psychiatric hospital', while Mr Brian Poh presented a poster on 'Treatment of a novel specific phobia using cognitive–behavioural therapy: Case study on sinoglossophobia (phobia of Chinese language)'.

In the future, MAC will be looking into better integration of its services with other services within DCAP, the evaluation of the effectiveness of psychotherapy interventions, as well as the harnessing of advancements in information technology to benefit the patients. In addition, initiatives in the area of trauma work, selective mutism and obsessive–compulsive disorder (OCD) treatment programmes will be explored.

2010 — Expansion and Development of Specialised Forensic Services

In the past, the psychologists provided mainly intellectual, personality and neuropsychological assessments for remand cases, but today, the scope has expanded to include the provision of services to long-stay forensic wards, forensic outpatients, Mandatory Treatment Order, emergency room and the remand ward. Services have become more specialised, including ADHD and ASD assessments, treatability, dementia assessments, diagnostic personality assessments, second opinions on diagnosis, psychopathy assessments, malingering assessments, risk assessments and capacity assessments. Collaboration with the State Courts, Attorney-General's Chambers (AGC) and MSF has increased with psychologists providing consultation and independent assessments for these agencies. Psychologists were also required to provide expert witness testimony on the stand.

In order to provide the specialised knowledge and skills required for the service, a group of psychologists were given training and received certification to do risk assessments, as well as to run the Reasoning and Rehabilitation 2 programme, a structured, group-based UK-developed programme to increase prosocial behaviour in participants. Plans are in place to roll this programme out to the long-stay, outpatient and correctional settings. To develop the area of forensic psychology, Dr

Gwee Kenji was awarded a HMDP for postgraduate studies in Clinical Forensic Psychology, and upon his return, he has been involved in a number of high-profile cases, and presented local data on psychopathy at the International Conference on Applied Psychology in 2013.

2010 — FRIENDS (Forensic Rehabilitation, Intervention, Evaluation and Network Development Services) at the Child Guidance Clinic

The Forensic Rehabilitation, Intervention, Evaluation and Network Development Services, or FRIENDS, was established in 2010 with funding from MOH. Led by Dr Parvathy Pathy, Senior Consultant Psychiatrist, as Programme Director, and co-led by Ms Carolyn Kee, Principal Psychologist, the programme was set up to assess and treat children and youth who had been identified to have or to be at risk of abuse-related trauma, juvenile offending or serious conduct issues using a systemic multimodal approach to intervention. In order to be equipped with the necessary skills in the assessment and intervention of this target population, the multidisciplinary team of psychiatrists, psychologists and medical social workers underwent training in a diverse range of courses including Sexual Offending, Trauma-Focused Cognitive–Behavioural Therapy, Eye Movement Desensitisation Reprocessing, motivational interviewing and therapeutic play skills.

In addition to being an early detection, intervention and prevention program, FRIENDS engaged extensively in outreach programmes such as meeting with the Courts, SPF and MSF to streamline services, giving presentations to external agencies about their programmes and training community partners such as staff from the Voluntary Children's Homes. In 2013, psychologists Mr Shyon Loo and Ms Clare Kwan conducted a six-session run of the BEARS (Building Emotional and Affect Regulation) programme with eight children from the Pertapis Children's Home and plans are in place for Mr Loo and Ms Fiona Tan to run the programme within CGC. Mr Kenny Liew was also involved in running a Violence Prevention Programme with probationers in MSF.

The FRIENDS team is currently in the process of starting a diversionary programme for sexual offenders in collaboration with AGC and SPF to provide intervention to youth arrested for offending behaviours of a sexual nature.

2011 — Specialised Neuropsychology Service

The specialised neuropsychology service started in November 2011 to better meet the needs of individuals with cognitive difficulties. Ongoing standard neuropsychological assessment services provided by psychologists evaluate an individual's cognitive functioning to answer a specific referral question (e.g. assessment for dementia). The additional specialised neuropsychology service aims to provide holistic care that includes comprehensive cognitive profiling to ascertain an individual's cognitive strengths and weaknesses, followed by a feedback session on the cognitive assessment results with the individual, family and caregivers, as well as members of the multidisciplinary team, as appropriate. Involving family and caregivers is necessary not only for the purpose of psychoeducation (i.e. explaining the impact of an individual's cognitive difficulties on daily functioning), but also aid family and caregivers to better understand how and what they can do to help the individual. Importantly, a set of strategies tailored according to the individual's cognitive profile is provided as part of one-to-one cognitive rehabilitation aimed at compensating for cognitive weaknesses and building on cognitive strengths. The goal is to enable the individual to better cope with cognitive difficulties, work towards achieving personal goals, and improve overall functioning.

In order to advance the development of this service, Ms Huang Wanping was awarded a HMDP scholarship to pursue postgraduate studies in Clinical Neuropsychology. As part of continuous learning and development of knowledge and skills in neuropsychology, she gave poster presentations at the College of Clinical Neuropsychologists Annual Conference in November 2011 and the International Neuropsychological

Society's 41st Annual Meeting in February 2013. She also presented a case report of a patient seen in the service as a poster presentation at the Royal College of Psychiatrists International Congress in July 2013.

In October 2012, the specialised neuropsychology service was extended to the new outpatient adult ADHD service. The specialised neuropsychology service receives referrals from the adult ADHD service to clarify diagnosis and inform management. Specifically, following neuropsychological assessment, psychological interventions are provided to address the impact of cognitive difficulties on the socio-occupational functioning of adults with ADHD.

2012 — Mood Disorder Unit

The Mood Disorder Unit (MDU) was established in 2012 with the aim of providing specialised services to those suffering from mood disorders. By adopting a clinical microsystems approach, MDU is redesigning processes to improve quality, add value and reduce variation and improve morale in the way mental health care for mood disorders is delivered. One of the highlights of MDU is a holistic day programme offering patients opportunities to engage, gain support and learn skills for coping with their mental health concerns. Clinical Psychologist Ms Chermain Wong, together with Occupational Therapist Ms Áine Boyle, work closely with MDU nurses to equip them with the knowledge to help patients practice these skills during their stay on the ward. Our outpatient Affective Disorders Service also works closely to manage treatment resistant mood disorders.

The team went for skills-upgrading in September 2012. Visits to the following centres were arranged to study best practices in the treatment of mood disorder: the Mood and Anxiety Programme, Centre for Addictions and Mental Health (CAMH), Canada; Mood Disorders Centre, University of Exeter, UK; and the Affective Disorders Service, Institute of Psychiatry, South London and Maudsley National Health Service (NHS), UK.

In 2014, MDU built a dedicated inpatient ward which has expanded the extend of its service.

2012 — Expansion of Inpatient Services in DCAP

The 20-bed dormitory-style inpatient service for children and adolescent psychiatry was developed in 1993 and caters to acutely ill patients with a mix of diagnoses and severity. As part of a multidisciplinary team that works together in the management of the patient, psychologists provide a range of services including but not limited to psychotherapy services and psychometric assessments for intellectual testing and adaptive functioning.

Currently, with the appointment of a full-time inpatient Clinical Psychologist, Ms Haanusia Prithivi Raj, since 2012, the inpatient services were extended to provide a more intensive and step-down care to the patients. Services that are provided include individual and group therapy for inpatients, training to nursing staff and staff from residential homes as well as consultation and support for agencies managing the patient (i.e. family, school, residential homes and MSF). Psychological services also include specialised programmes such as the Intensive Inpatient/Day Programme for Treatment of Moderate to Severe Obsessive–Compulsive Disorder, Inpatient Transition Programme for Inpatients Moving to Residential Children Homes and Inpatient School Refusal Programme. Arrangements are also made for discharged patients to be seen as outpatients to ensure smooth transition and to reduce and minimise the risk of relapse.

Moving forward, the team is looking to increase research and expertise in inpatient psychological services by networking with other acute child and adolescent inpatient services both local and overseas, as well as looking to provide attachment opportunities for local and overseas students.

Intervention Programs and Interest Groups

2008 — Eye Movement Desensitisation Reprocessing (Training and Clinical Practice)

Another evidenced-based treatment identified to benefit our patients was Eye Movement Desensitisation Reprocessing (EMDR). From organising the inaugural seminar in 2007 by Mr Sigmund Burzynski for IMH staff, subsequent workshops also attracted participation from the various restructured hospitals and agencies.

2009 — Child-Centred Play Therapy

Child-Centred Play Therapy (CCPT) was initiated and developed as a new service in DCAP in 2009, by Dr Ann-Marie Lo Castro, Principal Clinical Psychologist. The project included the introduction of a fully equipped and renovated Play Room at the Child Guidance Clinic.

In 2010, 12 staff members attended weekly two-hour professional sharing and practice sessions over 14 weeks initiated by Dr Lo Castro. A second fully equipped Play Room, a new service at the Sunrise Clinic at IMH for outpatients and plans for the introduction of play media and services for the inpatient ward were added to the service.

In 2011, a further development was introduced to the REACH programme. This initiative, led by Ms Grace Soo, incorporated the development of a Mobile Play Therapy Kit which allowed the Play Therapy initiative to be introduced to schools by clinicians.

IMH now offers two programmes, namely CCPT and Non-Directive Therapeutic Play Skills, which share a similar purpose, but with extended application and skills. A further 12 staff are currently engaged in professional sharing and practice sessions, in order to incorporate Non-Directive Therapeutic Play Skills as part of their therapeutic repertoire.

Future plans include an increase in the scope of programme to include Parent and Group Play Therapy work, research and publications and to invite HMDP experts in the field to network and train with practitioners. An increase in training opportunities for specialist Therapeutic Play skills, such as Sand Tray work, is also an important part of future plans.

2010 — Creative and Expressive Therapies Project

The Creative and Expressive Therapies (CET) Project was initiated and developed as a new service in DCAP in July 2010 by Dr Ann-Marie Lo

Castro. The objective was to broaden the scope of therapeutic practice at IMH by introducing evidenced-based, creative, and experiential techniques, as alternative applications to and in support of more traditional talking therapies. The aim was to provide youth and adolescents with a variety of modalities which might assist them with creative, fun and imaginative ways in which to engage and respond to their experience and treatment at the CGC.

Future plans include the consolidation and continual update of resources to allow for growth of the programme and to keep abreast of international research and practice in the field.

2011 — Dialectical Behaviour Therapy Interest Group and Intervention Programme

Fuelled by an interest in working with youths diagnosed with emerging borderline personality disorder, the Dialectical Behaviour Therapy (DBT) training programme was started in May 2011 led by Senior Clinical Psychologist Dr Sharon Sung.

After training was completed, a DBT therapist consultation team was formed and meetings were conducted fortnightly for psychologists to discuss cases, support one another in conducting DBT and review the skills they have learnt.

In October 2012, the first DBT skills training group for adolescents was offered at CGC. It was conducted by psychologists Ms Clare Kwan and Ms Shannon Peh under the supervision of Dr Sharon Sung. Over eight sessions, the group of participants consisting of adolescents ranging from 14 to 19 years of age learnt a variety of skills such as mindfulness, distress tolerance and emotion regulation to complement the individual therapy they were receiving. Ms Kwan shared the findings from the group therapy program by presenting a poster titled 'A novel attempt at adapting Dialectical Behavioural Therapy for Adolescents (DBT-A) in outpatient group treatment at a Singapore psychiatric hospital' in August 2013 at the 4th Asian Cognitive Behaviour Therapy Conference in Tokyo.

2012 — Acceptance and Commitment Therapy Interest Group

Acceptance and Commitment Therapy (ACT) has increasingly been incorporated into the work of psychologists since 2012 when psychologists attended training in the treatment modality. It has been used with both child and adult patients diagnosed with a variety of disorders including mood disorders, OCD and schizophrenia. Psychologists Ms Jade Jang and Mr Wong Chin Meng have organised interest group meetings for the psychologists with the aims of building our knowledge of and competency in using ACT, as well as to promote awareness and acceptance of ACT as a useful therapy. Mr Wong Chin Meng has also started propagating interest in ACT by presenting information on ACT to the multidisciplinary staff from other departments. In 2012, Ms Grace Soo presented as poster titled 'Switching from CBT to ACT for adolescents with Depression: Case studies in Singapore' at the 6th Australian and New Zealand Conference of the Association for Contextual and Behavioural Science in Melbourne, Australia. It is hoped that this would eventuate in more research studies looking into the feasibility and efficacy of use of ACT in the local population and for different clinical populations.

2012 — Selective Mutism (Research and Treatment)

Psychologists at CGC use Behavioural Therapy to treat patients with Selective Mutism (SM) as it is the most researched mode of therapy for this condition and studies have found strong support for its use with SM. CCPT is also available as an alternative form of intervention at the clinic.

In 2012, Ms Clare Kwan, Clinical Psychologist from CGC, worked collaboratively with lecturers and students from the School of Digital Media and Infocomm Technology in Singapore Polytechnic to improve the Quietroom (www.quietroom.com.sg) online portal, first started in 2003 by Dr Daniel Fung to provide patients and parents with resources to help support children and adolescents with SM. This collaboration with the community and educational institution played an important role in increasing awareness on the nature of SM and the difficulties faced by students who are affected by the disorder.

In April 2012, Senior Clinical Psychologist Dr Sharon Sung coordinated a symposium for a group presentation on SM by international speakers at the 32nd Annual Conference (Anxiety Disorders Association of America) held in Arlington, Virginia. At this symposium, Ms Kwan presented on 'Recent advances in the assessment and treatment of children with SM'. Currently, a study in collaboration with NTU is underway to explore the use of a virtual reality exposure task for SM. The use of the Quietroom online portal and engaging patients in treatment with the use of computer games was also a topic presented at the Serious Games & Social Connect 2013 Conference in August 2013, which was held in Singapore.

Moving forward, there are plans in place to harness social media and the possibility of increasing accessibility of the online portal through other online platforms, e.g. mobile devices/ tablets. In addition, there has been initiative in exploring the effectiveness of CCPT treatment with SM patients.

2012 — Research Activities and Interest Group

To build interest and capability amongst psychologists to adopt a research-informed practice and practice-informed mindset, bimonthly Research Interest Group meetings were initiated in August 2012. There are several notable research activities that the psychologists are involved in. Together with the IMH Research Department, Ms Huang Wanping is actively investigating the role of cognitive reserve in predicting neuropsychological outcome in schizophrenia. She is also a co-investigator in a three-year epidemiological study, looking into the well-being of the elderly population in Singapore.

Plans are also made to conduct research into the efficacy of psychological interventions. A research project headed by Dr Patricia Yap seeks to develop a culturally relevant form of psychotherapy that derives from a unique understanding of Asian families and their individual, family and socio-cultural systems that can contribute to family harmony.

Following a study on 'Families' experience of harmony and disharmony in systemic psychotherapy and its effects on family life' (Yap and Tan, 2011) published in the *Journal of Family Therapy* in 2011, Dr Yap is currently collaborating with systemic psychotherapists in IMH (Ms Magdalene Foo, Principal Medical Social Worker) and in the community, to develop a theory of family harmony that explains how therapists help families negotiate disharmony to maximise harmony.

Training and Supervision

2007 — Psychology Observational Programme

The Psychology Observational Programme (POP) was an initiative by the Department of Psychology in response to enquiries of internship opportunities by Psychology undergraduates from the National University of Singapore (NUS). Strictly observational in nature, the programme was designed to provide participants the opportunities to observe clinical psychologists at work with people having mental health concerns. Held twice-yearly during the academic semester breaks of our local universities, each run is conducted across a span of 2 to 3 weeks. The initial programme included topical psychology-related discussions, lectures and clinical case presentations conducted by various psychologists as well as group observations on a live recording, taped video or audio session with a fellow patient. Other activities included opportunities to attend Clinical Teaching Sessions, inpatient multidisciplinary team meetings and Continuing Psychiatric Education sessions at IMH.

Over the recent years, the POP has evolved continuously to meet the growing demands and educational needs of Psychology students, based on their feedback on the POP. One of the enhancements made included offering more hours, from 30 to 50 hours, in particular observations during clinical sessions. This exposure experience is presently extended to various disciplines and subspecialties of Psychology to include participation from fellow psychologists from DCAP, Addictions Medicine Department and Early Psychosis Intervention Programme (EPIP).

One future initiative currently being explored is to enhance the exposure of participants by incorporating possible volunteer opportunity in the programme. Moving forward, POP hopes to continually serve as a valuable motivating platform for future generations of aspiring clinical psychologists and to cement their passion in service of the mental health of the public in years to come.

2009 — Placement Programme for Masters in Clinical Psychology

With the introduction of the Masters in Clinical Psychology programme by NUS in 2008, IMH became a key player in offering internships to increase the pool of clinical psychologists in Singapore. Dr Matthew Woo who sits on the clinical faculty at NUS, has been coordinating the placement programme at IMH. Since the internship programme started in 2009, 30 interns were placed at IMH, offering a range of opportunities that exposed interns to a wide range of patient population, from children and adolescents right up to the elderly, as well as a range of settings from inpatient, outpatient and the community.

2009 — Training and Supervision of Supervisors

In the interest to maintain the highest standards of patient care, clinical supervision was identified as a key driver. At the 2009 Psychology Department retreat, Mr Siva Penchaliah led a discussion on supervision and its importance on the enhancement of quality of care for patients. In 2010, he provided a two-part workshop to all psychologists within the department on the principles of good supervision. Subsequently in 2011, Dr Patricia Yap mooted the idea to start supervisors' meetings so that supervisors could be supervised and continually develop their supervisory skills. Dr Yap was particularly cognisant of the work of Caldwald and Diamond (1996) that pointed to the lack of evidence to suggest that supervisors improve as they gain more experience. While supervisees continually improve in their clinical practice as they benefit from supervision, supervisors may stagnate in their supervision practice because they do not get supervision on their supervisory skills. In addition, ensuring a sense of safety and trust in the relationships between supervisors and supervisees were thought to be important issues to be addressed.

To increase their capability in supervision, Dr Yap went on a part-time course in 2011 and 2012, attaining a Diploma in Clinical Supervision, after which she was tasked to be the supervision lead for the Psychology Department. Supervision of Supervisors (SOS) became an integral part of the Department's supervision framework, the primary objective of which is for supervisors to continually improve in their supervisory practice. Since late 2011, supervisors, including those who were slated to become supervisor, attended supervisors' meetings which were intended to serve as a platform for discussion of supervisory issues, for sharing of multiple and differing views on supervision, as well as an opportunity for training of supervisory skills. In addition, four supervisors, Dr Yap, Ms Carolyn Kee, Ms Mavis Seow and Ms Shannon Peh, were chosen to champion SOS and attend specialised training in clinical supervision with the Counselling and Care Centre (CCC).

Future plans are for each supervisor to have access to a supervisor who will help them develop their supervisory skills in either an individual or group format. The primary responsibility of the supervisor's supervisor is best supervision practice.

Mental Health Education Initiatives

2002 — Stories for Parents and Children

Stories for Parents and Children is a series of books with themes that centre around how some children experience and cope with various problems that they may encounter at home or in school. This project was initiated by Ms Carolyn Kee, and the stories were written by psychiatrists, psychologists, social workers, an occupational therapist and a nurse from CGC. The objective was to help parents and children know that they were not alone in facing these problems and to provide education and information about the various mental health conditions commonly faced by children and adolescents. Written in the form of stories targeted at primary school-aged children, the books also provided tips on how to overcome and cope with such conditions as well as useful information on agencies that could be of help. Titles in the series include *My Secret*, a book about Obsessive–Compulsive Disorder, written by Ms Ong Li Min; *Bobby's Day Out*, an interactive book about making choices, written by Ms Joyce Leong; and *I Miss My Ah Kong*, a book about dealing with grief, written by Dr Patricia Yap.

2011 — The 'Mind This Voice' Trilogy

The concept for the '*Mind This Voice*' book trilogy arose from a discussion between Dr Patricia Yap and Mr Daryl Chow on how getting patients to write their stories and, with their permission, share their stories with other patients facing similar circumstances, was therapeutic both for the patient who shared, as well as for the patient who read the story. With the aims of enhancing the therapeutic potential of patients sharing stories with other patients, and as well as to destigmatise mental health concerns with the wider audience of the general public, they garnered support from the hospital (who sponsored the copy-editing costs) and the Health Promotion Board (HPB, the main sponsor) for this project. In October 2011, in conjunction with World Mental Health Day, the editing team comprising Dr Patricia Yap, Mr Daryl Chow, Ms Sharon Lu and Ms Brenda Lee, launched the first book *The Write to Recovery*, so-titled to privilege the recovery stories of our patients.

The response from readers was very encouraging, especially after media coverage by the English, Chinese and Malay newspapers and a Chinese radio station. Ms Diana Tan, who is certified to conduct writing workshops, offered her voluntary help after reading about this initiative, and began to conduct writing workshops for interested participants.

A new editing team comprising Dr Patricia Yap, Ms Chermain Wong, Ms Goh Zhengqin and Mr Shawn Ee, was assembled in 2013 to work on the second book *From Hurtful to Helpful*, which highlights pivotal relationships that our patients have that are hurtful or helpful. The book aims to share how to transform hurtful relationships into helpful ones when someone is struggling with mental health concerns. *Mind This Voice: From Hurtful to Helpful* was launched in October 2014, in conjunction with World Mental Health Day. It is envisioned that the last book in the trilogy, tentatively entitled *Bright Tales from the Dark Side*, would bring to light the positive amidst the negativity that people with mental health concerns struggle with.

Future Direction of the Psychological Services at IMH

In line with the IMH Vision to be a tertiary centre of excellence and global leader in mental health care, the Psychology Department has worked out its own vision at the department retreat in 2013 to be a respected global leader in innovating quality, accessible and affordable mental healthcare. To achieve this vision, three drivers have been identified:

1. To adapt evidence-based treatment based on practice-based evidence by high-quality clinicians;
2. To right-site psychological treatment modalities accessible to everyone based on the level of mental health care required by the individual; and
3. To deliver cost-effective psychological treatment that optimises the clinical expertise of the psychologists and our community partners.

Through continual skills development and training, networking with local and international organisations, and the utilisation and integration of technological advances, the Psychology Department aims to establish themselves at the forefront of psychological research and practice. It is envisioned that now and in the years to come, the psychological services will continue to be a beacon of good practice that encapsulates the organisation's values of professionalism, collegiate practice, partnership, responsible stewardship and service to the public.

References

Caldwell K, Diamond D (1996). In the cauldron: A case study of training for clinical supervision. In: American Association for Marriage and Family Therapy (AAMFT), ed. *Readings in Family Therapy Supervision: Selected Articles from the AAMFT Supervision Bulletin*. AAMFT, Washington D.C., pp. 241–243.

Long FY (1987). Psychology in Singapore: Its roots, contexts, and growth. In: Blowers GH, Turtle AM, eds. *Psychology Moving East: The Status of Western Psychology in Asia and Oceania*. Westview Press, Colorado, pp. 223–248.

Long FY (2001). Psychological support in civil emergencies: The National Emergency Behaviour Management System of Singapore. *Int Rev Psychiatry* **13**: 209–214.

Wikipedia (2016). History of Clinical Psychological Services in Singapore. Available at: http://en.wikipedia.org/wiki/History_of_clinical_psychological_services_in_Singapore

Yap P, Tan BH (2011). Families' experience of harmony and disharmony in systemic psychotherapy and its effects on family life. *J Family Ther* **33**: 302–331.

Psychological Services in Other Hospitals

Jimmy YAP

Introduction

For a long time, most psychologists in Singapore were employed by Woodbridge Hospital, the predecessor to the Institute of Mental Health (IMH). However from around the late 1980s, the various public hospitals in Singapore began employing their own psychiatrists and psychologists and setting up their own departments of psychological medicine. In many cases, both psychiatrists and psychologists worked together in the same department, but this was not always the case. Quite often, the different hospitals tell a similar story: starting with just one psychologist before slowly adding more to the team over time. Likewise, the services provided usually expand from doing cognitive assessments to eventually managing cases. Over time, the psychologists also began getting more and more referrals from other specialties. In addition, instead of merely referrals, the psychologists in hospitals also actively began working in teams with other specialties to support particular types of patients such as those with diabetics, the elderly, those undergoing bariatric surgery, as well as programmes such as addiction, weight management and cardiac health.

Tan Tock Seng Hospital

One of the oldest psychology departments, outside IMH, was set up at Tan Tock Seng Hospital (TTSH). It traces its roots to 1987 when Ms Alice Yeoh, a psychologist at Woodbridge Hospital, was sent on secondment to TTSH's Department of Psychiatric Medicine, which had been set up a few years before. Psychologists at TTSH continued working under this department until 2000 when the hospital was privatised. Today, psychologists work in the Department of Psychological Services, which comes under the umbrella of the Division of Allied Health Services and Pharmacy, while psychiatrists work in the Department of Psychological Medicine, which comes under the Division of Medicine. The Psychological Services Department have expanded to now include seven full-time psychologists, supporting the hospital. It was headed by Ms Yeoh from its inception until December 2015 when she retired.

While Ms Yeoh was only seconded to TTSH in 1987, she had actually been working with the hospital before that. As a junior psychologist at Woodbridge, she had been going to TTSH weekly, visiting the rehabilitation department to do cognitive assessments on patients. At present, there is now a smaller psychology unit made up of another four full-time psychologists who are based at TTSH Rehabilitation Centre in Ang Mo Kio to meet the needs of the patients there.

Back in the late 1980s, the main referrals were from psychiatrists. Ms Yeoh handled most of the cases, handing over some back to Woodbridge if there were security issues or if someone back in Woodbridge had expertise in a particular area. After privatisation, the psychologists started getting referrals from other departments, for example, helping cardiology, neurology and rheumatology, although these were then, and still are, a minority of cases.

At present, the psychologists at TTSH accept inpatient and outpatient referrals from doctors in all medical disciplines and clinics. However, besides psychiatry, they do work closely with some specific medical disciplines and run satellite outpatient clinics at these departments, which is separate from the main psychology outpatient clinic. For example, they work closely with the Geriatric Medicine Department (to do neuropsychological assessments for early detection of dementia, conduct workshops and run group cognitive remediation programmes) and the Pain Management Clinic (to help patients better manage their chronic pain as well as run ad hoc group programmes). There are also satellite clinics at the National Skin Centre and Specialists outpatient clinic J, of which the latter outpatient clinic is mainly to provide psychological support for patients with HIV. Psychologists at the department also do assessments to see if particular patients are suitable for bariatric surgery and to help these patients manage their lifestyle post-surgery. They also work closely with the inpatient trauma team to provide early screening for post-traumatic stress disorder. With the growth of the Psychological Services Department, in the past few years, it has also started to take in and train psychology interns who are enrolled in postgraduate psychology programmes.

Apart from therapy and assessments, the psychologists at TTSH have been active in providing help to health care workers at the hospital, if called upon. This began in an ad-hoc way, together with psychiatrists and medical social workers, during the SARS outbreak in Singapore in 2003. It has since evolved and is now helmed separately by the hospital's Staff Supporting Staff (3S) unit, with psychologists being called in to help when needed. Some of the psychologists are also part of the CARE team, and will be called in to support patients and families in times of a serious civil or national emergency.

National University Hospital

The Department of Psychological Medicine of the National University Hospital (NUH) was established at the Singapore General Hospital (SGH) in 1979. The Department moved over to NUH in 1986, a year after the hospital was established in Kent Ridge.

The first psychologist joined the Department a few years before the big move to its new home in Kent Ridge. Currently, the team has expanded to meet the increasing demands of health care. The psychologists provide clinical services to the outpatient, inpatient and community psychiatric programmes, with individual and group psychotherapy services for psychiatric patients, and psychological assessments, mainly intelligence testing in the early years. Over the years, in tandem with the department's growth, psychology services have evolved to cover across every age group, from the young to the elderly, and throughout the severity spectrum. The department focuses both on preventive work and specialised interventions for acute and chronic conditions.

Child psychology services include assessment for early developmental, learning, emotional and behavioural disorders in children and adolescents, and interventions in the form of specialised therapies for this group of patients, including parenting interventions and family therapy. These services are supplemented by the REACH (Response, Early Intervention and Assessment in Community Mental Health) West programme. NUH has a team of psychologists who go into the primary and secondary schools and junior colleges in the western region of Singapore to do early psychological screening and interventions, which are often conducted in collaboration with the school counsellors of the respective schools. More severe cases, notably Attention-Deficit/Hyperactivity Disorder (ADHD) and Autism Spectrum Disorder (ASD) in children and adolescents, are referred to the hospital services.

Adult psychological services span across the inpatient psychiatric ward, the outpatient service and the consultation liaison service which cater to the mental health needs of patients in the various disciplines including general medical, surgical, obstetrics and gynaecology, cancer and cardiology. Apart from individual therapy for a range of disorders from mood to anxiety to personality disorders and trauma, group therapy is offered for anxiety and depression, and mindfulness-based group therapy is offered for relapse prevention of depression and anxiety. Couple therapy is a key feature of the adult psychological services and addresses communication difficulties and marital conflict in couples.

Assessment services cover not only intelligence assessment (which is also offered to certain pre-enlistees to the Singapore Armed Forces before enlistment into National Service), but also diagnostic personality assessments. Neuropsychological assessments services have also expanded to include cognitive characterisation, neurological and psychiatric diagnostic clarification, acquired brain injury and tracking cognitive changes from interventions such as chemo- and radiotherapy.

Psychologists at NUH are also a part of the Women's Emotional Health Service, a specialised service of the Department established in 2008 that caters to the emotional health needs of women in the perinatal period and those suffering from gynaecological cancers. Services by psychologists include individual and couple therapy, parenting workshops, infertility counselling, foetal loss support and public seminars and roadshows for promoting mental health awareness. The psycho-oncology service provides psychological support for cancer patients and their caregivers, including mindfulness groups and caregiver support groups, and public talks on the subject.

Ageing medicine is a growing service that is in line with the national growing needs of the ageing population. The memory clinic was formally established in 2007 to provide early diagnosis and treatment of dementia. Psychologists at the clinic provide assessment of the patients. The G-RACE (Geriatric Psychiatry Out-Reach Assessment, Consultation and Enablement) Service was set up in 2012. It is an outreach service to provide psychiatric assessment and treatment for elderly with mental health conditions, living in the western region of Singapore. Psychologists in this service provide psychological therapy and neuropsychological assessment, as well as training and support for community partners who cater to the mental health needs of the elderly at the community level.

On the training and research fronts, psychologists are key faculty members, contributing towards teaching undergraduate medical students and Psychiatry Residency training on topics related to clinical psychology. The Psychology Observation Programme for psychology undergraduates has an annual intake and provides an exposure to the job scope of clinical psychologists in the clinical setting. The department also provides clinical internships, led by the senior psychologists, for Master's students in NUS and James Cook University clinical psychology programmes. Psychologists also provide inter-disciplinary training to nurses and other allied health professionals of the hospital, based on the needs on the ground.

In the pipeline is the expansion of the psychological rehabilitation service for patients with acquired brain injury, in collaboration with the hospital's Department of Rehabilitation. Services planned include cognitive rehabilitation and group therapy for the psycho-education of caregivers, as well as mood and cognitive groups for patients with brain injuries. The services are also expanding to include groups for depressed adolescents and their parents, and emotional regulation skill groups. Specialised assessment and therapy services for trauma and ADHD across the life span are also being planned.

The other department that employs a team of psychologists at NUH is its paediatric cluster. The paediatric cluster started collaborating with psychologists in 2008 to provide child and adolescent services. The psychologists in the team conduct cognitive and learning-related assessments, individual therapy and work with families. Much of the work involves behavioural and emotional issues such as somatic issues, eating disorders, depression, stress, anxiety, and difficulties stemming from acute or chronic medical conditions.

The department also has a group of psychologists at its Child Development Unit (CDU). This is a satellite operation located at Jurong Medical Centre. It is a multidisciplinary service staffed by paediatricians with developmental training and experience, and allied health professionals, to provide services for children under seven years old with developmental, learning or behavioural issues. Apart from educational psychologists, the other allied health colleagues who work with the children include speech therapists, occupational therapists, medical social workers, learning support teachers and physiotherapists. The CDU provides assessments, diagnostic and intervention services through a family-centred and community-based approach.

Singapore General Hospital

Presently the psychologists in SGH come under the Department of Psychiatry, Neurology and Respiratory Medicine. The Behavioural Medicine Unit under the Department of Psychiatry was set up in 2003. Prior to that, psychologists at SGH worked within various specific specialisations. In the 1990s for example, there was one psychologist in the Department of Paediatrics and another in the Breast Clinic and General Surgery team.

Currently, Ms Evelyn Boon is the senior principal psychologist within the department. She joined SGH in 1999 to provide services for three departments: Respiratory, Renal Medicine and Endocrine. She subsequently joined the Department of Psychiatry when it was set up and today, there are 10 psychologists in the department.

Psychologists at SGH have played an important role in various programmes such as the Eating Disorders Programme, Pain Management Unit, the IBS programme and the Obesity Management Unit (OMU) in the Department of Endocrinology. Ms Boon herself is one of the few psychologists specifically trained in diabetes management so she helps with the management of individuals with diabetes in the form of therapy and support group to help patients cope with the chronic lifelong condition.

OMU also boast to be different from other Obesity Management programme as SGH OMU has psychologists playing a vital role in providing pre-bariatric surgery assessment for suitability, proving therapy as well as facilitating the support group.

The SGH Smoking Cessation Programme under the Department of Respiratory was started by Ms Boon together to help individuals to quit smoking with a combination of psychological interventions and pharmaceutical aids

The Pain Management Programme is helmed by a multidisciplinary team with the physiotherapist, psychologist and anaesthesiologist. The psychologist's role in the team is to help individuals manage and cope with their pain through mindfulness and Cognitive–Behaviour Therapy (CBT) for pain.

During the SARS outbreak in Singapore, psychologists supported SGH health care workers, creating a de-stress corner with slides on self-care and coping and running crisis debriefing sessions for SGH health care workers to help with the psychological well-being of the health care workers.

Psychologists also played an important role in the development and running of the Eating Disorders Programme which is the only structured programme in Singapore and Southeast Asia. They provide individual therapy and facilitates the body image and motivation enhancement groups in the Eating Disorders Intensive Treatment (which is a day programme and step down care for individuals struggling in their recovery) as well as the Singapore Eating Disorders Support (SEDS) group together with the Singapore Association for Mental Health (SAMH).

Changi General Hospital

The clinical psychologists in Changi General Hospital (CGH) come under the Department of Clinical Support Services and the Department of Psychological Medicine. When the Department of Psychological Medicine started in 2001, psychological therapy and assessment were provided by locum psychologists until a fulltime clinical psychologist from Malaysia came on board in July 2002. She left the Department several months later and Dr Christopher Choo, the current chief psychologist, joined the Department in May 2003.

The team of clinical psychologists in CGH has grown considerably over the years, to its current strength of 15 members. Clinical psychologists in CGH function within a multidisciplinary framework, working very closely with psychiatrists, medical specialists, nurses, allied health professionals (e.g. physiotherapists, counsellors, occupational therapists, audiologists) in the hospital as well as health care partners in the community (e.g. polyclinic doctors and general practitioners). From mainly treating patients with Cognitive Behaviour Therapy (CBT) in the past, the team now also offers other additional psychotherapeutic modalities, such as Eye Movement Desensitization Reprocessing, Dynamic Psychotherapy, Mindfulness-based Therapies, Emotion Focused Therapy, Schema Therapy and Clinical Hypnosis.

The psychologists used to treat patients mainly from the Department of Psychological Medicine and chronic pain patients from the Department of Anaesthesia. Over time, psychological services have been extended to other patients and their families within and outside of CGH. In 2007, the psychologists became an integral part of two major services — the Community Psychogeriatric Programme (CPGP) and Psychosocial Trauma Service — that were set up in accordance with the National Mental Health Plan. Within the CPGP team, the psychologists work closely with elder care agencies (e.g. St Andrew's Community Hospital, St Luke's Eldercare, Apex Harmony Lodge) and family caregivers to increase their awareness of mental health issues among older persons, as well as to equip staff and caregivers with the necessary intervention skills through training sessions, case consultations and home visits. The Psychosocial Trauma service offers early trauma-focused assessment and intervention, and psychologists within the team are trained to provide specialized CBT and EMDR for patients suffering from post-traumatic stress symptoms.

During the following three years, the psychologists became members of multidisciplinary teams of several medical specialties. These medical patients — including patients from the Diabetes Centre and Integrated Sleep Service who present with poor compliance to their treatment regimen, or with difficulties coping with their illnesses — are referred to the psychologists for individual or group therapy. Patients from the Bariatric Surgery Services are also referred to the psychologists to assess their suitability for surgery based on their psychological state and, if found suitable for surgery, will be provided with the necessary psychological support before and after their surgery.

Psychodynamic Psychotherapy in CGH started off as an interest group amongst several psychiatrists, with a clinical psychologist coming on board in 2010. Currently, the team consists of more than 10 practitioners and supervisees, including two clinical psychologists. The team provides individual therapy, group therapy, psychodynamic assessment, and complex needs service. Recently, a complex needs service in the form of an intensive Therapeutic Community outpatient group was set up for patients with moderately severe personality disorders, and complex PTSD or those with impaired psychosocial functioning resulting from interpersonal and/or personality issues. This group meets weekly, with a psychologist serving as the main or co-facilitator.

The year 2013 saw a significant expansion of psychological services into a number of areas. The Adolescent Team (comprising a number of psychiatrists and psychologists) was formed to provide individual or group treatments to adolescents presenting with psychological problems, including mood and anxiety disorders, deliberate self-harm, autism spectrum disorders, school-related stress and interpersonal difficulties. The Changi Memory Service, a project funded by MOH, was set up to improve inpatient support services on dementia care. Through this service, the psychologists conduct regular case consultations and training for staff, in addition to providing dementia-specific individual therapy to patients in the wards. In the same year, outpatient service was also set up for patients with Chronic Obstructive Pulmonary Disease presenting with co-morbid issues (e.g. anxiety, depression, non-adherence to treatment regimen), with the psychologists providing individual therapy to these patients. Another exciting development that occurred that year was the launch of the the Health Wellness Programme (currently renamed as ASCAT, or Assessment and Shared Care Team programme), with Dr Andrew Peh (the current Chief Psychiatrist of CGH) at the helm. With the main aim of providing early assessment and treatment to individuals in the community with mild to moderate mental health issues, the psychologists have been active in rolling out a number of initiatives through the years to achieve this objective. These include providing individual and group therapy sessions in community clinics; equipping community healthcare partners (i.e. polyclinic doctors and general practitioners) with assessment and counselling skills through regular training seminars, workshops and supervisions; and contributing to various publications, journal articles, books and outcome research regarding this collaborative primary mental healthcare model and its effectiveness.

Modelling after Geisinger Health System's heart failure programme in the United States, the ValuedCare Heart Failure programme in CGH was launched in 2014 to provide high quality care to patients with heart failure through a highly integrated, multidisciplinary team approach. Clinical psychologists in this team attend to patients both in the wards and outpatient clinics who are not compliant with treatment. The factors for non-compliance are assessed and interventions such as motivational interviewing or advice are provided accordingly. Regular training and supervision are also provided to telephone-carers in the team on how to help people with various adherence and psychological issues.

The psychologists are also very active in other services. Within the Addictions Team, they work with patients who present with alcohol, benzodiazepine, gambling and other behavioural addictions (e.g. internet). In collaboration with the CGH Breast Surgery team, they assist the medical social workers in running breast cancer support groups. In the area of mental health promotion, psychologists are involved in conducting talks, seminars, workshops and public forums for hospital staff, the public, schools and external organizations on a regular basis. Senior psychologists also play the important role of being supervisors to clinical psychology interns on attachment and psychiatrist residents receiving training for CBT.

Khoo Teck Puat Hospital

Even though the Khoo Teck Puat Hospital (KTPH) in Yishun was only opened in 2010, psychological services were initially provided by locum psychologists when the hospital operated out of the premises of the old Alexandra Hospital. The locum psychologists' service ceased when Ms Teresa Foong joined in 2005 from IMH and she was the first clinical psychologist on staff. 'At that time, we only had one psychiatrist and both of us were handling the patients with psychiatric problems,' she recalled. There are currently nine clinical psychologists on staff and Ms Foong is the chief psychologist in the Department of Psychological Medicine.

The clinical psychologists initially focused on doing assessments and psychotherapy for adults and as more psychologists joined, they were able to expand their services. In 2006, psychological services were expanded to geriatric patients, offering dementia screening for all new patients and cognitive remediation groups in English and Mandarin for early-dementia patients.

In October 2010, the hospital recruited a child clinical psychologist and started offering child and adolescent psychological services for patients from seven years and upwards. These services included psychological assessments (e.g. IQ, autism, ADHD), psychotherapy for emotional and behavioural problems, and social skills groups for patients diagnosed with autism.

The clinical psychologists are also actively involved in other medical disciplines and programmes such as the weight management programme, cardiac rehabilitation, pain management, diabetes and palliative care.

'In recent years, we have turned our attention also to staff welfare and have conducted many initiatives to increase staff engagement with work, resiliency, finding meaning at work using principles from positive psychology and clinical psychology,' said Ms Foong. 'After a successful pilot study and numerous focus groups with staff, we are about to embark on helping senior groups of staff to create and enhance positivity in their work units.'

Based on surveys that indicate that there are many people who do not seek help in the clinic, the clinical psychologists developed self-help modules for six common psychiatric disorders that are accessible on the website to reach more people. They are currently exploring ways to provide therapy via the Internet for those who do not like to seek help on a regular basis in the clinic setting.

The department is actively involved in mental health promotion through talks and workshops to corporations, government ministries, schools and the public. The number of talks and workshops has increased steadily over the years. In addition, the department has produced a DVD aimed at patients and the public to teach them simple relaxation skills.

With emphasis placed on clinical quality and training, the senior clinical psychologists take on students completing their Master's in Clinical Psychology from the National University of Singapore (NUS) for their clinical internships.

Looking into the future, the psychology service is set to grow in strength and to work closely with other medical disciplines to meet the various needs of patients. There will also be a focus on mental health needs in the community and providing training to support other health professionals' work in the community.

KK Women's and Children's Hospital

The beginnings of psychological services at Singapore's leading and largest women's and children's hospital, KK Women's and Children's Hospital (KKH), can be traced back to the 1990s. One of the early milestones was the start of a programme in 1990 to provide psychological assessments of very low birth weight (VLBW) babies at the Neonatal Follow-up Clinic. This was led by Associate Professor Lim Sok Bee, former Head and Senior Consultant, Department of Neonatology (2001–2005) and Department of Child Development (2006 to 2016). VLBW babies received psychological assessment when they were two, five and eight years old.

In 1996, KKH set up a CDU to support the early detection and diagnosis of children with developmental problems. That was also the year when the Psychology Service became an independent service under the hospital's Allied Health Specialties Division. Then, the service was managed by several psychologists together with visiting psychiatrists. In 2006, KKH started a Mental Wellness Service, and the psychiatrists were transferred to this newly set up service.

Working closely with psychiatrists are also psychologists from the Psychology Service. Since 2006, the Psychology Service has grown from just three psychologists to a team of 13 currently. The team, currently headed by Dr Lois Teo, comprises Clinical Psychologists and Neuropsychologists, all equipped with either a Master's or Doctorate degree. The Psychology Service also focuses in training and education and therefore welcomes associate psychologists (with Honours), clinical/neuropsychology postgraduate students for their clinical placements and also has a one-week student observation programme for fourth year Psychology undergraduates.

KKH supports about 80% of the national cohort of preschool children with developmental needs under the Department of Child Development (DCD), led by Associate Professor Mary Daniel, Head and Senior Consultant. It is the biggest diagnostic centre for children with developmental needs in Singapore, and is the main hospital in Singapore with clinical, educational and neuropsychologists who manage children. In 2015, the DCD in KKH was awarded the National Clinical Excellence Team award by the Ministry of Health (MOH) for their outstanding contributions and achievements in providing integrated, family-centred and community-based outreach for preschool-aged children with developmental needs.

DCD is part of the national Child Development Programme (CDP) led by Professor Ho Lai Yun. It comprises a multidisciplinary health care professional team of medical doctors, nurses, educational and clinical psychologists, speech language therapists, occupational therapists and learning support facilitators, and manages over 3,000 new referrals and about 7,000 medical follow-up consultations in a year. The provision of psychological assessments, parents and caregivers' training, and psychological intervention provision have grown since the programme started in 2002.

Aside from clinical work at the hospital, the psychologists from DCD are also actively involved in development and consultancy work, helping to build both capacity and capability especially within the preschool landscapes across different agencies and ministries.

Today, the Psychology Service manages the psychological needs of both women (all ages) and children (aged three to 18) at KKH via inpatient and outpatient clinical services. It offers specialist psychological support and assessments for children and adolescents who present with a wide range of medical conditions as well as emotional/behavioural and learning concerns that have considerably impacted on their daily life and/or social functioning.

For women, specialist services are available for pre-and postnatal care (i.e. postnatal depression), diagnosis of gynaecological cancers and breast cancer, family medicine (i.e. menopause, weight management, sexual health and fertility-related issues), and coping with chronic medical conditions and mental health related disorders.

Currently residing under the Allied Health Specialties, the Psychology Service is also represented in a range of multidisciplinary teams such as cleft and craniofacial, neuro-rehabilitation, paediatric cancers, adolescent medicine/eating disorders, severe eczema and paediatric pain, etc.

As detailed above, the Psychology Service works closely with Psychiatrists where there is ongoing collaboration, easy discussion and referral of patients both ways, and/or joint clinic sessions when required so as to improve patient care and outcomes.

Apart from that, there has been increasingly more community, hospital and academic links today, compared to the past. Moving forward and in tandem with the needs of the population in Singapore, the Psychology Service is also constantly mindful in supporting this vision, in addition to upholding care that is of best practice, ethical and professional.

Trauma is a focus at KKH's psychological services. In 2007, the multidisciplinary Psychosocial Trauma Support Service (PTSS) was set up to provide trauma-focused support and intervention to children who present with acute stress and post-traumatic stress symptoms after a traumatic event (e.g. medical procedures, accidental injuries, extra-familial physical and sexual abuse). The team currently consists of psychologists, a medical social worker and a trauma counsellor.

In March 2014, Temasek Foundation Cares and PTSS embarked on a pilot programme, called Temasek Cares KITS (Kids In Tough Situations). This programme aimed to increase public awareness and knowledge about trauma, develop community-based therapy expertise in delivering trauma intervention within community agencies and schools, and develop local trainers in Trauma-Focused Cognitive Behaviour Therapy (TF-CBT). In addition, the programme aimed to conduct research to ensure that TF-CBT is culturally relevant and effective for Singaporean children. The therapists in the programme have reached out to more than 900 children and caregivers in various community settings and schools, who have been affected by traumatic events such as family violence, physical, emotional or sexual abuse. The collaboration between KKH and the Ministry of Education (MOE) also helped some children, who were affected by the Sabah earthquake in June 2015, to receive trauma support through the programme.

In May 2016, the PTSS team was presented the Public Service Distinguished Star Service Team Award in recognition of the contributions made in the area of trauma intervention and training in the hospital, community and schools.

Acknowledgements

Alice Yeoh Oon Eng (Tan Tock Seng Hospital);
Reshmi Karayan Kayanoth (National University Hospital);
Evelyn Boon (Singapore General Hospital);
Dr Christopher Choo (Changi General Hospital);
Teresa Foong (Khoo Teck Puat Hospital); and
Dr Catherine Cox, Dr Lois Teo, Mr Tang Hui Nee, and Ms Jean Kwek (KK Women's and Children's Hospital)

Occupational Therapists

TAN Bhing Leet, HO Soo Fung, IBRAHIM Kamaldin,
SIM So Sin, ANN Esther and Jovin HO

Prior to the relocation of IMH to our current premise, Mrs Sylvia Ng, the then Head of Occupational Therapy Department, designed the whole department's workshop facilities and rooms, in order to accommodate about four hundred patients. Sadly, she passed away shortly before the completion of the new hospital.

Moving into New Premises

The Occupational Therapy department vacated the old hospital for new premises in April 1993. It was a nice home, the old place. Madras thorn and angsana trees lined the department's open grassy field; a resplendent flame-of-the-forest, with its fiery red bloom, stood near the entrance. Patients grew tapioca, papaya, banana, cucumber, bitter gourd and long beans on our small farm. We left all this behind for our new two-storey building in April that year, a bit sad, but nevertheless, brimming with hope of a better future.

Soo Fung, one of the three occupational therapists during this critical period, was in charge of logistics. It was her task to identify equipment and material for the new department and to mark the obsolete ones for disposal. There were old sewing machines, typewriters, woodwork equipment, kitchen tools and a zillion other things to sort out, not to mention keys, tables and chairs. All needed to go, one way or the other. As a mark of respect and to remember our heritage, we brought along Mrs. Sylvia Ng's fine wooden display cupboard.

As an initiative to help patients reconnect with their colleagues, we ran 'Radio Rainbow'. Patients were invited to make song requests for their colleagues in other wards. A small team of patients, led by a Health Workshop Instructor, recorded the songs on cassette tape along with the accompanying goodwill messages. These were delivered to the wards for patients to enjoy. Reciprocal requests soon led to the re-development of old fraternal relationships.

Rehabilitation in Occupational Therapy Workshops

Our new department was vast. It constituted workshops, activity rooms, a forensic OT facility and a new IMH Day Centre within the campus. This translated into a major increase in our workload. Recognizing that our patients suffered as much from psychiatric illnesses as they did from social stigma and that the danger of being marginalized was all too real, our aims were to empower patients, strengthen their sense of personal identity, improve their social skills and, where possible, facilitate their return to work. Our approach was to engage patients via meaningful activities, a well-trodden path, towards good health. We envisaged the department as a dynamic community centre, yet one that provided stability in the midst of change.

In order to maintain clarity of purpose, we instituted three-monthly activity schedules. This allowed OTs to inject fresh ideas and maximize their creative potential.. Patients went on weekly trips to keep up with rapid changes in the community, for example negotiating the new MRT system and using phone cards. To reach as many patients as possible, OTs conducted groups in the department and at the wards.

Day centres continued to provide prevocational training and day care for outpatients. Choa Chu Kang Day Centre, our fourth day centre was opened in 1995. Barely a year later, it was relocated to Bukit Batok Polyclinic and aptly renamed Bukit Batok Day Centre. Several manufacturing companies regularly supplied assembly work, as well as employment opportunities for our patients. Mr Ang Tiong Beng, Health Attendant, remembers the vibrant social atmosphere that characterized the day centres. Senior Therapy Assistant Adam bin Salleh also said, "*The department was vibrant with lots of patients coming down daily to participate in activities run by OTs as well as therapy assistants (TAs)".* An article published in the Singapore Medical Journal noted that day centre patients "… are less socially isolated and have better occupational functioning." (Mahendran *et al.*, 1995)

Activities and Events

The administrators of Delta and Hougang Sports complexes kindly gave us free entry to their facilities, on condition that we came outside of their peak hours. Happily, we brought small groups of patients for weekly swimming sessions. Patients looked forward to roti prata and coffee afterwards. The 'Riding for the Disabled Association', were only too pleased to accommodate us when Els Van Malderen, our OT from Belgium, approached them for free riding lessons.

Pottery was a welcome throwback when Soo Fung reintroduced it in 2000. Her patients soon started producing quality items, many of which were later used as souvenirs for the hospital's esteemed visitors. Sheltered work activities continued to provide a healthy income. Earnings were ploughed back into programmes such as FAT-shop, an acronym for *'Friday Afternoon Teashop'*. Patients attending OT were given a 'bank-book' in which recorded the amount they earned in consideration of their participation in OT activities. These were used to make cashless transactions at the FAT-shop. Bernadette Fan, a returned scholar, later upgraded it into 'The Living Room'. She installed sofa sets, a decent library and an Internet kiosk. Looking back, Bernadette said, "*I treasure fond memories of the "FAT shop" at Block 7, the outings to the swimming pool at the Delta Swimming Complex where patients from the Alexandra Day Centre used to go on a weekly basis… "Why were these memories special?" you may ask. Because I could see the patients enjoy themselves and find meaning through the activities".*

We invested in sports equipment too. Sudev Sreedharan, one of the first OTs to graduate from Nanyang Polytechnic, School of Occupational

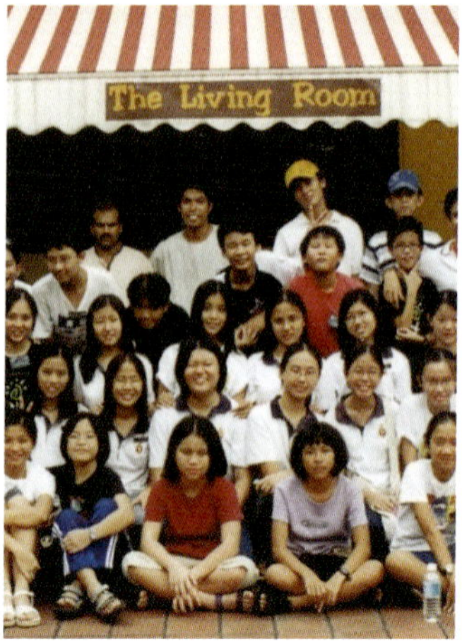

Kurunian, (Health Attendant) and Michael, (Healthcare Assistant) with a group of volunteers at 'The Living Room'.

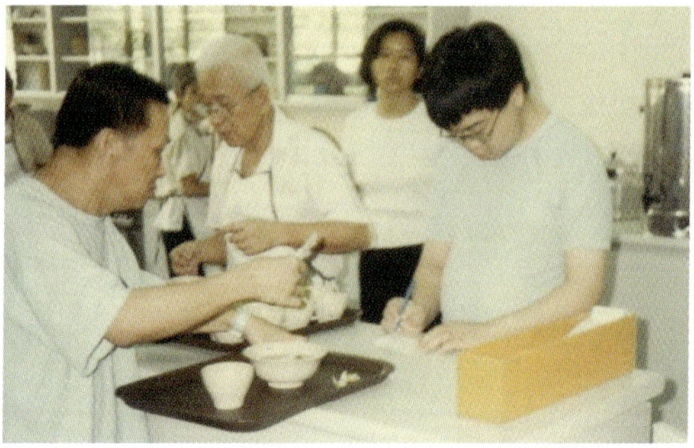

Ong Liang Cheak, OT watching over patients buying food at the 'FAT-shop'.

Therapy, organized a patients' soccer team. He acquired two complete sets of football uniforms, studded boots and all. A local football team agreed to coach our patients in exchange for free use of the hospital's football pitch. The culmination of our athletic programme was 'Sports Day'; the first in 1999, followed by another in 2000 and 2001. Contingents from Singapore Anglican Welfare Council, Singapore Association of Mental

Health, Sunlove Home and Woody Lodge came as invited guests and competed against teams from IMH for the 'OTD Sports Challenge Shield'. Scouts from 'Tanglin Special School' provided yeoman service. Senior Occupational Therapist Tan Peck Yan recalled, "*With smaller budget and less resources, we had to tap our creativity to make events interesting for our patients. A lot of effort went into the rehearsals but all of us from the staff to the patients had a great time doing it together.*"

In 1997, under Soo Fung's leadership, Andrea Lin, a Staff OT, and three Health Workshop Instructors conducted an overnight camp at Changi Chalet for about ten patients from Bukit Batok Day Centre. The team organized a rousing campfire and a sumptuous barbecue, the first and only overnight adventure ever held. We regularly took groups of patients for recreational visits to places such as Changi Airport, Singapore Zoo, Botanic Gardens and Sentosa. One December evening, patients were particularly delighted when five swanky air-conditioned coaches arrived to bring them for a night tour of the Christmas lights at Orchard Road, a treat given by our sheltered work sponsors.

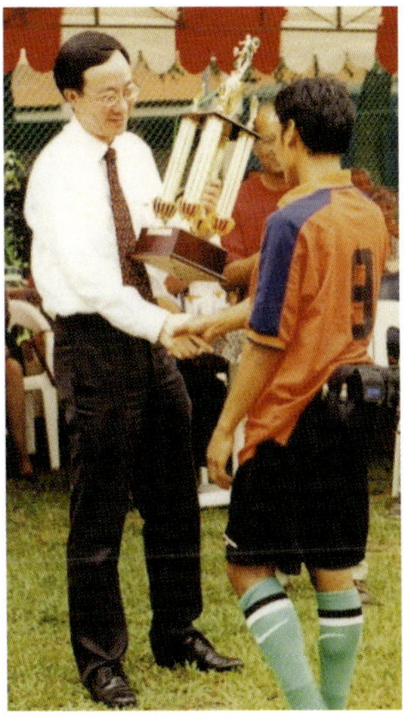

Mr Tan Tee How, former CEO of NHG, giving away the 'Soccer trophy'.

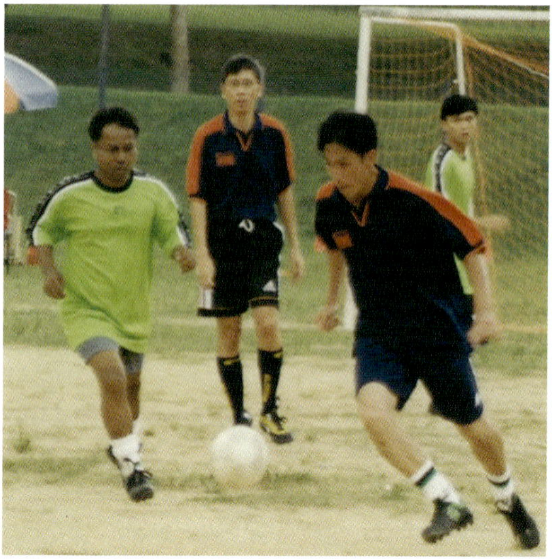

Dr. Eu Pui Wai watching Mr. Chua Kok Yeow, in blue T-shirt, scrambling for the ball.

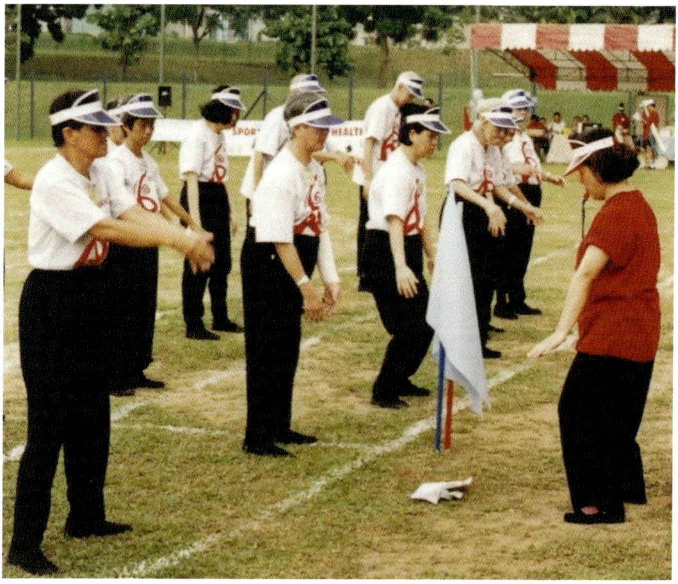

Vivienne Woo, Senior Therapy Assistant, leading a 'Tai Chi' group during Sports Day.

Vocational Rehabilitation in the 1990s

Vocational rehabilitation activities received close attention as well. Occupational therapist Tay Hwee Lin was largely responsible to supervise the 'Transitional Employment Scheme'. This scheme, which was started in 1997, gave patients a chance to work with the hospital's cleaning contractor in order for them to accumulate work experience. OTs upgraded the 'Worker Patient Scheme' by introducing formal assessments and instituting a new remuneration scale.

View Road Hospital was a major rehabilitation facility in those days. Carmen Tooren, an OT from Canada, and Soo Fung worked co-operatively with MSWs to support the 'Day Release Scheme', located there. They facilitated evening discussion groups, to accommodate patients who worked during the day, to let patients talk about the stresses they faced at work etc. In 2000, 'Bethesda Care', a Voluntary Welfare Organization, was awarded the contract to run the hospital laundry service. They provided several grades of sheltered employment exclusively to our patients with consultative assistance provided by OTs.

The OTs also assisted Singapore Anglican Welfare Council (SAWC) and Ministry of Community, Youth and Sports, (MCYS) in their endeavor to care for recovering psychiatric patients. SAWC eventually took over Mandalay Day Centre and later started both Hougang and Simei Care Centres. The MCYS included an 'Activity Hub' in their new Pelangi Village modeled after our department.

On average there were about 11 OTs in service between late 1993 and the beginning of 2003. OTs had large caseloads, usually a mixture of general psychiatry and one other sub-specialty. Everyone contributed towards the high daily patient attendance at the department. Wan Sau Peng, Senior Occupational Therapist said, "*All of us worked together for the benefit of our patients. It was hard work but enjoyable and meaningful.*" A word of gratitude must be reserved for our Health Workshop Instructors, Health Attendants, Health Care Assistants and administrative staff, without whom we could not have done as well as we did.

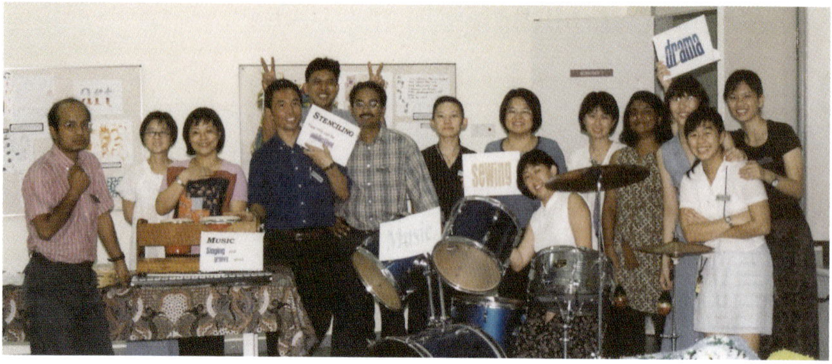

A motley group of OTs and TAs, 1998. Left to right: Kamaldin, Soo Fung Vivienne Woo, Abdul Rahman, Adam, Sudev Sreedharan, Corinne Hoo, Wan Sau Peng, Petra Lim, Sheila Dhamodharan, Sim So Sin, Yeo Jia Yeh, Sophie Chua & Pek Ling Ling (on drums).

Developing Vocational Rehabilitation in Mental Health (2003–2013)

In 2003, Ms Sheila Thamodharan took on the headship of the Occupational Therapy Department and set up 'JuiceWorks', a food and beverage outlet at the main lobby of IMH, to provide vocational training for patients. In addition, she also worked with the Institute of Technical Education (ITE) to run an ITE Skills Certificate in Food Preparation course, to enable patients to have a recognised certification which may facilitate job placement. Together with Senior Occupational Therapist Jayson Sudhasan, she also set up an in-house car wash service for IMH staff, to train patients in car washing.

In 2004, Sheila got married and left Singapore and Dr Tan Bhing Leet was transferred from National University Hospital to IMH to be the Head of the Occupational Therapy Department. She further developed vocational rehabilitation initiatives. In December 2004, she collaborated with The Salvation Army to set up a thrift store called 'Pick and Choose', to provide training for patients in retail. The store was officially launched in March 2005 by Minister of State for Trade and Industry, Mr Heng Chee How.

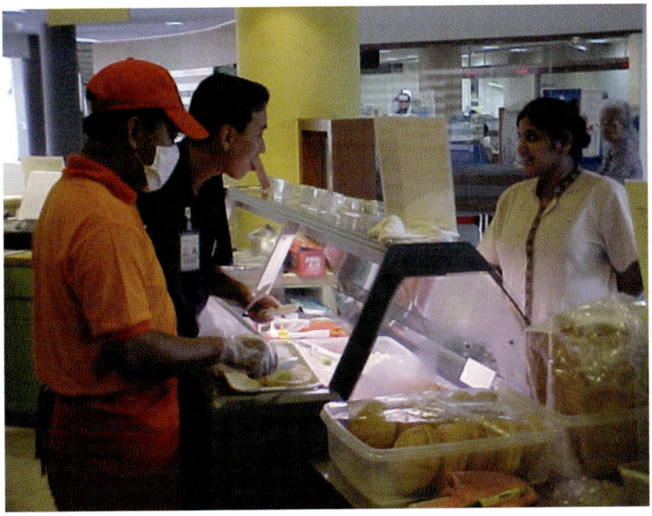

JuiceWorks, an OT-run sandwich and juice outlet.

Patients who completed this programme could either be employed by Salvation Army to work in other thrift stores, or obtain open employment in the retail sector. Subsequently, she also worked with a cleaning vendor to set up a cleaning training programme.

Sensing a demand for administrative work training among younger patients, training positions were also set up in the IMH Library and Occupational Therapy Department to meet such needs. These slew of training initiatives were then consolidated under the 'Outpatient Vocational Training Programme'. The Woodbridge Hospital Endowment Fund was also sought to co-fund this programme. In this programme, patients who were keen to be trained for work could be referred directly by psychiatrists, after which occupational therapists would assess patients before identifying a suitable training path for them. Patients have found such training useful for them. A patient who enrolled into the cleaning training programme said, "*The vocational training cleaning programme has assisted me to re-establish a good work routine, improve my physical endurance and work tolerance. These improvements have greatly benefited me in my current job as a cleaner*".

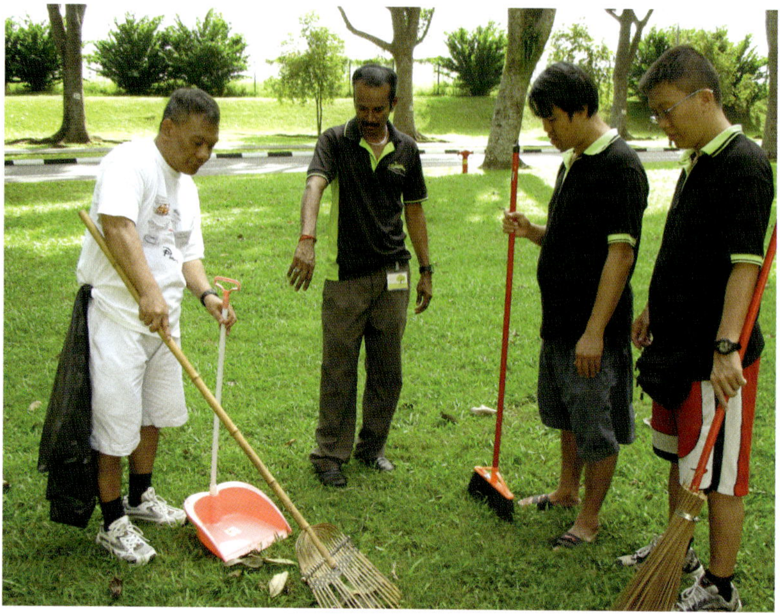

Health Attendant Kurunian conducting Cleaning Training programme.

In 2005, the department invited Professor Hector Tsang from the Department of Occupational Therapy at Hong Kong Polytechnic University for a series of staff training. Professor Tsang was an expert in vocational rehabilitation in psychiatry and a strong advocate of evidence-based practices. Both Professor Tsang and Bhing Leet saw the need to implement supported employment, which entailed job placement of patients in the open market, accompanied by job site support for both patients and employers. Such a model was more successful than fully focusing on in-house job training. Thus, occupational therapists started to job match patients who graduated from the Outpatient Vocational Training programme to open employment.

Occupational therapists in supported employment also negotiated with employers for worksite modifications and task adaptations. Besides that, they provided education and support to employers, to enable them to manage any difficulty with the employees. In order to encourage more employers to offer opportunities to psychiatric patients, a Fund-2-Work scheme was set up, using the Woodbridge Endowment Fund. This scheme was announced on 4 February 2006, at the launch of Silver Ribbon Singapore. The scheme provided financial incentives for employers to employ eligible persons by paying up to 50% of the person's salary for two months. This scheme attracted a few employers who had previously not employed people with psychiatric diagnoses. Many employers also found that once patients got the hang of the job, they remained loyal to the company and were very good employees. Thus, employers eventually did not see the need to utilise the Fund-2-Work scheme and it terminated a few years later.

Since 2003, JuiceWorks had provided a good showcase of psychiatric patients as being able to work in the service industry. However, IMH was not a place that was frequented by members of the public. Patients' exposure to working in a competitive environment could also not be simulated in JuiceWorks. Therefore, Bhing Leet collaborated with Ms Kala Karkal and Mr Christopher Lim to set up Dignity Links Ltd, a non-profit company that ran Barista Express, a social enterprise café. A/P Rathi Mahendran, then Vice Chairman of Medical Board, was also invited to be one of the company's directors. Barista Express was situated in Clifford Building, at the heart of the Central Business District. Senior Occupational Therapists Shirley Huang, Yogeswary Maniam and Tan Peck Yan were involved in the running of this programme.

The presence of this café raised the profile of people with psychiatric disorders tremendously. As this café was funded by the Social Enterprise Fund (SEF) administered by the then Ministry of Community, Youth and Sports (MCYS), many social entrepreneurs and business owners also came forward to support the cause. Barista Express even won 'The Pitch', a real-time contest for short-listed non-profit organisations to pitch their causes to a three-judge panel in front of a live audience, who would also get the opportunity to vote. This contest was organised by the National Volunteer and Philanthropy Centre (NYPC). Together with The Achievers voluntary group, Bhing Leet, Peck Yan and Dignity Links put up a video skit which won the votes of both judges and audience. Clinical outcome of this training programme was also positive. All the 25 patients who received training between 2006 and 2007 demonstrated statistically significant improvement in work behaviour before leaving the programme (Tan, 2009). Those who completed the training went on to sustain competitive employment for an average of 44 weeks.

Barista Express opened up many opportunities for occupational therapists to work with businesses and employers, one of which was Secret Recipe. Secret Recipe was a very supportive employer of psychiatric patients and eventually agreed to collaborate further by opening its kiosk at the existing JuiceWorks outlet.

The branding of Secret Recipe, together with the company's industry know-how, provided patients with a wide variety of training opportunities and enabled staff to have a different range of food choice. The Secret Recipe café was officially launched during Occupational Therapists' Day celebrations on 12 January 2009, by Mr Gerald Ee, chairman of National Kidney Foundation at that time. Secret Recipe also set up Laksania, a social enterprise laksa chain to provide employment opportunities for the disabled. The Laksania kitchen was located within IMH and patients were trained in the different stages of laksa preparation. Senior Occupational Therapist Tan Peck Yan was instrumental in the running of the F&B vocational training programmes. She had to learn new skills such as café operations and found herself spending time during weekends browsing at shops and cafes to study their layout and menus. She said *"the experience and exposure had made me more aware of the needs of our patients working in this particular industry. I find it heartening to see former patients who had graduated from the programme returning to thank staff for the training they had received after they have gotten a job"*.

In 2009, vocational rehabilitation in IMH took another big leap with the setting up of Job Club, a National Mental Health Blueprint programme funded by Ministry of Health (MOH). This was a joint collaborative effort between Medical Social Work and Occupational Therapy Department. Job Club was a supported employment programme, where a team of occupational therapists, medical social workers and job placement officers concentrated their efforts on work readiness assessments, job tasks analyses, workplace modifications, employer education and jobsite support (Tan, Li, & Tan, 2016). Staff would assess patients' job readiness before determining whether they could be immediately job placed or required vocational training. Referrals were accepted from both within and outside IMH. This programme was launched officially by Mdm Halimah Yacob on 4 November 2009. Every year, more than 200 job placements are made.

Part of Job Club's work was to partner with organisations that were working on the same cause. One of such organisations was BizLink, which had a long track record of developing enterprise services and job placement opportunities for the disabled. Eventually, BizLink also set up a café at the vacated Secret Recipe location and now has plans to develop a catering arm. Occupational therapists and Bizlink staff are currently working closely to develop the training process and continuum, as well as to ensure good job placement and tenure for patients who have completed the training.

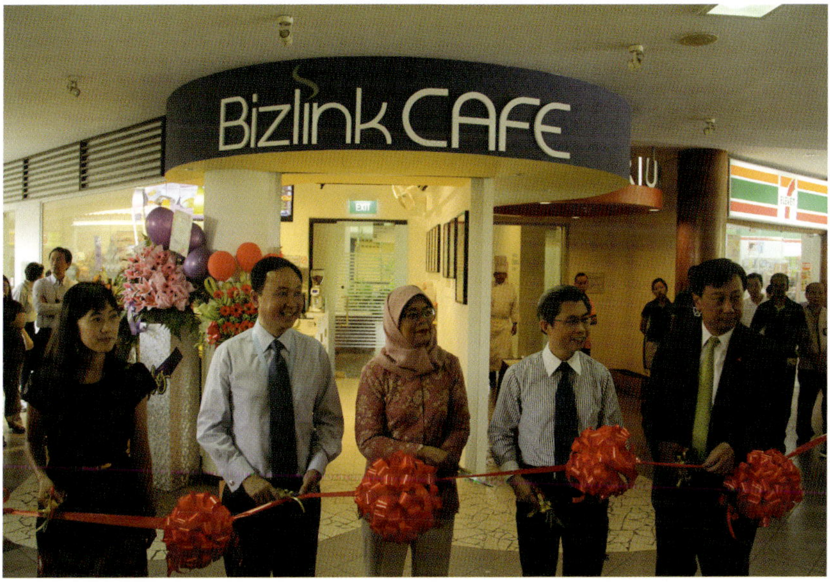

Launch of BizLink Café in January 2013 (Head of Department Dr Tan Bhing Leet on far left, with IMH CEO A/P Chua Hong Choon, Guest of Honour Mdm Halimah Yacob and Mr Alvin Lim, CEO of BizLink.

Rehabilitating Patients with Psychiatric Disorders

While reviewing rehabilitation services provided at IMH, the occupational therapists felt that therapeutic interventions had to keep up with advancements in the worldwide field of psychiatric rehabilitation, while meeting the cultural needs of the local population. The department had been running three day centres: IMH Day Centre, Alexandra Day Centre and Bukit Batok Day Centre. These day centres provided day rehabilitation as well as sheltered employment for adult patients with a variety of disorders. There was a need to provide treatment in a context of a recovery and wellness model. Thus, funding was secured to renovate new group therapy and individual treatment rooms within Occupational Therapy Department and IMH Day Centre was relocated there in 2007. In addition, the centre was also renamed 'Occupational Therapy: Activities, Vocation and Empowerment', or OcTAVE for short, to reflect a change in the model of rehabilitation. The centre focused on recovery and community integration. Patients were empowered through a range of clinical interventions and activities.

Craft Creates was set up to provide a structured programme of creative therapies for patients who required functional retraining. Patients were empowered to sell their craft products under the branding of Craft Creates. Lejia Society also kindly donated funds to set up Tranquil Garden outside OcTAVE, for staff to conduct gardening therapy with patients. Community living skills training, social skills training, lifestyle modification and support groups were also carried out.

In addition, a choir group called the 'Very Special Outstanding Performers' (VSOP) was set up in 2008, where patients were trained by a professional choir coach to perform at various public events. Senior Occupational Therapist, Mabel Shek, was in-charge of this programme and had led several performance and even two fund-raising concerts. She said, "The joy comes when VSOP members become more confident and start to interact with each other. Their vocal technique has also improved over the years. I hope that the VSOP fundraising concert will be held in the public one day". The VSOP programme has since expanded its repertoire to include fusion dance. Many people could see the transformation

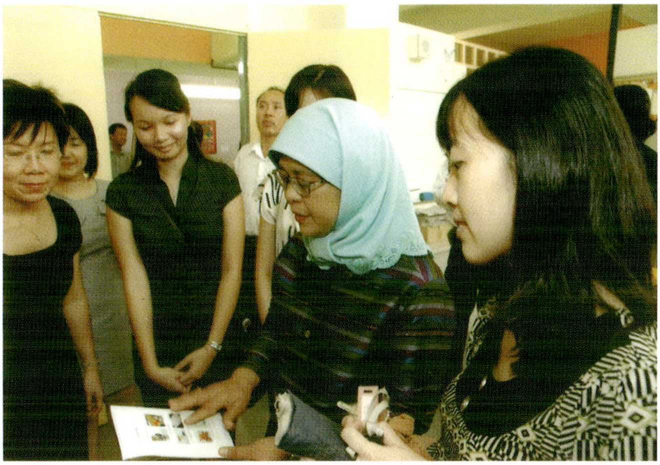

Tour of OcTAVE with Mdm Halimah Yacob, then Minister of State, MCYS (2009).

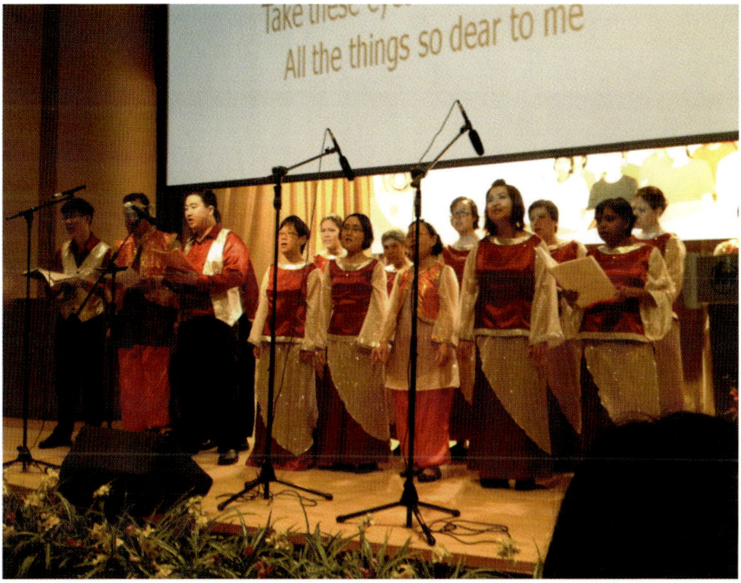

VSOP fund-raising concert at IMH.

of these patients, from being withdrawn and passive to become active and participative during song performances.

Cognitive remediation is an intervention to improve attention, memory and problem solving abilities of psychiatric patients and has gained much evidence for its clinical efficacy in the West. Thus, a research was embarked to test its efficacy within the local population. Results of the research showed that compared to a control intervention, participants who underwent cognitive remediation not only had improved cognitive functions, but also had better employment outcomes and greater community living ability over one year (Tan and King, 2013). We then invited an overseas expert to train occupational therapists in Neuropsychological and Educational Approach to Remediation (NEAR), a cognitive remediation programme developed in the United States. The NEAR programme was since conducted in the inpatient rehabilitation ward as well as OcTAVE centres. A patient who had undergone cognitive remediation commented, *"I find the fortnight bridging sessions on how to deal with cognitive challenges very useful. During the session, we will*

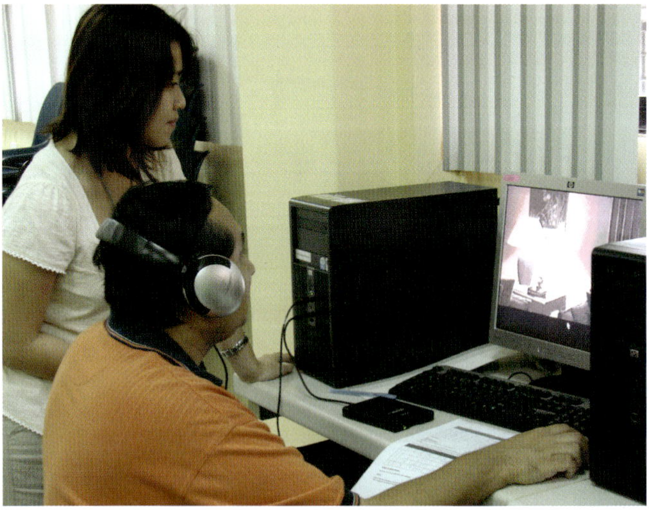

OT Jasmine Ong conducting Cognitive Remediation session at OcTAVE@IMH.

bring out the problems that we encounter in our daily lives. Therapist Wendy would try to discuss, provide us with the feasible solutions on how to deal with and solve these challenges".

Alexandra Day Centre was relocated to Cantonment Road in 2010 and was renamed OcTAVE@Cantonment, while Bukit Batok Day Centre underwent some renovation and was renamed OcTAVE@Bt Batok. Both also started to provide some interventions targeted at community integration. In addition, occupational therapists also conducted programmes at Community Wellness Centre @ Queenstown and held two art exhibitions to showcase patients' artwork.

In 2012, OcTAVE@IMH underwent a further revamp, to integrate with Vocational Training and Job Club, as well as to offer new clinical rehabilitation programmes such as Personal Effectiveness for Daily Living, Mindfulness-Based Stress Reduction, Illness Management and Recovery etc. Principal Occupational Therapist Wendy Chua was instrumental in this revamp. She said *"The outpatient service is now better able to meet patients' rehabilitation needs and also engage them in a variety of interventions to improve their independent living skills, thus enabling them to lead meaningful and productive lives"* Within inpatient wards, occupational therapists has also been redefining our services. Besides conducting group work, we have also focused on functional assessments, to assist the multi-disciplinary team in discharge planning. Occupational therapists have also provided more targeted intervention for specific groups such as the early psychosis inpatients as well as patients within the mood disorders unit. Senior Occupational Therapist Wan Sau Peng started an art service for the inpatient population, while Principal Occupational Therapist Ho Soo Fung is providing art therapy intervention for inpatients in the addiction ward as well as outpatients of various age groups. Senior Occupational Therapist Koh Hwan Jing, then inpatient team leader, was also working with the team on using sensory modulation and Integrated Psychological Therapy as part of their intervention for the inpatient population. This has certainly improved the quality of OT treatment.

Specialised Occupational Therapy Services

Occupational therapists are also instrumental in the treatment of children and adolescents with developmental and psychiatric conditions. In 2003, the Occupational Therapy gymnasium was set up at Child Guidance Clinic@ Health Promotion Board, where a variety of interventions such as sensory integration, gross and fine motor intervention, play and socialisation programmes and oral motor interventions could be carried out. In 2005, another Occupational Therapy gymnasium was set up, using donated funds from Jardine Cycle and Carriage. As such, occupational therapists were able to run outpatient clinics at both sites. Over the past years, group therapy programmes that improve body awareness, social skills and feeding problems are also implemented. Mr Ashley Jayapaul, who leads the Child Psychiatry OT team commented, "*When I first joined the team, I was amazed to see the wide range of talents each colleague possessed and their eagerness to acquire knowledge. It was very encouraging to see how each staff was trying his/her best to help the children and family*

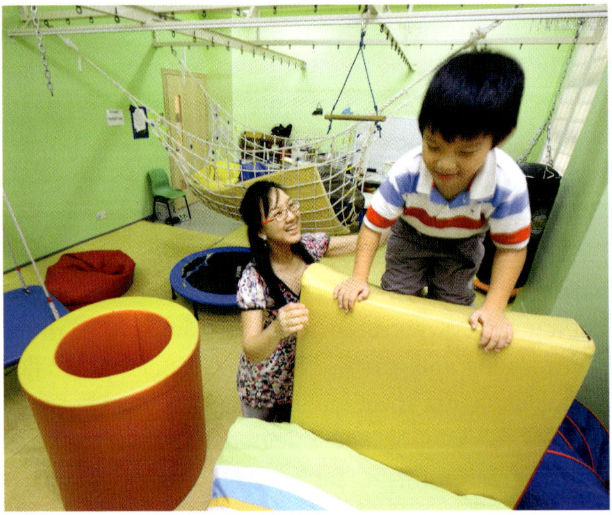

Senior OT Hannah Loh providing OT intervention for a child.

under their care. As a team, we managed to implement new therapeutic interventions and obtained additional manpower and physical resources to meet increasing demands for our services. I am very thankful that we have supportive colleagues and Head of Department who are guiding us positively in developing this specialized service."

We are also crucial in the rehabilitation of children and adolescents admitted to the inpatient wards. We run an inpatient cum day hospital programme that focus on activities of daily living, vocational exploration and creative expression. Occupational therapists also form part of the Adult Neurodevelopmental Service team, which treats adult patients with autistic spectrum disorder and moderate to severe intellectual disabilities. Working with this patient group is indeed challenging, but morale of the team is high, due to good teamwork and mutual support. Ng Zhuo Wei, Senior Occupational Therapist reflected, "*It was definitely tough at the start, but my passion for Occupational Therapy grows as I work more with this population. A lot of adults with intellectual disability drop out of the system after finishing special school as there is not enough day services for them. Loss of routine is the start of problem behaviour. This has also exposed them to higher risk of mental health issues. We are not only helping the patient but also the family member in regaining their quality of life by identifying the triggers of problem behaviour and providing intervention.*"

A new sensory integration gym and multi-sensory room were also set up in 2014 to treat this challenging group of individuals. Dr Tan Bhing Leet applied for funding through Mindset Care Limited and obtained support to convert an old workshop space into a sensory gym and physical exercise gym. This allows occupational therapists to carry out sensory work with adult patients with sensory issues, before working with them to address functional performance.

Occupational therapists have also started offering their interventions beyond forensic wards within IMH to the Singapore Changi Prisons. Occupational therapists and therapy assistants are deployed to the Prisons Psychiatric Housing Unit, where they conduct groups and provide therapeutic support to facilitate offenders in improving functional skills and attaining

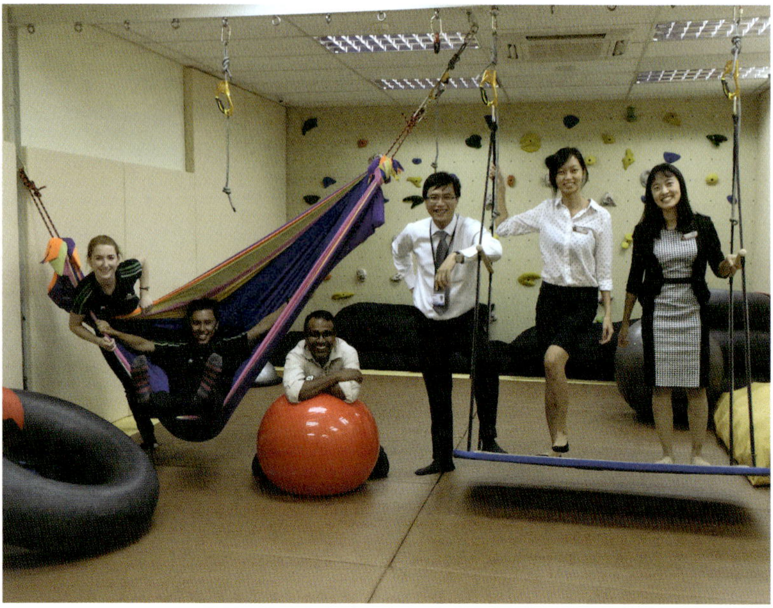

The ANDS team, during launch of Mindset Gym in 2014, from left: Ms Mairead Cushen, Mr Tang Wei Kiat, Mr Ashley Jayapaul (ANDS OT team leader), Dr Wei Ker Chiah (Chief of Community Psychiatry), Ms Yang Suyi and Dr Tan Bhing Leet (Head of OT Department).

pro-social behaviour (Tan, Kumar, & Devaraj, 2015). "*It was with some anxiety and apprehension that I took up the challenge to work in the Changi Prison Psychiatric Housing Unit programme in 2011. It has, however, turned out to be a rewarding experience providing treatment to offenders with psychiatric illnesses, despite the challenging and constrained environment.*" Senior OT Vasanth remembers. Occupational therapists are also members of community outreach teams such as Community Mental Health Team (CMHT) for adults, Response, Early Intervention and Assessment in Community Mental Health (REACH) for children and adolescents and Aged Psychiatry Community Assessment and Treatment Service (APCATS) as well as the Early Psychosis Intervention Programme (EPIP). Principal OT Joycelyn Neo was also the team leader for the REACH-South team.

Heads of Occupational Therapy Department	Years of Appointment
Mrs Sylvia Ng	– circa 1970–1990
Ms Lilian Leong	1991–1992
Mr Kamaldin Ibrahim	1993–2003
Ms Sheila Thamodharan	2003–2004
Dr Tan Bhing Leet	2004–2016
Ms Joycelyn Neo	2016–

Heads of Occupational Therapy Department since the 1980s.

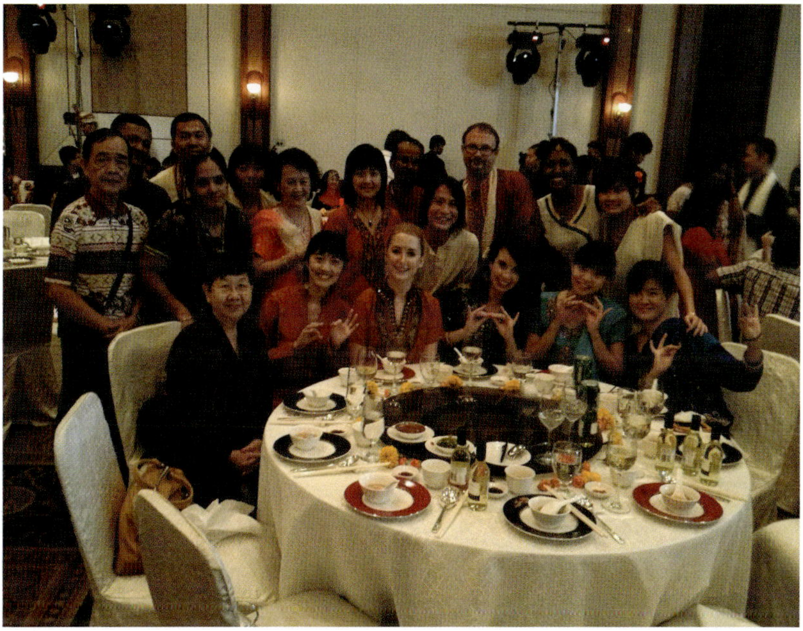

OTs and support staff at Dinner and Dance, November 2012.

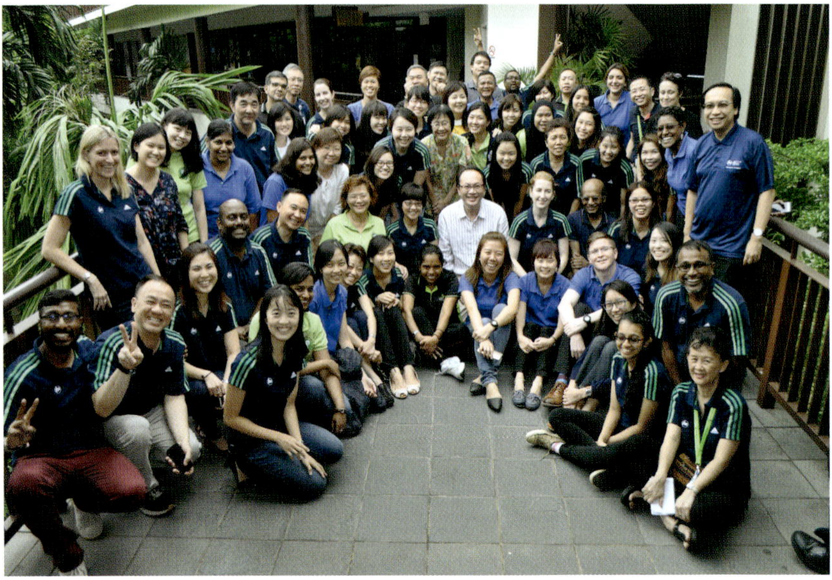

OT-Retreat March 2013

Besides the above services, we have also been running day programmes for acute and long stay psychogeriatric patients in Octave@IMH (Inpatients). Senior Occupational Therapist Carmel Tso has also put together a reminiscence therapy kit and manual and has worked with a psychologist and Institute of Technical Education to devise a cognitive stimulation software for elderly with cognitive difficulties.

The occupational therapy department has indeed come a long way from a decade before. It has now expanded to encompass more than 50 occupational therapists and more than 20 support staff. Its services have ranged from functional assessments and group work in inpatient wards, to specialised interventions within outpatient rehabilitation facilities and gyms, as well as community-based rehabilitation in outreach teams. Furthermore, occupational therapists have also been involved in research projects, clinical education and training for undergraduates and professional staff as well as mental health promotion. We have also been collaborating actively with community agencies to build up capability in psychiatric rehabilitation within the community. It is hoped that with these efforts, patients will have better rehabilitation outcomes and able to lead productive lives within the community.

OT Services in Restructured Hospitals

In the 1990s in National University Hospital (NUH), occupational therapists ran the day hospital programme in the psychological medicine ward. Dr Tan Bhing Leet, who was then at NUH, started outpatient service in year 2000 and conducted weekend stress management groups. She also provided stress management sessions for patients receiving cardiac rehabilitation. When Bhing Leet left for IMH, Senior Occupational Therapist Esther Ann went on to establish OT activity groups. Functional skills assessments, Activities of Daily Living training as well as lifestyle modification were also provided. From 2005, senior occupational therapists Esther and Wong Su Ren started providing services within the Women Emotional Health Services (WEHS) and adolescent weight management programme. Today, the ward programme has evolved to occur on a daily basis from Monday to Friday. The ward OTs conduct three groups which consist of the open art studio, a life-skills group as well as an activity group. From 2010, OTs Su Ren and Ngooi Bi Xia started to provide trigger point release and pain management services to patients with pain issues as well as stress management and lifestyle modification services to female patients seen in the Women's Heart Health Clinic. NUH OTs Eng Jia Yen and Esther Tai are also involved in the community outreach teams such as G-Race (for the elderly) as well as REACH-West.

At Changi General Hospital, occupational therapists were running inpatient groups twice weekly, which progressed gradually to weekly hydrotherapy sessions and twice weekly outpatient clinic services. Senior Occupational therapist Sim So Sin, with previous experience at IMH, started these services. The ward programme eventually becomes a daily one which are mostly skills-based, expressive-based or psycho-education in nature.

From year 2003, there were initiatives to develop psycho-geriatrics as a sub-specialization. There were also outpatient groups running on some weekends, mainly stress and anxiety management groups. In 2004, the occupational therapists started an outpatient service, named PREP, to serve the patients who were in recovery from their mental illness or those who were transiting from inpatients to outpatients in the community. They also began to be involved in corporate and outreach work. In 2007, OT services in psycho-trauma services and psycho-social trauma were developed at Kandang Kerbau Hospital (KKH), as part of the National Mental Health blueprint. Subsequently, the psycho-trauma services at CGH evolved to providing cognitive rehabilitation for patients with traumatic brain injury, as well as trauma-specific therapy for those with post-traumatic stress disorder, while the services at KKH evolved into OT outpatient mental health clinics at KKH Rehabilitation department.

Senior OT Koh Hwan Jing, then at CGH, also played a crucial role in the CPGP (Community Psycho Geriatric Program), a national mental health blueprint outreach programme for dementia care. In year 2010, the psychiatric occupational therapists became involved in liaison psychiatry work, where it expanded to service cardiopulmonary wards, rehabilitation wards as well as the stroke unit. As of 2013, the establishment of psychiatric OT stood at 7 staff and they were launching new services such as psychosocial wellness group for post-stroke patients and cognitive groups for patients with cognitive impairment.

In Singapore General Hospital, Occupational Therapist Florence Chiang was involved in OT intervention for people with eating disorders as well as provision of therapy for psychiatric inpatients.

OT Services in Voluntary Welfare Organisations

At Singapore Association for Mental Health, Occupational Therapy was provided at Oasis Day Centre for the period of 1997 to 2001. The Occupational Therapy services included contract work, skills training and therapeutic sessions, aimed at increasing trainees' level of functioning, insight, self-concept and social relationships, thereby reducing the rates of relapses. Opportunities were also given for the trainees to showcase their talents in performances. Together with the other team members, the Oasis Day Centre organized its first camp for the trainees and it was an invaluable experience for both the staff and trainees.

Occupational Therapy was provided at Activity Hub (AH) in Pelangi Village from 2002 to present. The objective of the OT Services is to enhance the quality of life of residents in PV by focusing on three components of occupational performance, namely Activities of Daily Living (ADL), leisure and vocational engagement. These include basic self-care and preparation of meals. Sensory and cognitive programmes include sensory awareness, current affairs, cognitive and reality orientation, reminiscence, table top activities, oral Tamil and cultural groups. There are also physical health programmes and social and recreational activities.

There are two vocational-engagement categories in AH — the Residents' Earning Scheme (RES) and Sheltered Workshop. The RES is a programme for residents to gain training and experience working in jobs that they might do in the community, such as cleaning and gardening. The Sheltered Workshop receives contract-based work from external organisations which usually involve packing and soft industrial work. Occupational Therapists from the Activity Hub provide job site support, skills training, problem solving to residents who are placed on external employment. The therapists act as mediators between the employers and residents in order to minimise any misunderstandings and to help both sides understand how to work with one another. Furthermore, education of employers and supervisors will also be carried out on site to help them accommodate to the needs of their new employees."

Next to IMH at Hougang Care Centre as well as at Simei Care Centre (run by Singapore Anglican Community Services), Occupational therapists have also been employed to provide psychosocial rehabilitation services, particularly in the area of vocational rehabilitation. They work closely with

IMH and other general hospitals to take over the care of the patients when they are discharged to their residential programmes.

Conclusion

Occupational therapy services have indeed come a long way and the last ten years have been especially exciting, with development of various services across the different organisations. The senior OTs are also glad that young OTs have been interested to specialize in mental health over the past few years, thereby growing our professional pool. The mental health occupational therapy family is a close knitted one and everyone is keen to contribute to the professional development in this area as well as to offer valued services for mental health users, both within hospitals and in the community.

References

Mahendren, R, Ibrahim, K & Tan, Y.P. (1995). Psychiatric day centres — the Singapore experience. Singapore Medical Journal, 36(6), 644–646.

Tan, B.L. (2009). "Hybrid Transitional-Supported Employment Using Social Enterprise: a Retrospective Study". *Psychiatric Rehabilitation Journal.* 33(1): 53–55.

Tan, B. L., Kumar, V. R., & Devaraj, P. (2015). Development of a new occupational therapy service in a Singapore prison. *British Journal of Occupational Therapy*, 78(8), 525–529. http://doi.org/10.1177/0308022615571083

Tan, B. L., Li, Z., & Tan, C. H. (2016). Evaluation of a national supported employment programme for people with psychiatric conditions. *British Journal of Occupational Therapy*, 79(5), 270–274. http://doi.org/10.1177/0308022615615891

Tan, B.-L., & King, R. (2013). The effects of cognitive remediation on functional outcomes among people with schizophrenia: a randomised controlled study. *The Australian and New Zealand Journal of Psychiatry*, 47(11), 1068–80. http://doi.org/10.1177/0004867413493521

Case Managers

Margaret HENDRICKS

Introduction

Case Managers were first introduced in the Institute of Mental Health (IMH) in 2000 for specialised programs, namely the Early Psychosis Programme and the Community Addiction Management Programme. The service extended to our general wards, namely the Acute, Rehabilitation and Forensic departments in 2003, the Psychogeriatric department in 2005, and the Community Psychiatry Department in 2007. Clinicians in the acute ward setting and Emergency Department proposed to extend Case Management services to these areas due to the need for close monitoring and provision of after care services to patients upon their discharge. A proposal was sent to Senior Management to recruit Case Managers to service departments deemed necessary by Psychiatrists. With their approval, a Senior Consultant Psychiatrist led the Case Management team in administrative and training matters, and the specific Psychiatrist of the various departments oversaw the clinical supervision of the Case Managers.

Today, the general Case Managers are also found in specialised programmes, namely the Mandatory Treatment Order (MTO) Programme, the Integrated Patient Assessment and Continuous Engagement (IPACE) Programme, the Mood Disorder Unit (MDU), the General Practitioner Partnership Programme (GPPP), the Aftercare Programme and the Obsessive Compulsive Disorder (OCD) Clinic. Besides these programmes, they are also involved in the Adult Neurodevelopmental Service (ANDS) and the Psychotherapy Service. Our Psychiatric Case Management Unit has grown from the initial three case managers to the present fifty-four.

Definition of Case Management, the Model We Use and What Do We Do

Psychiatric patients, especially those with severe psychotic illnesses, frequently default their treatment and follow-up. Some of the contributing factors include the lack of patient insight and poor family support. Therefore, to reduce patients' non-adherence to treatment, it is essential for adequate coordination, transition and continuity of care for patients from the inpatient hospital setting to the outpatient community setting.

The Case Management Unit adopted Thornicroft's definition of Case Management, which is the '*coordination, integration and allocation of individualized care within limited resources*', in planning the delivery of care (Mueser *et al.*, 1998). This formed the foundation for the formulation of a psychosocial needs assessment, individualised care plans, referrals and linkages to appropriate community services and resources, monitoring of patients' mental states and response to treatment, treatment adherence and side effects, the establishment and maintenance of a therapeutic relationship, as well as the provision of counselling, support therapy and psychoeducation (Thornicroft, 1991).

There are many models of Case Management, for example, Clinical Case Management, Strength Case Management, Rehabilitation Case Management, Assertive Case Management, and Intensive Case Management (Stein and Diamond, 1985). However, the Case Management Unit adopted the Brokerage Model of Case Management and adapted it to suit the Singapore context. The main objectives of this Model were to provide holistic care to patients and the appropriate utilisation of resources.

In the initial stages of development, the Case Management Unit prepared a set of inclusion and exclusion criteria for referral to the service to ensure appropriate referrals by the hospital staff. However, today all patients admitted to the inpatient ward are assessed by the case manager unless they are managed by other specialised programs. Clinical outcome measures such as the monitoring of patient treatment default rates and readmission rates were introduced to assist in the review of the service.

Although the primary role of Case Managers is to coordinate care and ensure a smooth continuity of care for patients upon their discharge, the Case Manager's role may differ across specialized programmes due to their different emphasis. The following table showcases the difference in Case Management roles across the disciplines.

INSTITUTE of MENTAL HEALTH

Loving Hearts, Beautiful Minds

Case Management Framework

ADDITIONAL SERVICES BY SPECIALTIES

FORENSIC CM	Rehab CM	COMM PSYCH CM	PSYCHOG CM
☐ Assess patients if they require assistance in legal aid and to assist when required	☐ Provide case management support to patients reviewed by the Intellectual Disable Service. This includes assessment of HONOS, ABC and Caregiver Burden of care scales	☐ Provide case management support for patients on the Psychotherapy program	☐ Visiting and training nursing home staff who have difficultes managing our discharged patients
☐ Track court outcomes of patients discharged to court	☐ Provide support to the CAC in the monthly audit of case notes	☐ Assist in case managing all black listed patients in the SOC	☐ Case manage patients who are discharged from the temporary long stay ward (Ward 64)
☐ Monitor patients under section 255 closely and remind them to come for their Visitors Board review		☐ Assist in the DUKE students' simulation patient practical exam	☐ Provide training to Advanced Diploma in Nursing students in Psychogeriatric Case Management
☐ Liaison work with prison services, subordinate courts, MCYS			

Training

The Case Management Unit has developed a training and supervision programme that equips new Case Management recruits with competent case management skills as well and provides them with continuous upgrading opportunities in their career. Four senior nurses were first recruited to the

Unit and since then, the Unit has expanded to a team of fifty-four Case Managers. When the Unit first started, the Case Managers were clinically supervised by their department psychiatrists, participated in attachment programmes to local hospitals, and attended a nine-month postgraduate polytechnic course in Case Management at the Nanyang Polytechnic. Today, our newly recruited Case Managers undergo a two-week intensive case management orientation programme conducted by their senior colleagues for knowledge and 'hands-on' experience. Simultaneously they receive continuous clinical supervision by their departmental psychiatrists, and mentorship by Senior Case Managers.

There are also Case Management retreats and regular bonding sessions held within the department to enhance communication and social interaction. To achieve international standards and to benchmark against the best in their field, the Case Managers participate in attachment programmes at international hospitals and clinics to study various case management systems. They also meet International Psychiatry Experts who visit IMH to discuss improvement strategies for their case management service.

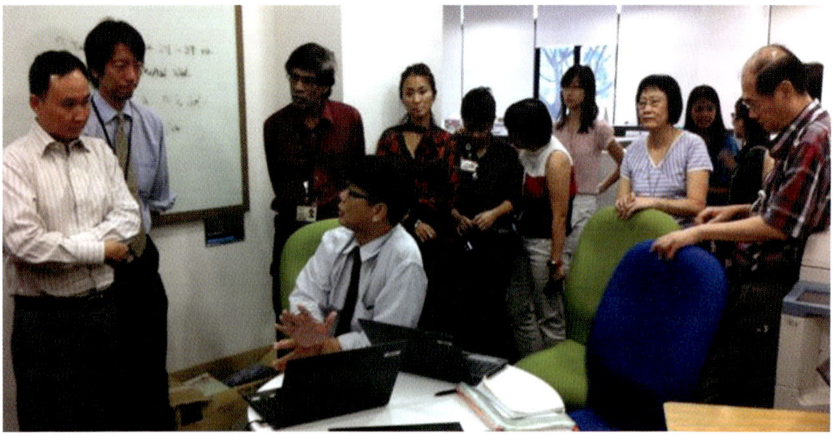

Launching of the iPACE system 2010.

What We Have Achieved

All Case Managers are encouraged to participate in oral presentations, poster presentations at local and international conferences and to publish papers on case management. To date, Case Managers have completed two research papers, eight Clinical Practice Improvement Programme (CPIP) projects, one Health Care Quality Improvement Project and done numerous service surveys. The Case Management Unit has published 13 journal articles in both local and international journals, presented more than 20 oral presentations and more than 50 poster presentations at local and international conferences. The Case Management Unit is currently in the process of completing one CPIP and six research projects.

The Case Management Unit has also won several awards locally and internationally, namely:

Ministry of Health Clinical Quality and Safety Poster Competition
First Prize, 2005, Singapore
Title of project: Clinical pathways and treatment algorithms enhance psychiatric care and improve clinical outcomes

Asian Hospital Management Award
Best Project Prize under Customer Category, 2007, Manila, the Philippines
Title of project: Reducing the rate of unplanned readmissions in the acute psychogeriatric ward

MOH Singapore Quality and Safety Poster Competition
Merit Award, 2007, Singapore
Title of project: Enhancing clinical and quality care through the reduction of unplanned readmissions in psychogeriatric unit

NHG Annual Scientific Meeting
Merit Award, 2007, Singapore
Title of project: Measuring clinical improvement outcomes in case management in a psychiatric tertiary hospital

NHG CPIP Award for IMH
Best Project Award, 2007, Singapore
Title of project: To reduce unplanned readmission in the acute psychogeriatric female ward by 50% within four months

11th Congress of the ASEAN Federation for Psychiatry and Mental Health
Third Prize, 2008, Bangkok, Thailand
Title of poster: A four-year review and outcomes assessment of case management in a tertiary psychiatric hospital

11th Congress of the ASEAN Federation for Psychiatry and Mental Health
Third Prize, 2008, Bangkok, Thailand
Title of poster: Implementing clinical pathways in a tertiary psychiatric hospital — a five-year review

NHG Annual Scientific Meeting
Merit Award, 2008, Singapore
Title of poster: The effectiveness of clinical pathways in psychiatric rehabilitation

NHG CPIP Award
Sustainability Award, 2008, Singapore
Title of poster: To reduce unplanned readmission in the acute psychogeriatric female ward by 50% within four months

Asia Hospital Management Award
Most Outstanding Award under the Internal Customer Category, 2011
Title of project: Re-engineering case management service to improve inpatient and outpatient follow-up care

Asian Hospital Management Award
Excellence Award (Runner Up) Project Prize under Internal Customer Category, 2012, Hanoi, Vietnam
Title of Project: Promote improved integrated care through the reduction of patient rejection referrals to the Community Mental Health Services

Awards

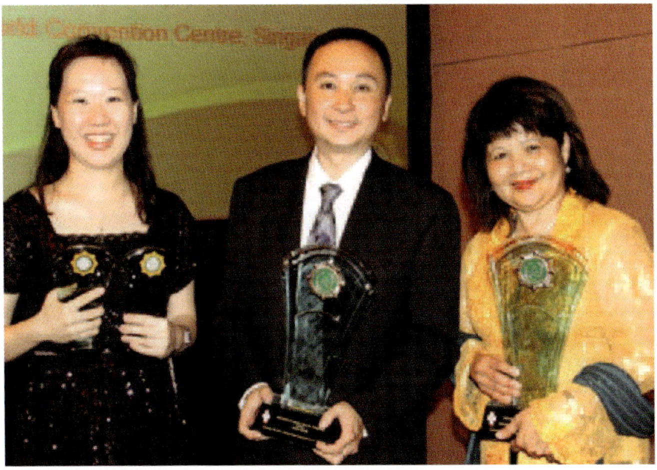

(From left) Dr. Goh Yen-Li, Dr. Chua Hong Choon, and Margaret Hendriks, receiving the awards for Mental-Health GP-Partnership Programme, Hospital of the Year, and Case Management Services, respectively.

The Asian Hospital Management Awards recognise and honour hospitals in Asia that implement best hospital practices. In 2011, IMH clinched the inaugural Grand Award for the Hospital of the Year, one Winner and two Excellence Awards. 'Re-engineering case management service to improve inpatient and outpatient follow-up care' won the Most Outstanding Project in the Service Improvement for Internal Customers Project Category, while 'An effective primary care model of stable psychiatric outpatients within the community — the mental health-general practitioner partnership programme' won the Excellence Award in the Operational Customer Service Project Category and the Marketing, PR or Promotional Project category. These projects were chosen from more than 300 submissions from 84 hospitals across 11 countries.

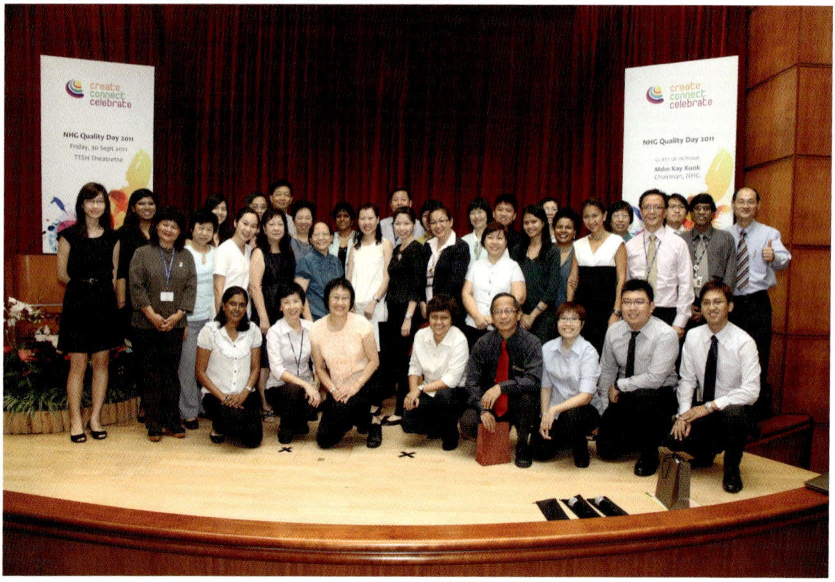

IMH Case Management Unit after receiving the NHG Team Excellence Award 2011 (Photo credit: NHG Group Corporate Communications).

The Case Management Unit won the National Healthcare Group (NHG) Excellence in Action Award 2011 (Team Award). This award honours outstanding teams who performed well in sustaining service excellence as well as contributed to the betterment of work practice and standards.

In the following year, The Asian Hospital Management awarded one of IMH's CPIP projects entitled 'Promote improved integrated care through the reduction of patient rejection referrals to the Community Mental Health Services' with the Excellence Award (Runner Up) in the Service Improvement for Internal Customers Project Category at the ceremony in Hanoi held on 13 September 2012. There were 363 entries from 89 hospitals across 12 countries vying for the coveted award.

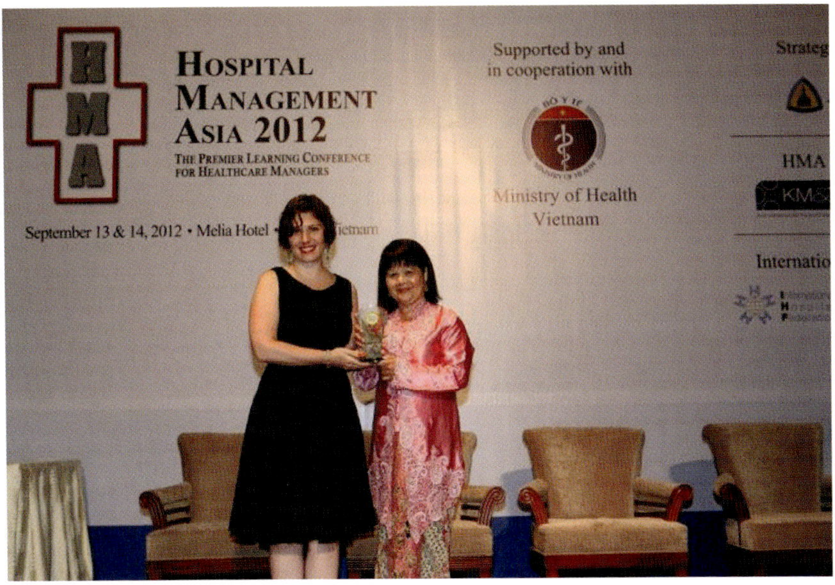

Ms Margaret Hendriks (right), Head of IMH Case Management Unit with Miss Lindsay Rothstein, Assistant Director of Marketing & Communications, John Hopkins Medicine International.

The Case Management Unit team, who led the project, noticed that in one of the acute psychiatric wards, 45% out of 34 patients who were referred to the Community Mental Health Team (CMHT) rejected the service. Hence, they developed the project with an aim to reduce the percentage of patients rejecting CMHT's services by refining the selection process and providing more patient education. The multidisciplinary team (MDT) developed materials on CMHT services for easy reference, checklists for Case Managers to use prior to making a referral, and posters and handouts for patients and their caregivers. They found that referring the right patient for CMHT services led to a decrease in rejection rate by more than half.

How Do Our Patients View Our Services?

'My name is Chan, a patient in Geylang IMH, I wish to formally thank Mdm Tay Sim Eng for making so much efforts [sic] to contact me to further my treatment. I have been going through a lot of problems and just when I lost all hopes, and faith in humanity, the said Mdm Tay went out of her way to contact me, making sure I get further treatments; someone does care about my well-being. I explained to her my reasons for not coming back for further treatments, and she convinced me I do have options. I have to admit, I was hesitant in coming back, due to my finance situation and also it seems pointless for me to continue since even the government is not even helping me. But her efforts in trying to contact me, really touched me. So I decided to write in to thank her. Thank You Mdm Tay Sim Eng.'

— Chan, patient from Community Wellness Clinic (Geylang)

'Ms Margaret Hendriks, Head of the Case Management Unit, has been there to help me in my time of need. Since my enrolment in polytechnic this year, I have felt inferior and faced many personal problems initially. In fact, I failed my exams due to my learning disability. However, Ms Margaret lent me a listening ear, and she called me regularly to make sure I was ok. Thank you all so much for providing me ample support when I most needed it.'

— Huang F., outpatient

'Hi Seok Siew,

I have met up with one of your attending patients: Ms PEK yesterday. She wishes to compliment you for your personalized and excellent services rendered to her. She suffers from depression and often needs a listening ear. She is very glad that you are always there for her and offer good advices to her. She feels very comfortable with you and appreciates your attentiveness in her case. She told me she feels better now and on the path of recovery. She wants me to convey her appreciation and send her regards to you. Great job done!'

— Janice Tang, Executive, Patient Relations Office

'To: IMH CEO

I am grateful to Mr. Raymond, Senior Case Manager who came to my house at my house Holland Road to my parents. Even now he takes care of me very well. Even got the MSW to get me a rental flat. Even he strict to me he gives me firm advice. I appreciate his concern for me. I hope he will be health always and I always will remember him in my years to come.'

— Toh Kok Wai

'To: Benjamin Tay

Thanks for being my kind case-manager! Thanks for giving me a listening ear! Thanks for all your help! May the Lord Jesus Christ bless your life abundantly and fill you with lots of love, joy and peace throughout this Christmas and the year ahead! Merry Christmas! And a Happy New Year! God Bless.'

— Rachel (Tip Eng)

'Dear Benjamin,

I greatly appreciate the generous assistance you have rendered. Thank you very much for all that you have done, especially with you concern, understanding, encouragement and guidance.'

— Tan Lay Eng

'Through her case management, my mum is coping well and taking ownership of her condition. I have reconnected with her and I thank Gemma (Fernandez) for that.'

— Mr R, caregiver

'I would like to thank Serlina Eng for her support and encouragement. My son had refused treatment for more than 10 years, and I've been feeling helpless. When my son got admitted, Serlina provided me with her handphone number and reassured me that I can contact her 24/7 if I was experiencing difficulty managing my son. I am really appreciative and thankful for Serlina's assistance.'

— Mdm Chua, caregiver

What Our Team Members Think of the Case Managers

'Case management has made a noticeable difference in our overall patient care.'

— Dr. George Fernandez, Senior Consultant Psychiatrist, IMH

"'Case management unit has growth from strength to strength in terms of numbers as well as expertise in Solution Focused Brief Therapy (SFBT) and Motivational Interviewing (MI). Case manager have also proven to be a dynamic and vital force in providing coordination to community mental health services and ensuring that resources are tapped effectively. This is evident in the recognition and multiple awards the department has won.'

— Dr Leong Jern Yi, Senior Consultant Psychiatrist, IMH

Case Managers at Work

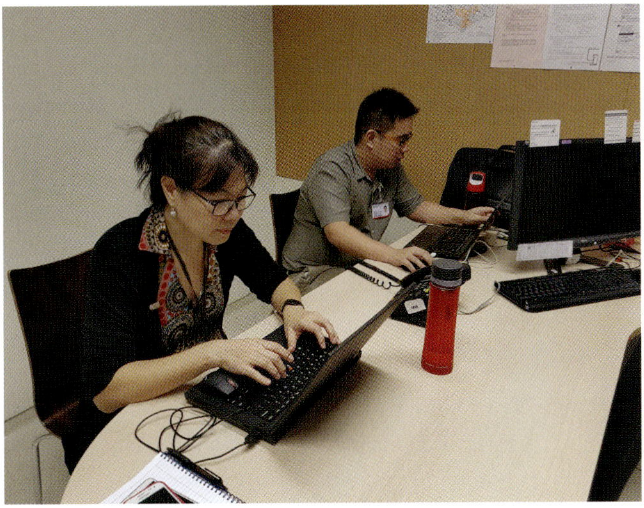

Case Managers documenting entries in c-doc after meeting their patients in the clinic.

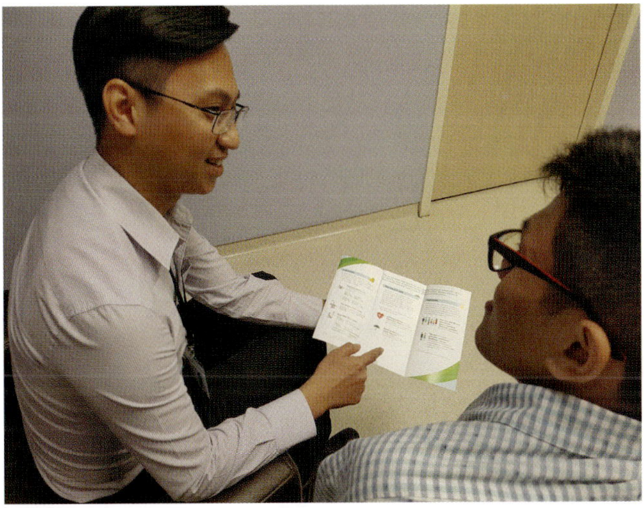

Psychoeducating patient on mental illness.

Conclusion

Psychiatric Case Management has indeed become a cornerstone to successful discharge, continuity of care and reintegration of patients to the community. The gradual expansion of the service has led to the presence of Case Managers in all acute admitting wards and different departments within the hospital, such as the Forensic Department, the Psychogeriatric Department and the Community Psychiatry Department. Case Management will continue to be a vital service for our patients as they progress in their recovery journey.

References

Mueser KT, Bond GR, Drake RE (1998). Models of community care for severe mental illness: A review of research on case management. *Schizophr Bull* **24**: 37–74.

Stein L, Diamond J (1985). A program for difficult-to-treat patients. *New Dir Ment Serv* **26**: 29–31.

Thornicroft G (1991). The concept of case management for long-term mental illness. *Psychiatry* **3**: 125–132.

Changi General Hospital: From Service to Department

YAP Hwa Ling and TAN Sheng Neng

About Changi General Hospital

Changi General Hospital (CGH), formally known as New Changi General Hospital, was formed on 15 February 1997 from the merger of Old Changi Hospital with Toa Payoh Hospital. The then Deputy Prime Minister Lee Hsien Loong officially opened the hospital on 28 March 1998. It became part of the Singapore Health Services (SingHealth) cluster in 2000 when the public health care system was restructured. In 2005, CGH became the second hospital in Singapore to receive the Joint Commission International accreditation. On 1 April 2011, the hospital became legally independent of SingHealth and, on 18 November 2011, became one of the founding members of Eastern Health Alliance.

CGH, in the eastern part of Singapore, has a comprehensive range of more than 23 medical services (from general surgery, internal medicine, cardiology, ENT, orthopaedic surgery to psychological medicine and sports medicine). In 2001, CGH had about 800 beds and served a community of 750,000. Today, it has more than 1,000 beds, serving a community of 1.4 million.

As part of its service expansion, the Psychological Medicine service was set up in July 1997 to meet the mental health care needs of the population in the east. It became the Division of Psychological Medicine in 2001 and a department in 1 February 2008.

Facilities

The psychiatric ward began with 27 beds but the number was reduced in 2014 to 17 due to the pressing need for more medical beds. There are rooms for interviewing patients, tutorials, family/group therapy and occupational therapy. The ward is equipped with facilities to perform electroconvulsive therapy.

Staffing

The department began in July 1997 with one full-time and one part-time psychiatrist, both of whom were seconded from the Institute of Mental Health (IMH)/Woodbridge Hospital. In April 2001, CGH decided to recruit its own psychiatrists. There are currently 14 psychiatrists and 6 Visiting Consultants. They are supported by a team of clinical psychologists, a medical social worker, an occupational therapist, psychiatric nurses and Advanced Practice Nurses (APNs).

Range of services

The department provides inpatient, outpatient, consultation-liaison psychiatry and psychogeriatric services.

In addition to general psychiatry clinics, the department has subspecialty clinics, catering to the needs of CGH patients and services, namely, Addiction Medicine Clinic, Insomnia Clinic in the Integrated Sleep Service, Adolescent Psychiatry Clinic, Bipolar Disorder Clinic, Psychodynamic Psychotherapy Clinic and Neuropsychiatry Clinic. The number of outpatient visits has increased from 2,081 in 1998 to 19,433 in 2014. Referrals from medical and surgical departments in the hospital for consultation-liaison psychiatry consults have grown from 600 referrals in 1997 to 1,241 referrals in 2014.

The Psychogeriatric Service was set up on 1 Jan 2013 with its own Director. Before its inception, psychogeriatricians were already supporting existing geriatric services in CGH. Community psychogeriatic services were extended to the community through the Integrated Framework of Healthcare of the Elderly during the period of 2001 till 2004. In 2007, the

Community Psychogeriatric Programme (CPGP) was set up under the funding from Singapore's Ministry of Health (MOH). This further strengthened its capabilities in providing elderly mental health care through training, consultation and support of the family practitioners and community eldercare agencies. Clinical services for home bound elderly with mental disorders or dementia was also provided under this programme. In 2010, the CPGP became involved with the National Dementia Strategy to develop and initiate, coordinate and integrate dementia care for the Singapore population.

Teaching, Training, Research

The department is active in the teaching of medical students from Duke-NUS Graduate Medical School and Yong Loo Lin School of Medicine. It is also a training site for the National Psychiatry Residency Programme. The department also offers training for the SingHealth Family Medicine Residency Programme. Currently, the department is able to provide teaching, training and exposure on multiple aspects of psychiatry to our residents at all levels of their training. The psychiatrists are also involved in giving lectures to nurses in the Advanced Diploma in Nursing (Mental Health) programme.

In addition to a strong teaching culture, the department is also strongly involved in both standalone research and collaborative research. General psychiatry has been involved in open labelled and phase 3 drug trials. The Psychogeriatric service is active in multiple areas of dementia research and it is constantly looking into more innovative ways to develop better dementia care. It is currently involved in an international multi-centre phase 3 drug trial. Research done by Addiction Medicine has been presented in overseas conferences.

In recent years, the department has placed increasing focus on Medical Education as well. There are frequent meetings and regular sessions to upgrade the teaching skills of its staff from residents to consultant psychiatrist.

The Future

The department is cognisant of changes in mental healthcare delivery. From the being institutional or hospital based to one with a community focus, the idea being to right site the delivery of mental health services. The department set up the Health Wellness Programme at Bedok Community Health Centre in 2012 to provide community-based mental healthcare as well as support persons with chronic medical illnesses who need psychological interventions. The department continues to explore different ways in which we can contribute to capacity building in the community.

National University Hospital System: The Journey of Academic Psychiatry in a University Hospital

TENG Jia Ying and John Chee Meng WONG

Founding of the Department (1979–1994)

The Department of Psychological Medicine was established in September 1979 to provide education in undergraduate and postgraduate psychiatry, clinical training and conduct research. Before 1979, the psychiatry teaching programme for University of Singapore medical students was held at Woodbridge Hospital (WH).

Dr Tsoi Wing Foo, the founder of the department, was then the medical superintendent at Woodbridge Hospital. Dr Tsoi was invited to set up the Department of Psychological Medicine at the Department of Medicine, University of Singapore. This was located at the current Singapore General Hospital campus. Over the next three years, Dr Tsoi recruited Dr Kok Lee Peng and Dr Kua Ee Heok, as well as administrative staff, to support the department.

In 1985, the department moved to the new National University Hospital (NUH) in Kent Ridge. The department had its own inpatient unit in Ward 12, which was the first general hospital psychiatric ward in Singapore. The inpatient service was supported by full medical laboratory and imaging investigation facilities for complex medical psychiatry patients. It provided a patient-focused and family-friendly treatment milieu. This helped to facilitate greater social and occupational rehabilitation for a range of psychiatric conditions.

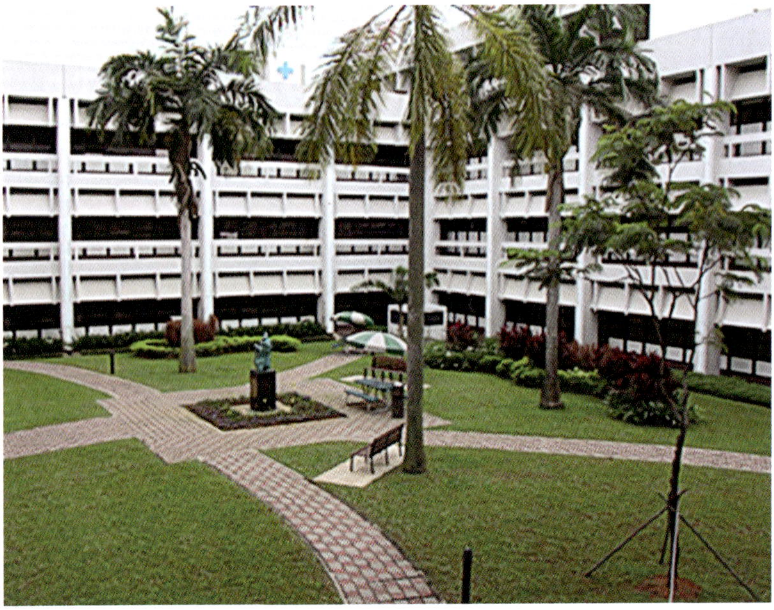

Garden of NUH Ward 12.

'The new psychiatric ward gave patients an alternative place for treatment. This ward gave hope to many patients, because it helped them to allay their fears of receiving psychiatric treatment.'

Dr Tsoi Wing Foo,
Founder and Head of Department from 1979 to 1994.

'The ward Sisters asked us to conduct daily morning Qi Gong for the patients. We initially dreaded it! They had to come up with a roster, and we learned the art of basic Qi Gong. After some time, it became one of the most enjoyable morning routines, to gather patients in the garden and perform Qi Gong to soothing music. My lasting impression of Ward 12 is the strong team spirit and camaraderie amongst the nurses, allied health professionals and the doctors.'

— Nurse-Clinician Mary Pui, joined Ward 12 as Staff nurse in 1987

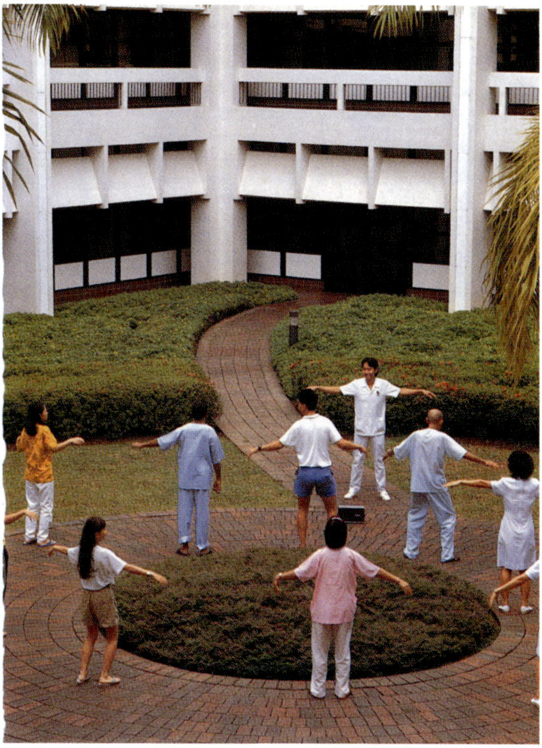

Ward 12 staff leading the morning Qi Gong exercises for patients.

Education and Training

Prior to 1972, the psychiatry teaching programme for medical students at the University of Singapore consisted of 20 hours of lectures, followed by a visit to Woodbridge Hospital. Later, the clinical postings were increased progressively to two weeks, and subsequently four weeks. A longer clinical posting was needed to help the students develop a better understanding of mental health issues. For example, being able to appreciate the impact that mental health has on a patient's physical health, and how to recognise early signs of psychiatric conditions so that early intervention can be provided.

With the increase in teaching staff and inpatient beds at NUH, medical students were able to have their clinical postings at NUH, in addition to Woodbridge Hospital. Another significant milestone was the first Postgraduate Examination for the NUS Master of Medicine (Psychiatry), which was conducted in August 1985 in conjunction with Woodbridge Hospital.

The department at NUH started to recruit psychiatry specialty trainees in 1986. The first cohort of trainees included Dr Ko Soo Meng, Dr Tian Cheong Sing, Dr Lee Ee Lian, Dr Brian Yeo, Dr Pamela Chan, Dr Anthony Ang, Dr Calvin Fones, Dr John Wong, Dr Tommy Tan and Dr Inez Pereira.

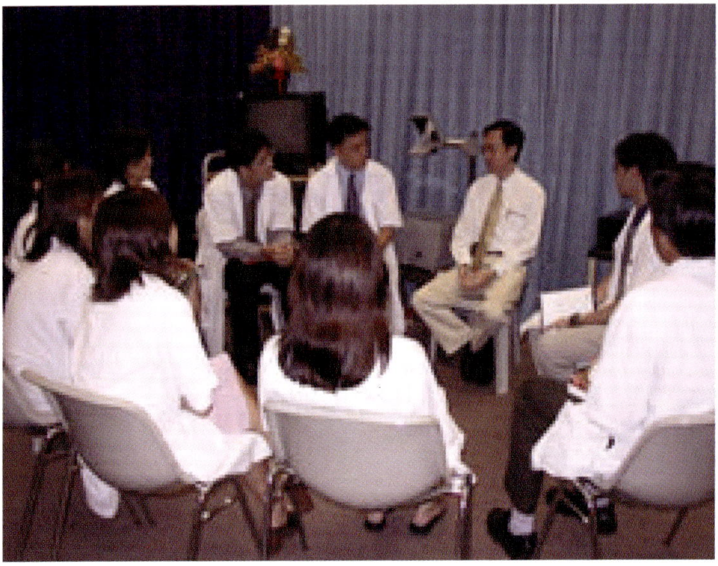

Dr Anthony Ang teaching undergraduate medical students.

Research

The pioneering members of the department were enthusiastic in research, and there was rapid development in this area. Dr Tsoi pioneered many studies in schizophrenia and transsexualism. Prof Kok Lee Peng conducted studies on suicide and Prof Kua investigated the area of alcohol use disorders and old age psychiatry. Dr Lionel Lim had a keen interest in psycho-genetics and obtained a PhD from the University of London under an NUS Scholarship. Dr Ko had a keen interest in cognitive behavioural therapy and the condition of obsessive compulsive disorder. Dr Yeo was involved in research on opioid drug addiction and psychosomatic disease. Dr Tian and Dr Ken Ung conducted studies in the area of child psychiatry and eating disorders. Dr Fones focused on anxiety and primary mental health services.

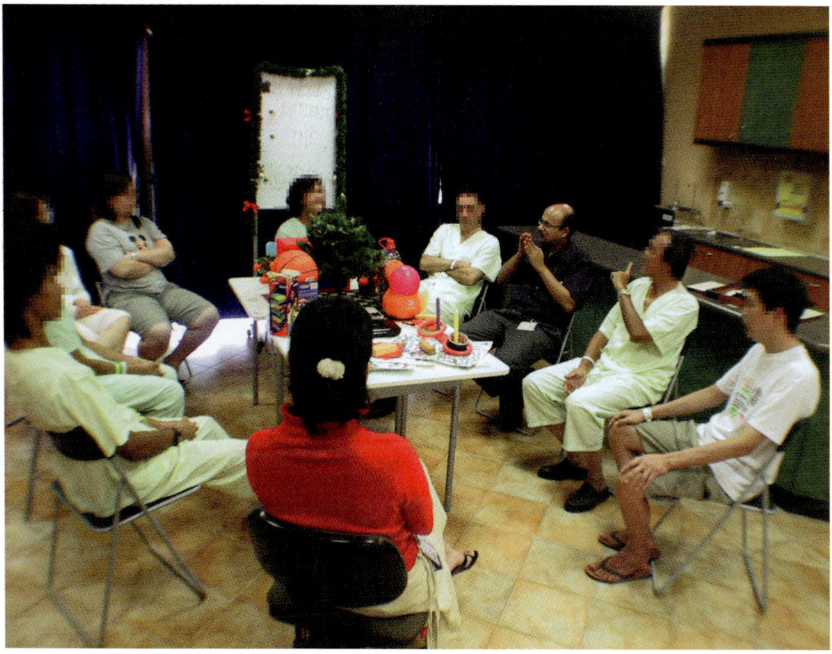

Group activity for patients led by Staff Nurse Noor at Ward 12 — time for holistic team-based psychiatric care and strong teaching.

'As one of the first batch of residents at NUH in 1986, we had lots of time — time which we could spend interviewing patients, the time to engage with staff, the time to not just focus on biological treatment, but psychological treatment.

We had time to reflect and think. The time to interact with staff and different disciplines. NUH management of psychiatric patients was a team-based approach. The team consisted of psychologists, occupational therapists, nurses and social workers. The contribution that each member of the team brought was highly valued. Everyone was given time to share their views.

That way with the team approach, it helps us to best manage and support the patient. So that even though we may not always find a cure — as they say cure is seldom, comfort often, but care always.

We had a wonderful team of teachers — Prof Tsoi, Prof Kok and Prof Kua. The team of these three professors impacted us a lot. It was not just about imparting knowledge, but inspiring us to ask questions. That led us to do research. We were asked to be engaged in research projects right from the start. The strong teaching has set for us models that we can follow, and models that we can become for the next generation — so that in the end, psychiatry can be brought to a higher level.'

— A/Prof Ko Soo Meng, Senior Consultant at NUH (1987 to 2004)

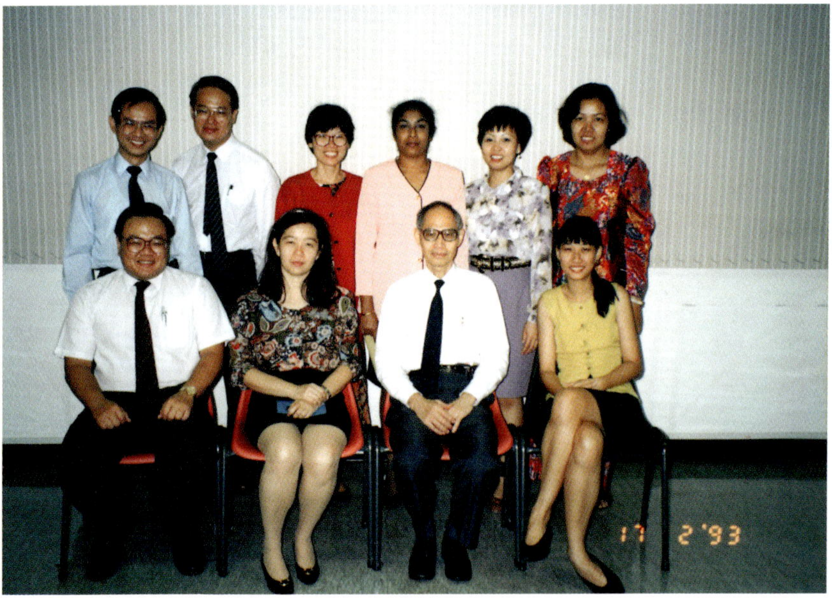

A group photo from the year 1993. First row (seated): Dr Brian Yeo, Ms Lydia Hoalim, Dr Tsoi Wing Foo, Ms Gina Tan. Second row (standing): Dr Ko Soo Meng, Dr Tommy Tan, Ms Lim Wee Cheng, Ms Vanaja Thangaraju, Ms Jasmine Tan, Ms Aminah Bte Rais.

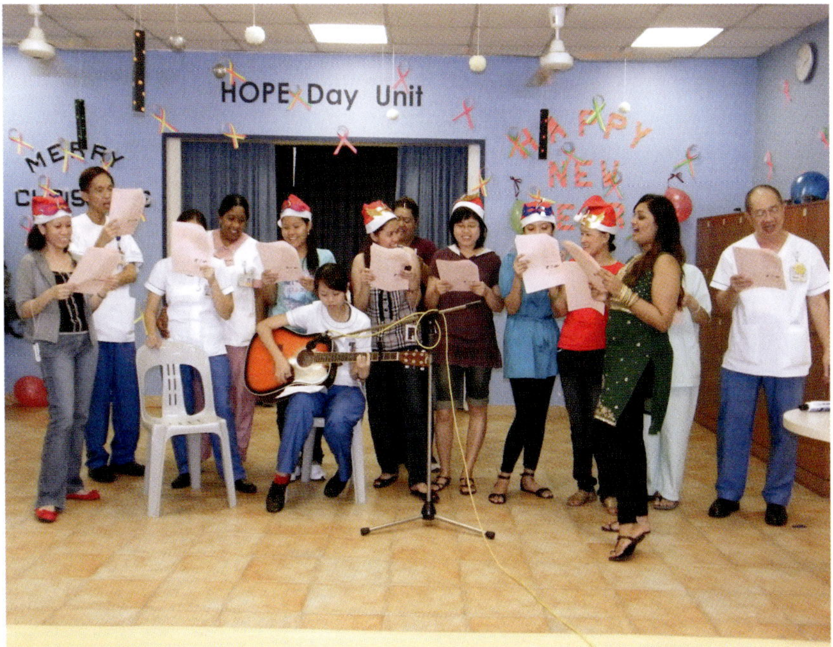

Christmas party at NUH Ward 12.

Development of Clinical Services (1995–2016)

After Dr Tsoi Wing Foo's retirement in 1994, Prof Kua Ee Heok became the Head of Department. The department's clinical services continued to expand. The Hope Day Unit at Ward 12 housed a day hospital programme, where patients who had been discharged from the ward could participate in ward activities. This allowed continued engagement of the patients and rehabilitation, to promote better re-integration back to the community.

The department grew under the leadership of A/Prof Calvin Fones, A/Prof Chandrashekhar Bhalchandra Khare, A/Prof John Wong and their faculty. It developed its scope of academic mission and clinical service delivery, to become a psychiatric centre of excellence both locally and regionally.

Specialised Clinical Services

The team at NUH re-organised the outpatient clinical services into consultant-led subspecialty clinics. These clinics provide care to patients with depression, bipolar disorder, anxiety disorders, psychosis and memory problems.

With a dedicated consultation-liaison (CL) psychiatry service, inpatient referrals are seen promptly, optimising multidisciplinary care for NUH patients with complex conditions and needs. This facilitates consistent care by the same team of doctors throughout the patients' hospital stay. The patients are also followed up at the CL psychiatry clinic after discharge, by the same team of doctors.

Specialist care services such as Psycho-Oncology, Psycho-Cardiology and Transplant Psychiatry were developed to support the national centres in cancer (National University Cancer Institute), cardiology (National University Heart Centre) and organ transplant (National University Centre for Organ Transplantation).

Improving Clinical Services and Teaching at Ward 33

The ward moved from the ground level of NUH at Ward 12 to level three of the Main Building in 2010. The planning of the new ward was led by A/Prof Khare, who was Head of Department from 2009 to 2010. This project was supported by A/Prof John Wong and Department Manager Carol Cheah. The new facility was designed to provide a safe and pleasant therapeutic milieu for our patients. The central location of the nursing station provides a 'bird's eye view' of the ward. Special teaching rooms with modern audio-visual equipment were also included, to enhance the experience of the undergraduate medical students who were posted to the department.

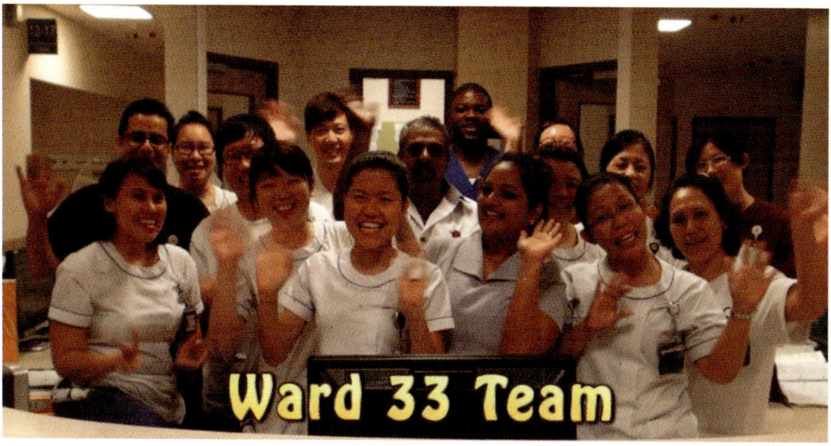

Ward 33 nursing team and allied health care staff.

Compassion for Our Patients

> *'You need to bring everything you have, and to work with compassion. They [the patients] don't have anything against you. Sometimes they are aggressive, and at times you're even afraid they will hurt you. We all must realise they really need our help. They're not here to hurt you, they can't control it. They need our support, and we need to be there with them 110%. We feel really glad when we see improvement in them.*
>
> *It's beautiful, to be a mental health worker.'*
>
> — Michael Olarewaju Ayeni, NUH Ward 33 Nurse Manager

Integrated Care in the Community

The team at NUH has progressed to build an integrated care system, with services stretching from the community to the hospital, and back. The community programmes provide holistic care to the patients at various phases of their illness. It also promotes recovery of their function within their natural environment.

Geriatric psychiatry out-Reach Assessment, Consultation and Enablement (G-RACE)

G-RACE is an outreach service that provides psychiatric assessment and treatment for elderly patients living in the western region of Singapore. Set up in 2011, the multidisciplinary team of health care professionals includes psycho-geriatricians, nursing-trained case managers, occupational therapists and psychologists. G-RACE aims to provide mental health services to the elderly who have difficulty accessing outpatient services. The other objectives of the service are to prevent unnecessary hospital admissions and reduce the length of stay for the patients. By providing

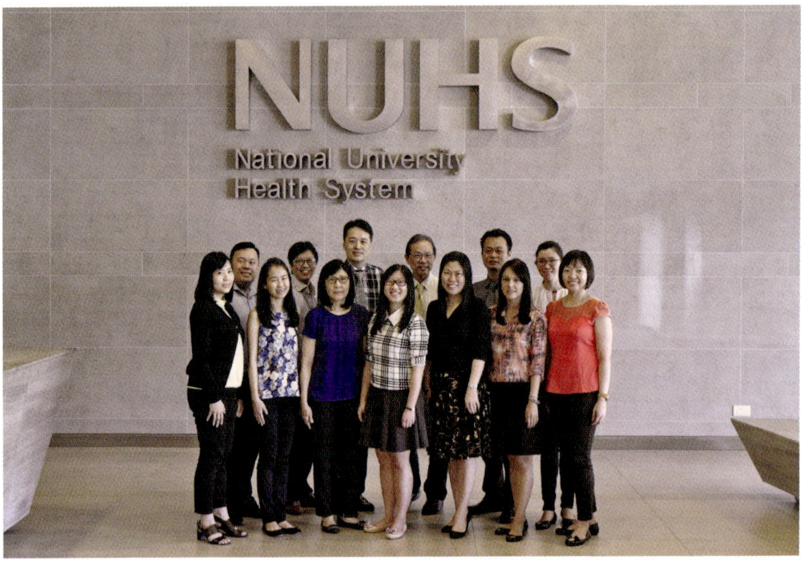

G-RACE team.

comprehensive care to the patients and their families, G-RACE hopes to improve the quality of life of elderly people in the community, and to alleviate the stress of their caregivers.

Women's Emotional Health Service (WEHS)

WEHS was started in 2007 at NUH, to work with the Department of Obstetrics and Gynaecology in looking after several high-risk populations. Initial outreach efforts were targeted at women during pregnancy and post-delivery, as well as women with gynaecological cancers. Over the years, the service has expanded to meet the psychological needs of women with diverse conditions. These include subfertility, foetal loss, premenstrual dysphoric disorder, peri-menopausal anxiety and depression, as well as breast cancer. The team takes on a multidisciplinary approach, and includes psychiatrists, nurses, psychologists, case managers and

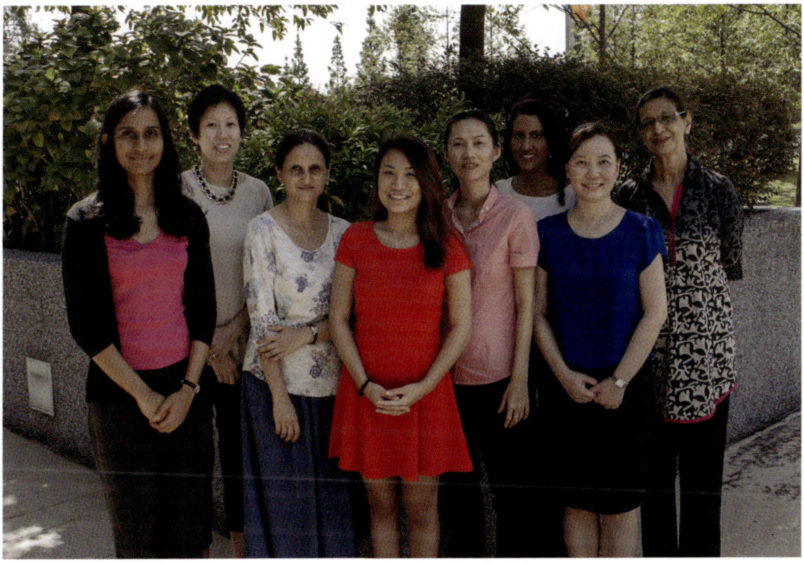

WEHS team.

occupational therapists. One of the team's research projects on perinatal depression studied the effects of the confinement experience of Singaporean mothers (Chee *et al.*, 2005).

Response, Early Intervention and Assessment in Community Mental Health (REACH) West

REACH West is part of a nationwide community-based mental health programme developed to support schools, community agencies and family doctors. Set up at NUH in 2011, the programme helps to screen and provide early intervention to school-going children and adolescents with emotional, behavioural and neurodevelopmental issues. It augments the hospital's Child and Adolescent Psychiatry Services.

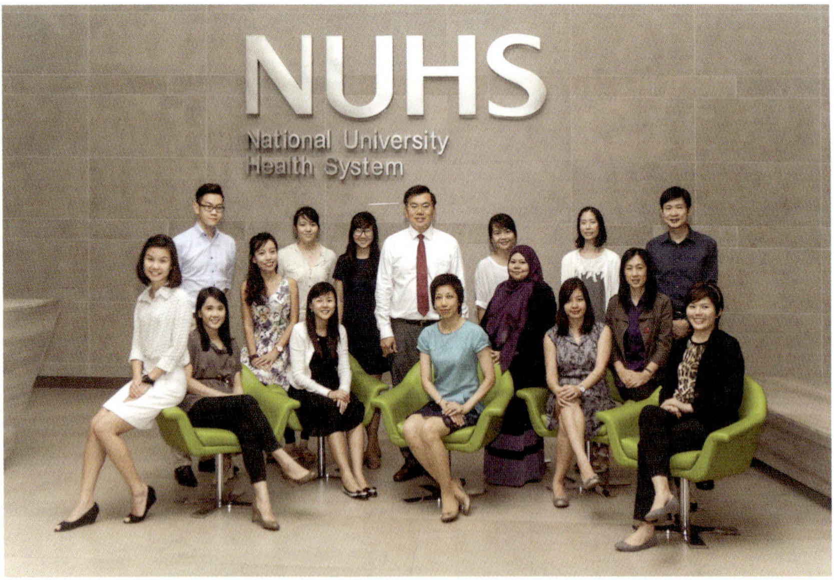

REACH West team photo.

Further Development of Research, Training and Education

In the past decade, the Gerontological Research Programme and Singapore Longitudinal Ageing Study group at NUH have attained international accolades for research on dementia and successful ageing. One of the research projects led by A/Prof Ng Tze Pin examined the effects of lifestyle activities in promoting active ageing. This provided an evidence base for recommending leisure activities in a public health campaign targeting senior citizens (Niti *et al.*, 2008). The department is also building strengths in research on maternal, child and adolescent mental health, and on rapid diagnosis and treatment for mood disorders. In all of this research, the emphasis is on clinical translation and public health impact. The department has also identified and nurtured new clinician scientists, who can continue with their efforts to advance knowledge in the fields of neuroscience, mind–body medicine and biological psychiatry.

Nurturing the Next Generation

Over the years, the department has helped to train new generations of psychiatrists in Singapore, by contributing to the Basic and Advanced Specialty Training programme, as well as the Residency programme.

The department continues to promote academic learning and clinical skills development amongst psychiatrists and allied health mental health professionals. The undergraduate education team has also taken on a leading role in the design and coordination of the Psychiatry teaching curriculum for the Yong Loo Lin School of Medicine students.

The Way Forward

The team at NUH is excited to explore innovative care solutions, such as e-mental health, new therapies in the form of new drugs, as well as new uses for old drugs. The development of updated, evidence-based clinical protocols is one of the essential elements in ensuring that patients receive high-quality treatment.

The field of Psychiatry in Singapore is rapidly moving forward, with the development of integrated services with community partners and primary care providers. This can be achieved through strong collaboration with the Regional Health System and Agency for Integrated Care. The contribution of academic psychiatry continues to be of great importance in this new health care paradigm.

It is, indeed, beautiful to be a mental health professional.

Acknowledgements

The authors would like to thanks Dr Tsoi Wing Foo, A/Prof Ko Soo Meng, Ms Mary Pui and Mr Michael Olarewaju Ayeni for the references and photographs provided.

References

Chee CY, Lee DT, Chong YS, Tan LK, Ng TP, Fones CS (2005). Confinement and other psychosocial factors in perinatal depression: A transcultural study in Singapore. *J Affect Disord* **89** (1–3): 157–166.

Niti M, Yap KB, Kua EH, Tan CH, Ng TP (2008). Physical, social and productive leisure activities, cognitive decline and interaction with APOE-epsilon4 genotype in Chinese older adults. *Int Psychogeriatr* **11**: 1–15.

Khoo Teck Puat Hospital

Chris CHEOK and CHAN Keen Loong

Pioneering Care in the North

The Khoo Teck Puat Hospital (KTPH) Department of Psychological Medicine (KTPH Psymed) was established in 2010 with the opening of KTPH in Yishun. Being a new department, KTPH Psymed had the opportunity to pioneer new models of care. Serving an existing population of 500,000 and with population growth projected in the future, the challenge was to build a department that could serve the community well.

KTPH Psymed pioneered care in the following ways:

a. Being a pioneer in leveraging on E-Health as a force multiplier;
b. Partnering community agencies to form a network of mental health providers in the north of Singapore;
c. A care model based on outpatient services which served the majority of our patients;
d. Innovative services to help special populations; and
e. Being a corporate member of society by volunteerism.

Community Programmes

KTPH Psymed operationalised one of the two pioneering community mental health services funded by the Agency of Integrated Care (AIC). Known as ASCATs (Assessment and Shared Care Teams), this was named THRIVE. Using a multi-pronged approach, THRIVE used e-cognitive–behavioural therapy, self-help programmes, rapid access clinics and community networks to help the residents of Yishun, Sembawang and Woodlands. In an attempt to reach caregivers and people with mental illness who do not wish to seek help, the THRIVE website tailored content specific to their needs. The website received about 2,000–3,000 unique visitors monthly who read 30,000 to 50,000 pages of content. The website can be viewed at www.thrive.org.sg. Another novel effort to promote health to the public was the use of positive psychology techniques. The programme Achieving Happiness in Singapore has reached over 60,000 people through books, e-books and talks. In recognition of the THRIVE programme, the International Society for Research into Internet Interventions (ISRII) award THRIVE the best presentation of the annual conference in 2014. Audits by the Economist Intelligence Unit commissioned by AIC also found that THRIVE met or exceeded international benchmarks for best practices in community mental health care.

KTPH Psymed has no inpatient facilities and all psychiatric care was provided on an outpatient basis. Leveraging on partnerships with Voluntary Welfare Organisations within the northern region, a comprehensive range of services including home visits, day care, community-based counselling and hospital-based medical care could be delivered. KTPH Psymed also had an integrated service where patients from age 7 to the elderly could be followed up in the same clinic. Clinical services included a child psychiatry service that partnered the REACH-North team, an adult psychiatry service and a geriatric psychiatry service. The SAF (Singapore Armed Forces)-KTPH Psychiatry service was also started to serve NSF with psychological disorders in the northern region of Singapore.

As a responsible corporate member of society, KTPH Psymed supported volunteerism in the department. Members of the team volunteered on various working groups and committees within the Ministry of Social and Family Development and they were a key supporter of the Law Society Criminal Law Assistance Service (CLAS). Under CLAS, KTPH Psymed psychiatrist volunteered to do pro-bono forensic assessments for people facing trial so that justice could be adequately served for those who could not afford to pay for psychiatric assessments.

KTPH Psymed also worked in partnership with the local police force and developed a micro-site to educate policemen about mental health issues in a neighbourhood. KTPH Psymed was recognized by the Ang Mo Kio Police Division for 'Public Spiritedness' in 2013.

Manpower Resources

Dr Christopher Cheok, the founding Head of Department handed over the department to Dr Chan Keen Loong in November 2014. As of September 2016, the department comprises six full-time and one part-time specialists.

Conclusions

As of September 2016, the Alexandra Health System comprises KTPH and the Yishun Community Hospital (YCH). As the Alexandra Health System expands to include the Admiralty Medical Centre (AdMC) in 2017, the Sembawang Primary Care Centre (SPCC) in 2019 and the Woodlands Integrated Health Campus (WIHC) in 2021, the challenge is to integrate mental health services across the different institutions and community partners.

Jurong Health Services: Psychiatry for the West

Michael YONG Kian Hui

When Jurong Health Services (JHS) first took over Alexandra Hospital in 2010, there were many other hospital matters which took priority and required immediate attention. It was therefore understandable that there was no urgency to develop a comprehensive psychiatric service at that time. In August 2010, National University Health System (NUHS) signed a service level agreement with JHS to provide coverage for in-patient psychiatric referrals on alternate mornings, and to run 3 out-patient clinic sessions a week.

By November 2010, with the arrival of JurongHealth's own psychiatrist, Dr Michael Yong, things started to change. This involved the gradual expansion of basic psychiatric services to include coverage of both inpatient referrals and the running of outpatient clinics.

This service, having been established from scratch, and being the "new kid on the block", had its fair share of challenges. The team was fortunate to have Dr Daniel Kwek, a senior consultant psychiatrist, with an impeccable track record both clinically and administratively, join us the following year.

In laying the foundations of the future of psychiatry in Ng Teng Fong General Hospital (NTFGH), we had to rethink how psychiatric services could be delivered in line with the ethos of JurongHealth, without being held back by tradition or "legacy" practices. In light of this, we decided that it was of foremost importance to inculcate a unique identity which would set us apart from existing institutions elsewhere.

Recruitment of manpower began with a strong focus on attracting local-trained psychiatrists, especially at the registrar level. We were making a very unique offer not seen anywhere else which was to allow our advance trainees to kick start their careers early, and to complete their sub-specialty training in the best centers in Singapore. While we were not yet an accredited training institution for psychiatry, our trainees had the privilege of doing psychiatry rotations in Singapore General Hospital, Tan Tock Seng Hospital, Changi General Hospital and the Institute of Mental Health. Best practices from each department were gleaned and incorporated into the core development of future psychiatric services in JurongHealth.

Since its inception, it has been JurongHealth's commitment to bring health into every home, and this includes mental health. We formed a small workgroup focusing on community mental health work and started to network with our future partners, the primary care physicians, in the West. Soon after, we partnered with the Agency for Integrated Care (AIC) and launched the first restructured hospital community mental health team in the west, the GP Partnership Program.

We also built working relations with the NUHS Department of Psychological Medicine, and established a mental health network covering the western region. This aimed to combine the expertise of both institutions to help promote, treat and maintain good mental health for the residents of Western Singapore.

In parallel with our community mental health efforts, we also started developing our intra-hospital capabilities to complement the strengths of our medical and surgical services. This process involved dismantling existing policies which were not working and creating new ones with fresh workflows. Training was conducted for various hospital teams to boost their knowledge and understanding of psychiatric conditions, staff mental health and systemic management of psychiatric emergencies. To date, we have trained clinicians from the medical, surgical and emergency departments, nurses, security officers and medical social workers.

As the service grew, we embarked on setting up our own psychogeriatric service, modeled after CGH's highly successful and comprehensive psychogeriatric services and tailored to fit JurongHealth's values and model of care. This service will meet both the in-patient and out-patient needs of NTFGH, as well as participate in the shared care of geriatric patients in Jurong Community Hospital. The next step will involve partnering with AIC and the respective stakeholders in the community to establish a dementia network in the western region.

Plans are also underway to develop our neuropsychiatric, psychosomatic medicine and psychotherapy services. This would not be possible without the support of our colleagues from the other medical disciplines. We have enjoyed a strong working relationship and trust with the Department of Medicine, forged over the five years during which Psychiatry was a part of the department.

An important issue in forming a new department is career planning for our young psychiatrists. Once a master plan that is aligned with the institution's vision has been established, resources must be set aside to enable our psychiatrists to complete their Health Manpower Development Plan (HMDP) posting. It is also crucial to keep vacancies open for future local-trained psychiatrists, so that we can remain nimble in a competitive manpower situation.

Our current team of eight will be sufficient when we make the move to the new hospital. The delay in the move proved to be a blessing, as it gave us more time to be better prepared. A major aspect of the move entails adapting to a completely new Electronic Medical Records system, which had to be configured for psychiatric work. Much effort went into planning, tweaking and testing before it was deemed operationally ready.

We have remained small in numbers compared to the more established psychiatry departments in other hospitals and this lacking in numbers dictates our need to work harder than our counterparts. There is simply no room to worry about the little things at work if we are to succeed in our goal as a department.

Overall, the journey of psychiatry in JurongHealth had seen its ups and downs. Many of us had to learn new ways of doing things as our brand new hospital was shaping up. Much may be written about what we have already achieved, but I prefer to look forward and draw your attention to the unwritten pages of our future endeavors.

The Birth of Psychiatry in Singapore General Hospital

WAN Yi Min and Leslie LIM

Established merely two years after the founding of Singapore by Sir Stamford Raffles in 1819, the Singapore General Hospital (SGH) is the oldest and largest tertiary hospital in the country. Yet, the origin of Psychiatry in SGH remains a moot point. It appears that the early beginnings of the specialty could be traced back to when SGH was known by another name, the Outram Road General Hospital. This was many years before the present Department of Psychiatry was officially inaugurated.

In 1953, psychiatric outpatient services in Singapore were first introduced in SGH, although these were eventually relocated to other centres in 1967. Moving into the late seventies, specifically 1979, Dr Tsoi Wing Foo (a former medical director of Woodbridge Hospital), who was later joined by Dr Kok Lee Peng, started a University Department of Psychological Medicine at the SGH campus. Under their guidance, the department flourished with other psychiatrists joining them subsequently.

Consultation-liaison work at SGH came under the auspices of the University Department. At that time there was no dedicated psychiatric ward and patients with psychiatric problems had limited access to only a few beds in the medical wards. Psychiatric services were mostly organised around the outpatient clinics.

In July 1985, the University Department of Psychological Medicine shifted from the Faculty of Medicine Building to the old Medical Unit II office at Bowyer Block, continuing to provide consultation-liaison services to all the other departments in SGH. Despite its duties to SGH patients and its location within SGH grounds, it was not considered a bona-fide department of SGH per se, but as part of the fledgling Department of Psychological Medicine of the National University Hospital (NUH). It eventually returned to the main building of NUH on Lower Kent Ridge Road in 1987, with the opening of its 28-bedded ward there.

From then onwards and up until the early years of the 21st century, all aspects of consultation-liaison work at SGH were handled by visiting psychiatrists from the Institute of Mental Health (IMH). A/Prof Teo Seng Hock helmed the SGH psychiatric outpatient clinic for many years, eventually succeeded by Dr Ng Li Ling. She subsequently passed the mantle to Dr Ng Beng Yeong in the year 2000 when she left for the Changi General Hospital (CGH). All urgent psychiatric inpatient referrals were also attended to by visiting consultants from IMH at that time.

In the year 2000, the senior management of SGH realised that, in order to enhance patient care, the hospital needed its own department of Psychiatry. One of the major proponents for this vision was Prof Woo Keng Thye, who was a member of the SGH medical board during that period.

In an interview, Prof Woo spoke about his considerations with regards to spearheadin the venture at SGH: 'The initial arrangement with IMH was not satisfactory, as patients had to wait a long time for the psychiatrists to travel to SGH. Reviews after the initial consult were infrequent and continuity of care was therefore compromised. For patients with suicidal tendencies, we had to send them away to IMH despite their having associated medical conditions which required the expertise of the SGH specialists. As Division Chair for Medicine at that time, I told myself that we must be self-sufficient. We must not rely on other hospitals to provide us with what I consider essential services required by patients coming to SGH. I wanted to develop specialties which we do not have in SGH to complement existing services. Psychiatric Medicine had been one of the earliest on my agenda. How could the largest tertiary hospital in Singapore not have its own Department of Psychiatry? Hospitals which were smaller in scale than SGH already had their own internal psychiatric services.'

Among the first psychiatrists to form the new Department of Psychiatry were A/Prof Leslie Lim, Dr Ng Beng Yeong and Dr Lee Ee Lian. Individually, these psychiatrists have their own specific strengths and interests, and together they laid the foundation upon which the department was built. Established on 1 April 2003, it was originally known as the Department of Behavioural Medicine.

> Its objectives were: '*...to provide more holistic care to patients, by offering a comprehensive, integrated, multidisciplinary service to manage patients with psychological and psychiatric disorders... [and] to support other clinical departments by helping patients manage conditions including anxiety, depression, eating disorders, psychosis, and organic brain disorders.' (SingHealth Annual Report 2003)*

A/Prof Leslie Lim, who was the inaugural Head of the Department, saw the formation of the new department as an excellent opportunity to provide psychiatric services to treat the mentally ill in the nation's flagship hospital. He had always relished new challenges. Indeed, prior to joining SGH, he had been a pioneer in launching community psychiatric services in IMH. In his own words, he had felt that 'SGH desperately needed its own psychiatry department for better continuity, consistency, and accountability of patient care'. He described his initiation into the SGH family as 'an experience difficult to forget', not least because it coincided with the horrifying SARS outbreak in Singapore. Together with the Tan Tock Seng Hospital (TTSH) in 2003, SGH was instrumental in stemming the tide of the SARS epidemic in the country.

Caught in the grip of SARS, SGH shuddered under the pall of death, while the psychiatrists, often forgotten at the sidelines in an epidemic, were called upon to provide solace to grieving family members and staff who had cared for SARS victims. They worked with the psychologists in conducting debriefing groups and providing individual counselling, as well as offering psychiatric treatment whenever necessary. Both A/Prof Leslie Lim and Dr Lee Ee Lian narrated how they were quarantined for at least 10 days due to their proximity and exposure to the families of SARS victims, as well as to the staff who had direct contact with them. It was a particularly difficult time when several of the health care staff at SGH succumbed to SARS as well.

Prof Woo spoke about his observations during that particular period: 'I was most grateful that, at the time [April to June 2003], SGH already had its own Department of Psychiatry on board to cope with the demands for psychosocial help and psychiatric support required by so many, patients and staff alike. The psychiatrists, even though they were all overworked and under great stress (as some had to be quarantined away from home because of their exposure to indexed cases of SARS), somehow managed to rally forth and provide succour to the many afflicted staff members, not to mention patients and some of their relatives as well.'

Initially, the SGH psychiatry office was situated in the Houseman Quarters which is itself located adjacent to the beloved Housemen canteen. The quarters, which were primarily intended for residential use, were converted into offices for certain administrative departments, including the Department of Psychiatry.

'The smell of food welcomed you whenever you exited the building. As it was located in the lower floor of the split-level building, entering the office meant that one had to descend a flight of ancient rickety stairs, built to allow only one lean person to use at any one time,' recounted A/Prof Lim in a nostalgic moment. 'There were only three psychiatrists and one full-time psychologist in the team serving the 1,500-bed hospital. We attended to around 12 to 17 inpatient referrals from other departments daily, with the busiest periods occurring on Mondays and after public holidays.' Eventually, the psychiatry headquarters shifted to level 2 of Bowyer Block, and then finally to level 3 of the Academia Building in June 2013.

At first, psychiatric inpatient services were limited to only five beds in Ward 64, carved out from the Rehabilitation Medicine ward during this period. Recognising the urgent need for an inpatient unit tailored specifically to cater to patients with psychiatric disorders, the administrators helped to search for a suitable space to house the psychiatric ward. For this purpose, part of ward 46, then occupied by Endocrinology and Gastroenterology patients, was renovated and renamed Ward 46A.

After refurbishments, it was officially opened on 18 February 2005. Although the 15-bedded ward was not considered large by general hospital standards, it meant that at least there was a place where a committed team of trained staff could attend to those with psychiatric problems. The multidisciplinary team included the psychiatrists, the nursing staff as well as the allied health professionals. Initially there were no psychiatrically trained nurses. After the nursing staff sent for formal training in psychiatric nursing returned with tertiary qualifications, it marked a key milestone in the development of psychiatric care of the mentally ill in SGH.

Another defining moment in SGH psychiatry history was when the appellation 'Department of Behavioural Medicine' was formally changed to 'Department of Psychiatry'. In an effort to combat stigma, the SGH psychiatrists felt that the word 'Psychiatry' should be borne proudly by those who served in its name. As Dr Lee Ee Lian reflected, 'I have always felt that we should be apologists, not apologetic.' SGH is therefore the first restructured hospital to title its psychiatric department 'The Department of Psychiatry'.

One of the key services offered by the Department is the landmark Eating Disorder (ED) Programme, established by Dr Lee Ee Lian in 2003 under the Singapore National Mental Health Plan, a government-funded initiative. 'Patients with eating disorders are best treated in a general hospital, due to the myriad of medical complications associated with the illness. It was my primary reason for starting the programme at SGH,' she explained when asked regarding her views during those early days.

When it was launched in July 2003, the programme outline was rudimentary at best, initially offered only on an outpatient basis, before expanding to inpatient service once Ward 46A was opened. At first the team consisted only of Dr Lee, the ED specialist, along with a psychologist (Ms Evelyn Boon), and a family therapist (Ms Anita Foo). During the SARS outbreak, the team decided that for the sake of minimising the risk of infection, ED inpatients and outpatients who were attending the ED Programme should not mingle in the event of possible future epidemics, which meant that a dedicated space was needed for treatment of patients with eating disorders.

Thus began numerous meetings and discussions between the department and the senior management of SGH as well as the administrators of the SingHealth cluster, all of whom Dr Lee described as 'incredibly supportive of the ED programme'. The Bowyer Block, despite being ramshackle at the time and said to 'house mostly moulding mattresses and rusting metal bits', was recognised as an appropriate location. 'But the space was large and it would be a waste for it to only cater to patients with ED,' Dr. Lee explained. 'We decided that its use should be expanded to include the treatment of patients afflicted with illnesses which were largely related to lifestyle issues.' Acknowledging the potential of the Bowyer Block to become a one-stop centre for patients requiring lifestyle intervention, the ED team partnered with the Department of Endocrinology to help implement this project.

And so, it came about that the SGH Lifestyle Improvement Fitness Enhancement (LIFE) Centre was officially opened in 2008. It was described as one of the proudest moments for the ED team. Dr Lee Ee Lian, who was the founding Clinical Director of the LIFE Centre, personally ensured that there were individual rooms tailored especially for the use of each allied health professional during patient consultations. In particular, the kitchen, fitted specifically for the treatment of patients with eating disorders, was a source of pride and joy. The Centre offers not only the services of the ED Programme, but also that of Obesity Management, Bariatric Surgery, Lipid and Metabolic Programme, Osteoporosis and Bone Metabolism Programme, as well as Lifestyle Modification Programmes.

In 2004, Dr Lee Huei Yen joined SGH, and eventually took over the mantle of Director of the Eating Disorders Programme from Dr Lee Ee Lian in 2008. Over the past decade, the ED Programme scaled even greater heights. Not only did it flourish into a renowned national programme, it also expanded into a regional one, serving the needs of all who were afflicted with eating disorders.

Dr Ng Beng Yeong was appointed to the Headship of the Department on 1 July 2006, succeeding A/Prof Leslie Lim. Under his guidance, the Department of Psychiatry expanded in multiple directions. With a keen interest in Organic Psychiatry and Neuropsychiatry, he ran clinic sessions in the Sleep Disorders Unit (SDU), as well as in the Urology Centre where he treated patients with sexual concerns. A/Prof Leslie Lim is himself a visiting consultant to the Department of Palliative Medicine at the National Cancer Centre. Dr Sin Gwen Li, a consultant psychiatrist, has a special interest in the mental health needs of the elderly. Another consultant psychiatrist, Dr Chan Herng Nieng, attends to the care of patients at the Pain Management Centre and at the Obstetrics and Gynaecology Centre in SGH.

With the advent of the Duke-NUS Graduate Medical School in 2007 on a site adjacent to SGH, training and research in psychiatry progressed at an even greater rate. A/Prof Lee Tih Shih, a Visiting Consultant at the Department of Psychiatry at SGH, is a principal investigator in the Neuroscience and Behavioural Disorders Programme at the school. With the collaboration between SGH and Duke-NUS, research relating particularly to Neuropsychiatry advanced into new and exciting areas. For instance, one of A/Prof Lee's projects involved using Brain–Computer Interface systems to treat patients with Attention-Deficit/Hyperactivity Disorder (ADHD), as well as to support cognitive rehabilitation in the elderly.

As more psychiatrists joined the ranks of the department, new services were developed. Since 2009, for instance, SGH has started an early intervention programme for the management of anxiety and depression among patients with irritable bowel syndrome (IBS), as part of the National Mental Health Blueprint (NMHB) 2007–2012 in Singapore. The SGH psychiatrists and gastroenterologists worked together in an integrated, multidisciplinary approach in the treatment of these patients.

In light of the shifting focus from institutional to community psychiatric care, the SGH–General Practitioner (GP) partnership programme was introduced at the beginning of 2013. Its main purpose is to transfer patients who are in stable condition to the care of GPs in the community, for improved accessibility, convenience and cost-effectiveness.

Prof Woo described his vision for the future of SGH psychiatry thus: 'I would like to see it eventually burgeon into a regional centre for

Psychiatry with a full array of related services. We need to continue to build the eating disorders unit and to develop geriatric psychiatry to cater to immediate needs. Our staff at all levels, from doctors to paramedical staff need to have dual appointments for teaching and research with Duke-NUS so that they can catch the headwind of academia and propel the Department into the future. We need to recruit and train clinician scientists. Interested staff should be encouraged to engage in research. It is through teaching and research that we advance in our onward journey to achieving first-world excellence in the delivery of Psychiatric medicine. Our main focus should be in the development of staff capability and progress. We may have the buildings and necessary infrastructure, but without human capital, new ideas and technology to harness the resources of the new millennium, we will lack the wherewithal for our voyage into the future.'

Conclusion

From the brief chronicle depicted above, it is evident that the Department of Psychiatry has come a considerable way from its humble origins over a decade ago. Despite encountering numerous hurdles along its journey, there have been various accolades received by the Department and its staff. With its main focus on a few key areas in Psychiatry, such as eating disorders, psycho-oncology, neuropsychiatry and sleep disorders, the Department seeks to continue developing its services in SGH and ultimately advance the cause of Psychiatry in Singapore.

Acknowledgements

The authors wish to offer their special thanks to Prof Woo Keng Thye, Emeritus Consultant and Advisor, SGH Department of Renal Medicine, for his efforts in convincing the hospital management of the necessity to set up the department of Psychiatry, and for his unwavering support of the work of our Department. We are also immensely grateful to A/Prof Ng Beng Yeong, Senior Consultant and incumbent Head of

Department, for his valuable contribution regarding the formation of the department of Psychiatry at SGH. Our warmest appreciation also goes to Dr Lee Ee Lian, Visiting Consultant and former Director of the SGH Eating Disorders Programme, for providing insights into the advent of the Eating Disorder programme and the inauguration of LIFE centre. Thanks also to Ms Evelyn Boon, Principal Clinical Psychologist in SGH, for supplying the photographs; and to Ms Toby Huynh, curator of the SGH museum, for granting us access to archival information.

References

Institute of Mental Health (2007). National Mental Health Blueprint Singapore. 2007–2012. Available at: https://www.imh.com.sg/uploadedFiles/Publications/IMH%20National%20Mental%20Health%20Blueprint.pdf

Kua EH (2004). Focus on psychiatry in Singapore. *Br J Psychiatry* **185**: 79–82.

Lee HY, Hoodbhoy Z (2013). You are worth more than what you weigh: Preventing eating disorders. Ann Acad Med **42**(2): 64–65.

Lum WMA *et al.* (2010). The successful collaboration between psychiatrists, a mental health institution, and general practitioners in primary care. *Singapore Fam Physician* **36**(4): 19–20.

Ng BY (2000). *Till the Break of Day: A History of Mental Health Services in Singapore, 1841–1993*. Singapore University Press, Singapore.

The SGH Newsroom — news clippings 2003–2012 and press releases of the Mind-Body Link.

Singapore General Hospital 50th anniversary publication 1926–1976.

Singapore General Hospital. Annual Reports 2003–2012. Available at: https://www.sgh.com.sg/about-us/newsroom/pages/annual-reports.aspx

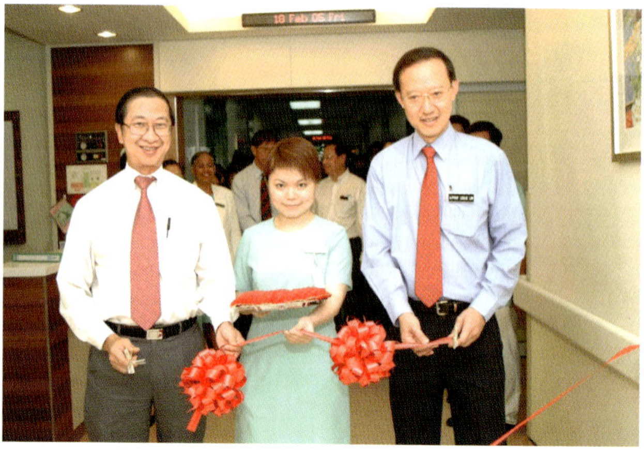

Prof Tan Ser Kiat (left) and A/Prof Leslie Lim (right) at the opening ceremony of Ward 46A in 2005 (Photo credit: Ms Evelyn Boon).

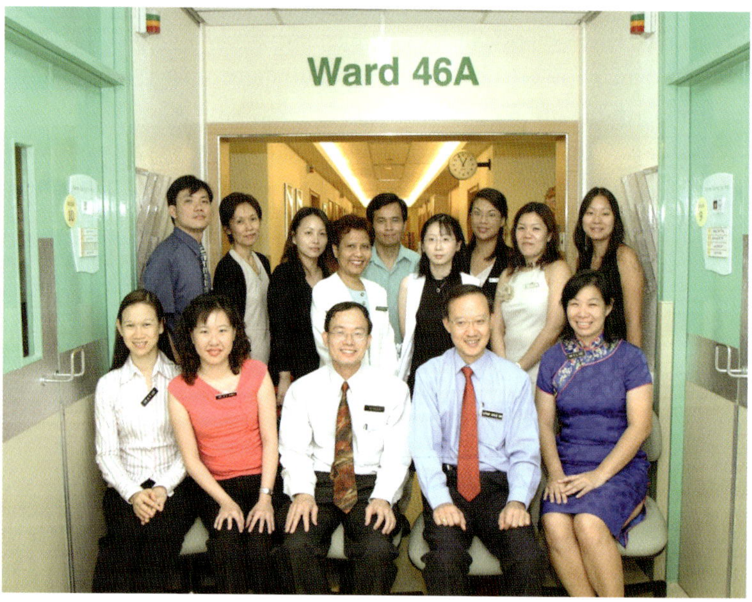

The Psychiatric team at the official opening of Ward 46A. (Seated from left to right): Dr Goh Yen Li, Dr. Lee Huei Yen, A/Prof Ng Beng Yeong, A/Prof Leslie Lim, Dr Lee Ee Lian (Photo credit: Ms Evelyn Boon).

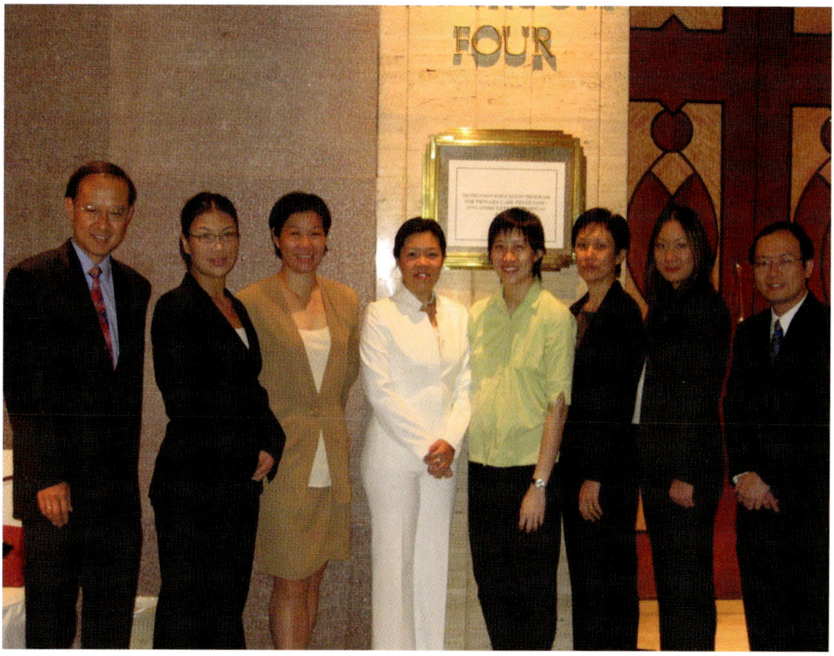

The Psychiatric team at the first public forum on depression organised by SGH on 3 August 2003. (From left to right) A/Prof Leslie Lim, Ms Evangeline Tan, Dr Lee Ee Lian, Ms. Evelyn Boon, Dr Tham Wai Yong, Ms Janis Lim, Ms Esther Tan, A/Prof Ng Beng Yeong (Photo credit: Ms Evelyn Boon).

A Brief History of the Department of Psychological Medicine, Tan Tock Seng Hospital

Aaron ANG Lye Poh

In the Beginning

In 1982, the Singapore Government Health Plan mooted the decentralising of mental health treatment (*The Straits Times*, 1985). Prior to this, all mental illness was treated solely at Woodbridge Hospital. Unfortunately, over the years, the stigma of mental illness resulted in people being reluctant to be treated there. As the stigma of mental illness not only affected its sufferers but also the mental healthcare workers, another objective of setting up an off-site psychiatric unit was to reintegrate the community of psychiatrists into the larger medical fraternity.

In December 1985, the Ministry of Health (MOH), Singapore, announced plans for a psychiatric unit to be set up outside the premises of Woodbridge Hospital. This unit would be a self-contained service to treat patients with mild psychiatric illnesses, such as depression, obsessions, hysteria, phobias and even mild schizophrenia (*The Straits Times*, 1985; 1986). The unit would provide not only inpatient services, but outpatient services (twice weekly, Wednesdays and Saturday morning clinics) as well as day care facilities. Patients were expected to stay for a much shorter period of 3 to 6 weeks, compared to the months or even years that patients were spending at Woodbridge Hospital.

The Tan Tock Seng Hospital (TTSH) was earmarked for this revolutionary project and renovation work was started in February 1986. On 1 August 1986 (*The Business Times*, 1986), the 24-bed inpatient psychiatric unit at TTSH was officially opened. TTSH thus became the first general hospital in Singapore with specialised capabilities to treat patients with mental illness other than the academic psychological medicine unit at the National University. Of particular significance was that both male and female patients were housed within the same ward which is unusual in modern psychiatric facilities throughout the world. This was the first mixed ward in Singapore, and it paved the way for the acceptance of mixed wards in the future.

Ward 13 was a part of a cluster of pavilion wards annexed a short distance from the TTSH main building and these wards were affectionately known as the 'Siberia wards'. It used to be a ward for patients who suffered from tuberculosis. It was specially selected because it was a single storey, stand-alone building with a small compound. This extra space was required for recreation, dining as well as group therapy that were essential for the treatment of mentally ill patients. Initially, the psychiatrists and psychologist who worked in the unit were seconded from Woodbridge Hospital. The pioneering team comprised Dr Ong Thiew Chai (*The Straits Times*, 1985) who headed the unit (part-time), together with Dr Yeo Seem Huat (psychiatrist, full-time) and Ms Alice Yeoh (psychologist, who is presently the head, Psychological Services, TTSH). At that time, manpower, resources and funding were limited. Even though psychiatric units in general hospitals were already present internationally in the 1980s, the Department of Psychological Medicine, TTSH was among the first of such units in Singapore. Therefore, local guidelines had to be carefully drafted for the management of psychiatric patients in the acute general hospital (in August 1985) and specifically, TTSH (in October 1987). The pioneering team had its work cut out for it, as it had to move away from the comfort zone of practicing psychiatry in a large institution (i.e. Woodbridge Hospital) to a new paradigm, where psychiatric patients were managed in an acute general hospital, in a consultation liaison setting, i.e. with other physicians and surgeons and in the community. Though this entailed taking a step into the unknown, there were bold plans to incorporate psychiatric facilities and services into the redevelopment of TTSH (*The Business Times*, 1987).

Developing Services

The years from 1986 to 1993 were when the Department was finding its feet in terms of developing new services and consolidating manpower. Dr Tay Woo Kheng, Consultant Psychiatrist, joined the Department in 1988 and was also instrumental to the Department in its formative years, strengthening the foundations. Some of the psychiatrists who spent their formative years in TTSH during this period included: Dr Ng Li Ling (then a Registrar, 1990–1991), Dr Chong Siow Ann (then a Medical Officer Trainee, 1990) and Dr Chua Hong Choon (then a Medical Officer Trainee, 1992). Dr Ng Li Ling is now a Senior Consultant in Changi General Hospital (CGH), and is generally acknowledged as a pioneer of Old Age Psychiatry in Singapore. A/Prof Chong Siow Ann is now the Vice-Chairman, Medical Board, Institute of Mental Health (IMH) and the leading researcher in Psychiatry in Singapore, while A/Prof Chua Hong Choon currently serves as IMH's Chief Executive Officer.

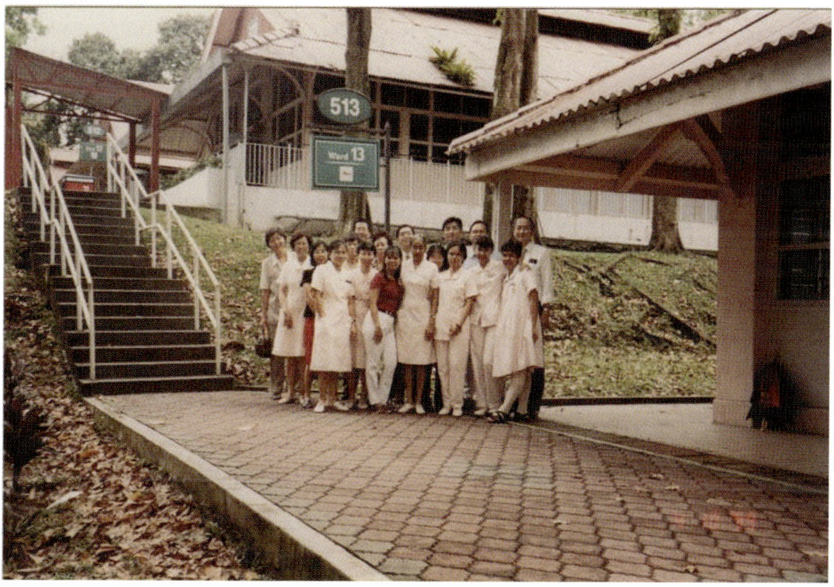

Staff of Ward 13, Department of Psychological Medicine, TTSH.

In 1998, A/Prof Ong crafted the mission statement of the Department to enshrine the dual purpose of the Department: to provide specialist psychiatric services in the community, as well as provide psychiatric support for the medical and surgical departments in the TTSH.

Even today, the core duty of the Department reflects this abiding mission. The goals, as encompassed in the mission statement are to:

- Provide a comprehensive psychiatric service at TTSH;
- Develop with and in support of the other medical/surgical departments in TTSH;
- Make the Department a niche for itself in psychiatry;
- Involve in teaching, training and research, in imparting knowledge, skills; and
- Achieve the highest moral, ethical and professional standards in patient care.

The Department's clinical workload increased significantly from its humble beginnings in 1986. In 1987, it started with 1,732 outpatient visits, of which 211 were new cases. A total of 419 consultation-liaison referrals were received. In 1993, there was a more than four-fold increase to 6,000 outpatient visits, of which about 8% (469) were new cases. There were more than 700 consultation-liaison psychiatry referrals. By 1997, outpatient visits had grown to more than 8,000 outpatient visits and 542 were new cases. There were more than 1,253 consultation-liaison psychiatry referrals in 1997.

Through this period, the Department was functioning with similar psychiatrist staffing as when they first started in 1986 (i.e. two Consultant Psychiatrists, one part-time, and a Registrar who was seconded from Woodbridge Hospital).

It was apparent that further manpower was needed. In 1996, A/Prof Ong joined the Department full-time. In 1997, Dr Low Bee Lee (1997–2007) joined the Department as its third Consultant Psychiatrist. The Department realised that it needed to recruit and groom purpose-trained consultants for the Department. As such, in the same year, Dr Daniel

Kwek Seow Khee (1997–2011) joined the Department as a Registrar. Dr Chan Keen Loong joined the Department as a second Registrar in 1998 (1998–2006). To bolster the clinical expertise and mentorship, private psychiatrists Dr Kok Lee Peng and Dr Tay Liam Kai joined the Department as Visiting Consultants (VCs) in 1999 (and are still VCs to this day). Dr Chew Wuen Ming, Nicholas and Dr Tang Hui Kheng (2001–2007) joined the Department as Registrars in 2001.

A/Prof Ong oversaw the transition from old TTSH to the new building in 1999. He was Head of Department from 1 August 1986 to 31 July 2002 (i.e. 16 years). During this period, senior clinicians in the Department received further overseas specialist training under the Health Manpower Development Plan (HMDP). Dr Low Bee Lee spent three months in 1999 in a fellowship programme for Depression at the University of Texas, Southwestern Medical Centre, Dallas, Texas; Dr Chan Keen Loong spent 12 months in 2000 to 2001 in a fellowship programme for Neuropsychiatry at the University of Iowa's Health Care and Department of Psychiatry, College of Medicine, Iowa; while Dr Kwek Seow Khee, Daniel spent 12 months in 2001 to 2002 in a fellowship for Psychosomatic Medicine at both the University of Manchester, UK and Rikshospitalet, Univesrilectsklinikk in Norway.

Severe Acute Respiratory Syndrome

Dr Low Bee Lee took over the headship from A/Prof Ong Thiew Chai, and was head from 1 August 2002 to 31 July 2006. Less than a year after she was appointed head, SARS (severe acute respiratory syndrome) hit Singapore with patient zero being admitted to TTSH on 1 March 2003. The country was in the grip of this medical crisis, with TTSH, having been designated as the SARS hospital, in the eye of the storm.

The frontline health care workers were fighting this deadly disease on two fronts: not only were they battling to save patients from the virus, but they were also labouring under tremendous psychological stress, having witnessed comrades infected with, and felled by the disease. The Department recognised the hidden emotional battle and worked behind the scenes to address the psychological needs of all the hospital staff (Kwek *et al.*, 2004).

The Department was recognized for their tireless efforts. Dr Low Bee Lee received the Commendation Medal (National Day Award) in 2003, while Dr Ong Thiew Chai, Dr Chan Keen Loong, Dr Daniel Kwek Seow Khee, Dr Nicholas Chew Wuen Ming and Dr Tang Hui Kheng received the Courage Star Award (Courage Fund) (Ng, 2004). As a result of SARS, the peer support groups were started, and have continued till today to support staff under emotional stress.

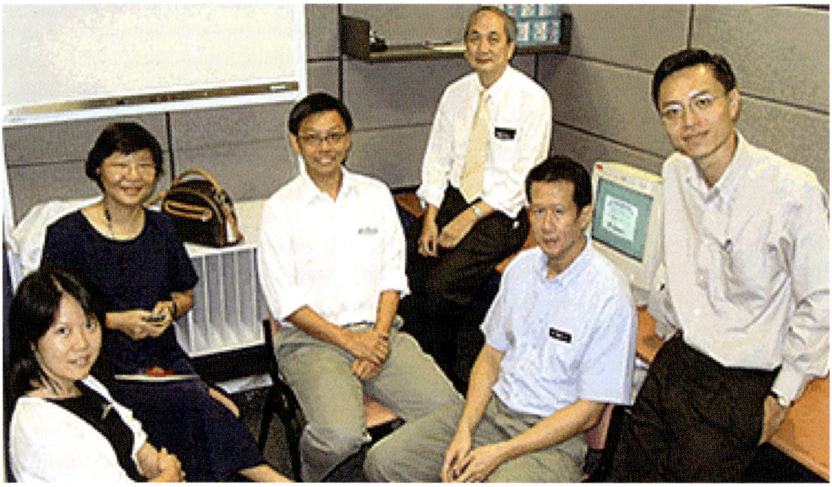

Department of Psychological Medicine, TTSH during SARS. (From left to right) Dr Tang Hui Kheng, Dr Low Bee Lee, Dr Chew Wuen Ming, Nicholas, A/Prof Ong Thiew Chai, Dr Chan Kheng Loong, Dr Daniel Kwek Seow Khee.

In her time as head, Dr Low had overseen the Suicide Prevention Programme, where the hospital underwent a systemic and extensive retrofitting, at significant financial cost, to reduce opportunities for patients to attempt suicide.

In August 2005, TTSH achieved accreditation by the Joint Commission International (JCI). The Department developed guidelines for quality and safety for procedures like Electroconvulsive Therapy, Usage of the Quiet (Seclusion) Room, etc.

Under the HMDP, Dr Nicholas Chew Wuen Ming spent 12 months in 2005 in a fellowship programme for Psychotherapy in General Hospital Practice at McGill University, Montreal, Québec in Canada.

Mental Health Blueprints and Other Programmes

Dr Daniel Kwek Seow Khee headed the Department from 1 August 2006 to 31 March 2011. During this period, Dr Tham Wai Yong and Dr Jaspal Singh joined the Department as Registrars in 2006 and 2007, respectively. In 2008, Dr Lynette Teoh Si Jing, Dr Kwan Yunxin and Dr Lynnette Tan Pei Lin joined the Department as Registrars. In 2009, Dr Chan Lai Gwen joined the Department as Registrar. In that same year, Dr Ang Lye Poh, Aaron and Dr Habeebul Rahman joined the Department as Consultant and Associate Consultant, respectively.

With the acknowledgement that there cannot be health without mental health, the National Mental Health Blueprint (NMHB) was formulated in 2007. The Department of Psychological Medicine, TTSH supported the NMHB by contributing two Integrated Hospital Teams: the HIV Psychiatry Programme and the Effective Mood Management after Stroke (EMMAS) Programme.

The HIV Psychiatry Programme sees a collaboration between the Departments of Psychological Medicine and Infectious Diseases, TTSH. Patients who were diagnosed with HIV were screened and managed for mental health issues. The programme has screened and managed more than 600 HIV patients to date. To better manage the programme, under the HMDP, Dr Jaspal Singh spent six months in 2012 in a fellowship programme in Conssultation Liaison and HIV Psychiatry, St. Vincent's Hospital, Sydney, Australia.

The EMMAS Programme sees the collaboration between the Departments of Psychological Medicine and Rehabilitation Medicine, TTSH, where patients suffering from acute stroke are screened and managed for depression. The programme has screened and managed more than 2,000 stroke patients to date.

The Peer-Support Peer groups, which had started de novo after SARS, were formalised during this period into the Staff-Support-Staff (3S) Programme. Dr Chan Oi Mei, Angelina (Consultant Psychiatrist, CGH) has supported the Department by providing training under the CGH Psychosocial Trauma Team, a NMHB Programme. The Psychological Services was also instrumental in the success of this programme.

In the same year, planning for the National Psychiatry Residency Programme was underway. The Department of Psychological Medicine was to be a training site for Inpatient Psychiatry Rotation, Consultation-Liaison Psychiatry Rotation, Continuity Clinic and Psychotherapy Rotation as well as Elective Rotations. Dr Nicholas Chew Wuen Ming and Dr Aaron Ang Lye Poh represented the Department in contributing to the planning and development of the National Programme. The Department received its first Psychiatry Resident, Dr Joshua Nah, in November 2010.

The Next Lap

Dr Aaron Ang Lye Poh took over the headship from Dr Daniel Kwek Seow Khee in April 2011. Dr Chan Yuen Sze and Dr Rochelle Kinson joined the Department as Registrars in 2011. In 2012, Dr Jason Lee Kim Huat and Dr Vanessa Mok Wai Ling worked as Registrars in the department from 2012 to 2015.

By this time (2011–2014), outpatient visits had grown to more than 15,000 patient-visits per year, with about 10% being new cases. In keeping with the tradition of TTSH being the pauper's hospital, 90% of its outpatients are subsidised by the Government. With the growth and development of the general hospital, consultation-liaison referrals have grown exponentially to more than 4,000 cases per year (most of them being subsidised).

The Department is presently (as of the end of 2014) 12-Specialist strong. The transitions across the past decade are nothing short of remarkable. However, the challenges ahead are equally daunting. Clinical workload is projected to remain high, given the aging population, as well as increased awareness and reduced stigma of mental illness.

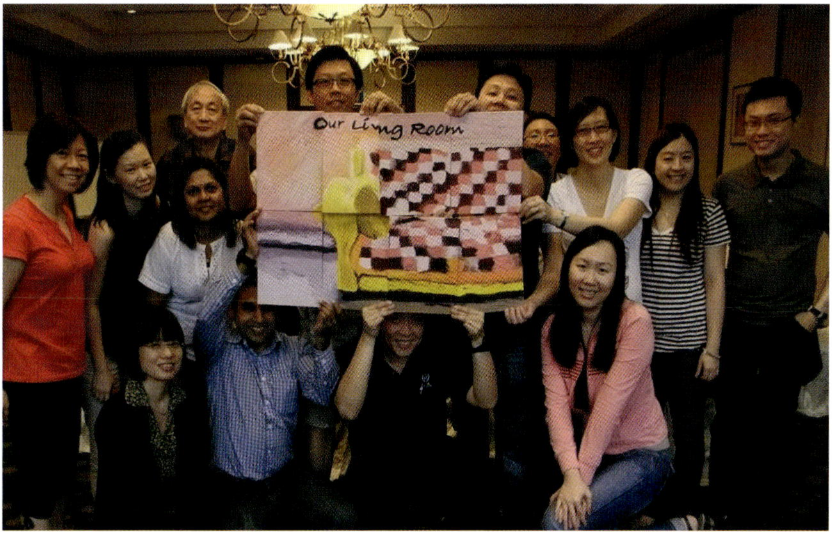

Departmental of Psychological Medicine Retreat, 2012.

Apart from the traditional medical education provided to the ever-increasing numbers of undergraduates at the Yong Loo Lin School of Medicine (YLLSoM), National University of Singapore (NUS), there are new and escalating demands on the Department. In the coming years, TTSH is positioning itself to develop into a centre of clinical and academic excellence. With the gradual gearing up of the Accreditation Counsel Graduate Medical Counsel-International (ACGME-I) Residency Programmes as well as Lee Kong Chian School of Medicine (LKC-Medicine) at the Nanyang Technological University (NTU), the Department will have to increase commitments to both medical education, as well as clinical research.

With the challenges of rising health care cost and retaining increasingly mobile clinicians by matching their aspirations, the Department needs new and innovative ways of delivering excellent psychiatric service for those under its care. In a sense, the Department has come full circle. With the pioneering spirit of the 1980s, it is again compelled to take that lead into this new frontier.

Acknowledgements

I would like to express my heartfelt thanks to A/Prof Ong Thiew Chai, Dr Low Bee Lee, Dr Daniel Kwek Seow Khee and Dr Nicholas Chew Wuen Ming for being witness to the history of the Department of Psychological Medicine, TTSH and so graciously sharing it with me (verbally, in writing and in historical materials) for the writing of this chapter. I hope I have been able to capture the struggles and joys accurately as you journeyed with the Department over the past many years.

References

Kwek SKD, *et al.* (2004). The psychological impact of SARS on healthcare providers. *Crit Care Shock* **7**: 99–106.

Ng WC (2004). *The Silent War: 1 March–31 May 2003*. Tan Tock Seng Hospital, Singapore, pp. 4–5.

The Business Times, 30 July 1986. 'Psychiatric unit to open next month', p. 2.

The Business Times, 16 March 1987. 'Government plans to provide more services for mentally-ill patients', p. 16.

The Straits Times, 29 December 1985. 'Removing the stigma of Woodbridge Hospital', p. 10.

The Straits Times, 25 July 1986. 'Tan Tock Seng to start unit for mild mental cases', p. 15.

Psychiatry Services at KK Women's and Children's Hospital

Helen CHEN Yu

Introduction of Psychiatry to KKH

The main maternity hospital in Singapore is a grand dame of 159 years in 2017. Past generations were delivered at the KK Women's and Children's Hospital (KKH), otherwise colloquially known as '*Zu Jiao Yi Yuan*'. In 1992, the maternity hospital moved from its old building located where now the Land Transport Authority (LTA) sits, to occupy the women's tower of the spanking new building across the road, along Bukit Timah Road. The children's hospital also came together at the same time, with all the various paediatric units from other hospitals coming in to form a single unit. Thus began the modern era of KKH.

The core obstetric and paediatric services soon created the need for psychiatric support, understandably as emotional and psychological issues were not uncommon in these populations. In the 1990s, KKH bought services from the Institute of Mental Health (IMH) for perinatal psychiatric support — Dr Pauline Sim, former consultant psychiatrist at IMH with special interest in perinatal psychiatry, would provide a session of ambulatory clinic service as well as blue-letter consultative-liaison service. She was instrumental in developing local interest in the area, having taught batches of trainees, including myself. Similarly, paediatric psychiatric services were provided by Dr Sharon Chan, former consultant child and adolescent psychiatrist at IMH, who too, has taught and inspired generations of psychiatric trainees, and to this day remains involved in teaching. In the late 1990s, she passed the baton to Dr Ng Koon Hock, child and adolescent psychiatrist in private practice, and he fronted the psychiatric needs of the children's hospital at KKH, running a short-term care and triage service, which was necessary with the limited resources over the next 15 years.

In 2005, Dr Pauline Sim, having already supported the service for 15 years, requested for a departure from the service to devote and focus more time to build her own private practice. IMH was approached to provide alternative support, and I was assigned to take over her role, after having just returned from an overseas fellowship in Nottingham, UK, in the area of perinatal psychiatry. The potential of developing a dedicated women's mental health service was soon apparent, and the pent-up needs clearly identified. Dr Pauline Sim had laid a good foundation for the women's hospital to recognise and be open to psychiatric care, and there was much support from the medical board to set up such a service. Furthermore, it was clear that peripartum women would hesitate to go to IMH, because of the stigma of severe mental illness, and the distance from their obstetric care — as such it was ineffective running a perinatal psychiatric service at IMH as the patients would present too late in their illness course. The timing was right: in July 2005, former Health Minister, Mr Khaw Boon Wan announced plans to expand KKH's role in women's healthcare services. With that, a dedicated women's mental health service was set up in May 2006.

KKH Mental Wellness Service (2006–2012)

Under the leadership of former Chief Executive Officer of KKH, Prof Ivy Ng, the fledgling service started mainly as a perinatal psychiatric service, catering largely to women with peripartum-onset disorders such as antepartum depression and anxiety, postpartum depression and anxiety, puerperal psychosis. Very quickly, with recognition of the special expertise, referrals would come in from other psychiatric units for management of women with pre-existing mental illness needing preconception counselling or antepartum management. Additional caseload included women with pregnancy loss issues, infertility and psychosexual problems. As the nature of the work in obstetric consultation-liaison psychiatry often involved challenges relating to ethical and moral issues, these would soon feature as a prominent component of casework. Apart from the perinatal psychiatric caseload, referrals were also received from oncology services for psychological disorders related to breast and gynaecological cancers, pain specialists, as well as the paediatric hospital for mothers of paediatric patients.

Mental Wellness Service — Pop or Real?

At the KKH medical board meeting in late 2005, when the feasibility of the new service was presented, senior members had argued for a patient-centric and acceptable name — thus was decided the name of Mental Wellness Service (MWS), suggested by Prof Chay Oh Moh, former Chairperson, Division of Medicine, KKH. This would later prove to be quite noticeable to the wider medical community and the public, although the psychiatric collegiate took a while to embrace this, something that would make me feel a little dissonant. Indeed, because of the concept of mental wellness, referrals for care were more willingly accepted by women, who would normally decline because of the stigma of psychiatric treatment. The 'mental wellness' title also soon proved to be quite acceptable, and similarly adopted for programmes and initiatives by other organisations. Thus KKH's MWS was born, on 1 May 2005, with a tiny inception team of one part-time consultant psychiatrist, one case manager and an executive administrative staff. A community psychiatric nurse would have been ideal resource, but it was challenging filling the position. A visiting consultant filled one session and provided cover when the lead psychiatrist was on leave. Despite the miniscule team, the service took off quickly. By October 2006, the KKH's MWS constituted two arms: the Women's Mental Wellness Service (WMWS) and the Child and Adolescent Mental Wellness Service (CAMWS). Although the latter really still consisted of the brave and lone Dr Ng Koon Hock, there was now a collective psychiatric presence in the hospital.

Early achievements and collaborations which helped the new service build its identity included developing the Carers' Support Network, a frontline peer counselling support system for staff, together with Prof Lim Sok Bee, former Head, Department of Child Development, KKH, who had championed the idea and lent her credibility in supporting the initial setup. This would in later years be handed over to the Peer Support Programme, which was funded under the National Mental Health Blueprint (NMHB), championed by Dr Angelina Chan of Changi General Hospital (CGH); this remains an ongoing programme, fronted by KKH medical social workers, which proved a better fit because of the concerns with stigma with mental health services, something that remains entrenched in our culture. Another notable achievement was the very first public forum on postnatal depression, held in Nov 2006, which brought much publicity to the new service.

Case management was the key model borrowed from the IMH Early Psychosis Intervention Programme (EPIP), and had never been used before in a perinatal mental health setting. As obstetric care is largely centred on medical interventions with advancing healthcare services in Singapore, this provided the means to cater to the emotional needs of peripartum women, who are particularly vulnerable at this time. Such a role would otherwise be filled by midwives and perhaps health visitors in other countries like the UK and Australia, as was also available in Singapore in the 1950s with domiciliary maternity services. Thus the MWS case manager formed an important link between psychiatrist and patient, providing support and continuity of care throughout the peripartum period, especially through phone counselling and monitoring of high risk mothers. Ms Ch'ng Ying Chia, Senior Case Manager, was instrumental in leading the development of perinatal mental health case management, and has been the longest serving staff since 2006.

It was with the Ministry of Health (MOH) NMHB funding that MWS really grew in 2008. Securing a grant of half a million under the Integrated Hospital mental health initiative, the Postnatal Depression Intervention Programme (PNDIP) kick-started in April 2008 with an additional headcount, increasing the manpower three-fold from the original number. Embedded in obstetric outpatient services, the programme provided free screening for postnatal depression for some 2,000 women annually, with key aims to identify cases early for intervention. The PNDIP provided a framework for the growth and development of the psychiatric services at KKH, creating a greater awareness and acceptance of mental healthcare, with wider reach into all other disciplines.

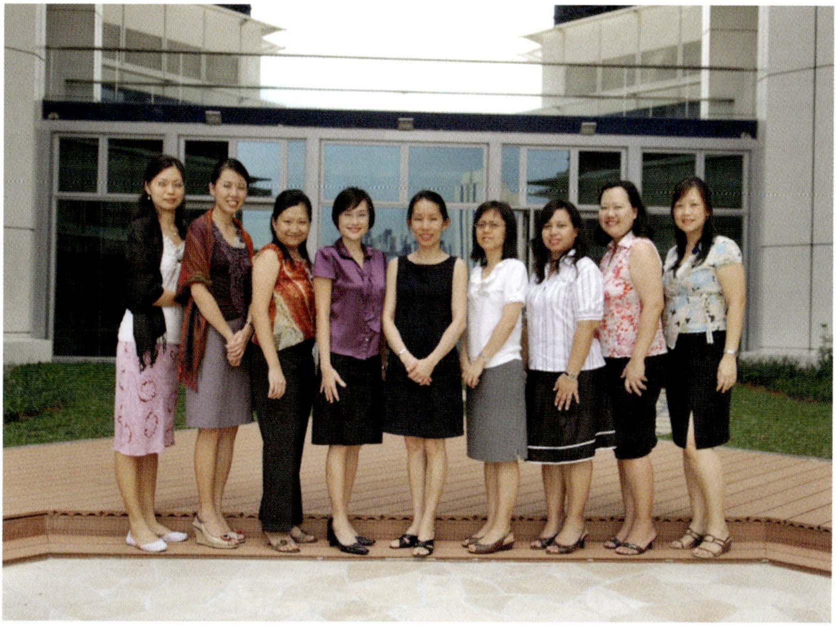

The team which set up the PNDIP in 2008. *From L to R*: Ms Susan Goh, Ms Jemie Wang, Ms Ch'ng Ying Chia, Dr Theresa Lee, Dr Helen Chen, Ms Lim Bee Moy, Ms Roshayati Mingoo, Dr Loretta Ang, and Ms Julia Ong.

By 2009, with increasing headcount, psycho-oncology services also developed, most notably through art as a modality of healing. The self-funding heART programme, under the direction of Dr Choo Chih Huei, Head and Senior Consultant, MWS, KKH, provided a means for cancer patients to explore their emotions through art expression, and find mutual support as they journeyed with cancer.

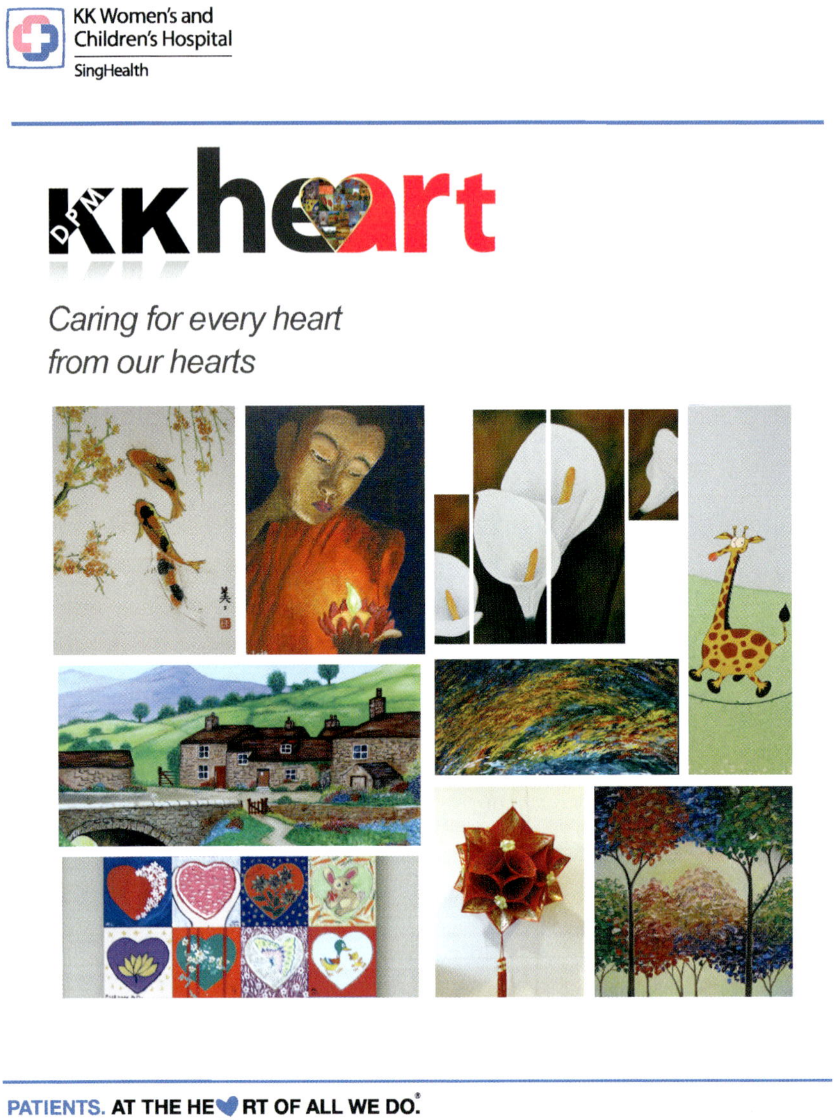

The KKheART Programme.

Becoming Department of Psychological Medicine, KKH

Even as MWS grew, it seemed apparent that the woman needed her child to grow. For indeed, WMWS was a full and stable service by 2010, CAMWS consisted of just the visiting consultant alone. An opportunity came in 2011, when IMH approached KKH to take over the east team of a school-based national child and adolescent mental health programme. An agreement was made for IMH to second a senior child and adolescent psychiatrist, Dr Ong Say How, to lead this programme, as well as to provide leadership to grow CAWMS into a full service. In Oct 2011, the Response, Early Intervention and Assessment in Community Mental Health (REACH) East team transitioned over to KKH; the 13 staff comprised eight psychologists, two medical social workers, an occupational therapist, a nurse and an administrative assistant. Thus with CAMWS having a lead specialist heading, as well as a resource nurse, dedicated case manager, and administrative staff, and the extended REACH-East team, MWS was positioned to become a department.

Choosing the name for the department was easier this time, for the medical board accepted the proposal of Department of Psychological Medicine (DPM), as was commonly used in other institutions. It was quietly reassuring, for it had been somewhat peculiar having KKH's MWS listed as affiliation alongside the other academic and standard affiliations in collaborative publications. Ironically though, the name MWS stuck as glue — colleagues from within the hospital and in the wider community would continue to refer to our team as such — it was after all just a name.

On 1 April 2012, the WMWS and CAMWS teams gathered, and thus the DPM, KKH, celebrated its inaugural meeting. That year, team-bonding and building a unified identity were the main focus, along with setting up the departmental infrastructure, and a dedicated clinic for psychiatric and psychological services.

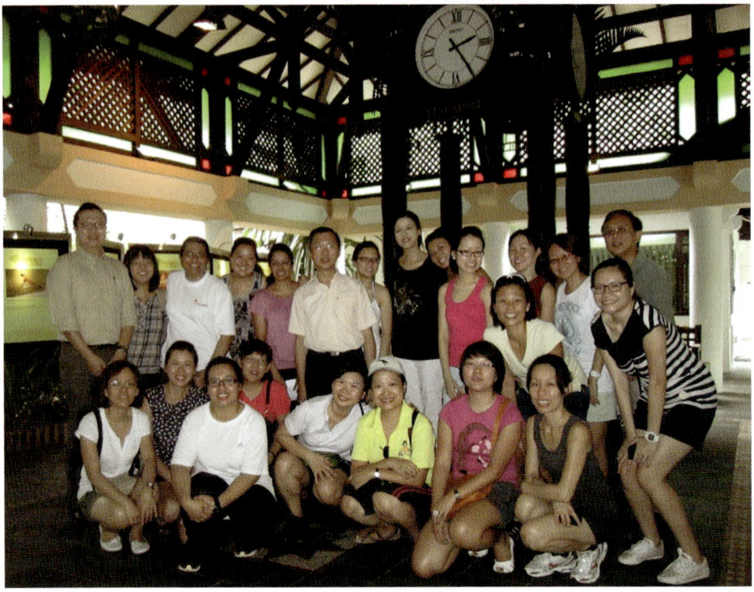

The inaugural team-bonding event for DPM was held at the Botanic Gardens in 2012.

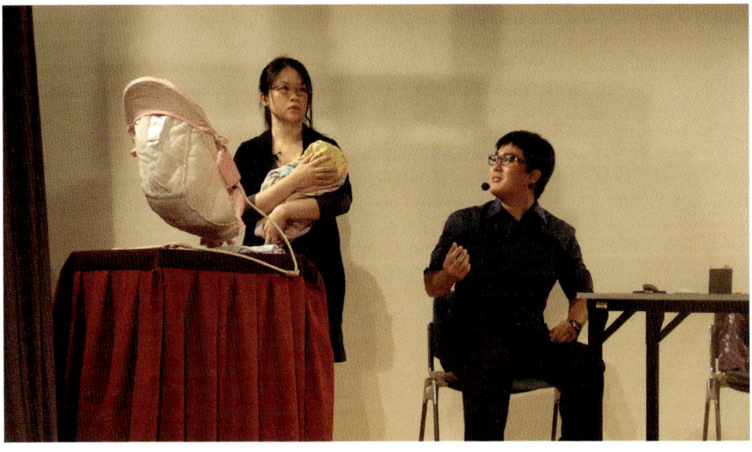

A theatre forum, *Love Out Loud*, was held in 2014. Dr Chua Tze-Ern and Mr Julian Lee are seen here in the photo, enacting postnatal depression.

By the following year, the department had settled, and celebrated its first anniversary with confidence, and embarked on the first retreat to plan ahead for the next year. Though small, and diverse, the team was unified and strong. Since then, DPM, KKH has sustained its steady progress, participating as part of an academic medical centre under the SingHealth group, and contributing actively to research, education, and evidenced-based medicine. In August 2016, Dr Chua Tze-Ern successfully completed her Khoo Clinical Scholar Programme in her area of research interest in duration of untreated illness for postnatal depression. With a keen focus on the needs of women, child and adolescents, programmes and initiatives have been designed accordingly. The shared belief of working for the family drives both services to collaborate and integrate resources, offering women and children interventions that address needs of both. Over the past three years, the department has successfully organised two forums focusing on mental health of women, children and their families. Special services targeting this unique group include reflective family therapy, parent-child psychotherapy, infant-led psychotherapy, attachment-based psychotherapy, hypnotherapy and art

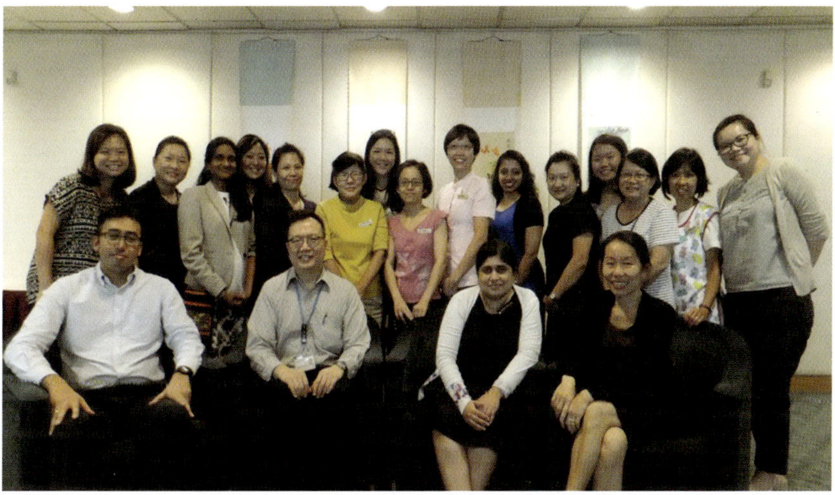

An appreciation lunch was held for DPM in 2016.

therapy. The case managers also developed mental health counselling as a cost-effective alternative intervention to psychologist-led therapy, and counselling clinics are available daily. The REACH-East team has also progressed under the leadership of principal psychologist, Dr Delphine Koh, moving on to develop services for the pre-school population, and providing group therapy, whilst maintaining their core work of providing consultancy in child and adolescent mental health in the east-zone schools. Clinic G, the dedicated clinic, has also established its presence as a valuable resource in the hospital. Our team has also been creatively working on public education and creating awareness to destigmatise maternal and child mental health, using a theatre forum and reflective short film as a modality of outreach.

Conclusion

This year, with a staff-strength of 41, and youthful spirit of a four year-old, and having had an incubation period of six years as MWS, DPM will be embarking on a journey to discover new perspectives — possibly in infant mental health. That chapter is yet to be written but possibilities are surely ahead.

References

Chen H, Lee T, Chee KT (2014). Perinatal psychiatry. In: Sim K, Sengupta S, Fung D, Chee KT, eds. *Essential Guide to Psychiatry*. Pearson, Singapore, pp. 353–368.

Chen H, Wang J, Ch'ng YC, Mingoo R, Lee T, Ong J (2011). Identifying mothers with postpartum depression early: integrating perinatal mental health care into the obstetric setting. *ISRN Obstetr Gynecol* **2011**: 309189.

Chua TE, Allen J, Ang L, Ong LL, Ch'ng YC, Chen H (2016). Patterns and predictors of treatment outcome for antenatal major depression. *PubMed J* doi: 10.11622/smedj.201610.

Lim CG, Ong SH, Chin CH, Fung SSD (2015). Child and adolescent psychiatry services in Singapore. *Child Adolesc Psychiatry Ment Health* **9**: 7.

Training for Undergraduates

Roger HO, Melvyn ZHANG, Aaron TIONG and Joel WONG

The Experiences at Yong Loo Lin School of Medicine, National University of Singapore: 1990–2015

From 1990 to 2010, the psychiatric education was divided into a four-week posting in the third year and two-week posting in the fifth year in the Bachelor of Medicine and Surgery (MBBS) curriculum. Medical students used a textbook, Psychiatry for Doctors edited by Prof Kua Ee Heok, A/Prof Calvin Fones and A/Prof Ko Soo Meng. For psychiatry, the medical students were required to pass both written and clinical examinations in the third year and a written year in the fifth year. Prior to 2007, the clinical examination was based on assessment of real psychiatric inpatients. Since 2007, the objective structured clinical examination (OSCE) was introduced and students were asked to elicit specific psychiatric symptoms or explain treatment to a stimulated patient.

In order to coordinate psychiatric education in a relevant, integrated and efficient manner, the psychiatric posting was combined into a six-week posting in fourth year of the MBBS curriculum in 2011. This allows the competency- and knowledge-based curriculum in psychiatry to be delivered in a seamless way. The challenges of the new psychiatric curriculum include the need to train a larger number of medical students, deliver most up-to-date psychiatric knowledge and to incorporate latest technology in teaching. Most medical students are interested in medical and surgical disciplines. We need to train and impress our future physicians and surgeons about psychiatry and hope they can apply psychiatric knowledge in their future practice.

Education Direction for the Future

Introduction

Medical undergraduates are posted for their clinical posting in psychiatry for a period of six weeks in their fourth year from July to December of an academic year. The main teaching objective is to help medical students to master the basic psychiatric knowledge and clinical assessment techniques. Medical students will be competent to manage common psychiatric disorders at the level of general practitioners. Weekly centralised teaching is held at the National University Health System (NUHS) to ensure standardisation. The clinical postings are conducted at the National University Hospital (NUH), Khoo Teck Puat Hospital (KTPH), Tan Tock Seng Hospital (TTSH), Changi General Hospital (CGH), Singapore General Hospital (SGH) and Institute of Mental Health(IMH) to provide broad clinical exposure. The teaching activities include foundation lectures, case-based discussions, small-group tutorials, observed clinical interview, clerking and presentation of a long case (bedside tutorial) and attachment to various community psychiatric services.

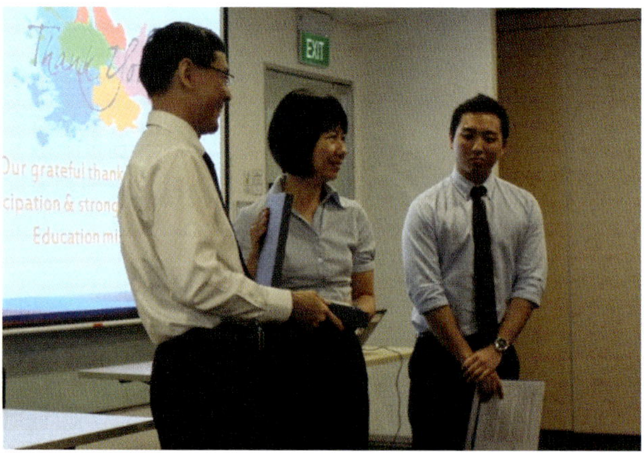

The Dean of Yong Loo Lin School of Medicine, A/Prof Yeoh Khay Guan presenting an award to A/Prof Chiam Peak Chiang, Vice-Chairman, Medical Board (Education), IMH. This awards recognises the commitment of IMH in undergraduate psychiatric education.

Teaching objectives

To conduct a systematic psychiatric evaluation using appropriate interviewing and communication skills to elicit signs and symptoms of common psychiatric disorders. At the end of the posting, the student will demonstrate an effective level of clinical knowledge, understanding and manage a psychiatric patient from a bio-psychosocial perspective relevant to a general practitioner in the following areas:

- General adult psychiatry
- Risk assessment
- Geriatric psychiatry
- Child and adolescent psychiatry
- Consultation-liaison psychiatry
- Addiction psychiatry
- Psychopharmacology
- Psychotherapy
- Local mental health legislation and forensic psychiatry

The following table summarises the topics of lectures and teaching activities.

Week	Topics for Common Lectures / Case-based Discussion at NUHS	Other Teaching Activities at NUH, CGH, SGH, TTSH and IMH
First Week	• Introduction to psychiatry • Classification of psychiatric disorders • Overview of psychiatric services in Singapore	• Daily ward round • Attachment to clinics • Attachment to liaison psychiatry team
Introduction week	• Psychiatric history taking and mental state examination • Psychopathology • Cognitive assessment	• Attachment to community psychiatric services (depending on availability at each hospital)

(*Continued*)

(*Continued*)

Week	Topics for Common Lectures / Case-based Discussion at NUHS	Other Teaching Activities at NUH, CGH, SGH, TTSH and IMH
Foundation lectures will take place on Monday and Tuesday during the first week.	• Psychiatric ethics and mental health act • Introduction to schizophrenia • Introduction to antipsychotics • Introduction to anxiety disorders • Introduction to psychotherapy • Introduction to mood disorders • Introduction to antidepressants, mood stabilisers and hypnotics • Research findings in Singapore and psychiatric epidemiology	• Bedside tutorial • Observed clinical interview • Tutorial with tutor
Subsequent weeks	• Assess and manage a patient who has abnormal illness behaviour	• Daily ward round • Attachment to clinics
(Week 2–5)	• Assess and manage a patient who is depressed or in grief • Assess and manage a patient suffering from memory loss	• Attachment to liaison psychiatry team • Attachment to community psychiatric services (depending on the availability of such service at each hospital)
Case-based discussion will take place on every Friday of Week 2–5.	• Assess and manage a psychotic patient • Assess and manage a patient with postnatal depression and psychosis • Assess and manage a patient with sleep problems • Assess and manage a manic patient • Assess and manage an anxious patient • Assess and manage a confused patient	• Bedside tutorial • Observed clinical interview • Tutorial with tutor • Grand ward round (depending on the arrangement of academic activity at each hospital) • Journal club (depending on the arrangement of academic activity at each hospital)

(*Continued*)

(*Continued*)

Week	Topics for Common Lectures / Case-based Discussion at NUHS	Other Teaching Activities at NUH, CGH, SGH, TTSH and IMH
	• Assess and manage a person with personality disorder • Assess and manage a patient with eating disorder • Cognitive–behaviour therapy • Assess and manage substance abuse • Suicide and deliberate self-harm • Forensic psychiatry • Brief dynamic psychotherapy and defence mechanisms. • Psychosexual medicine • Intellectual disability • Neuropsychiatric disorders	

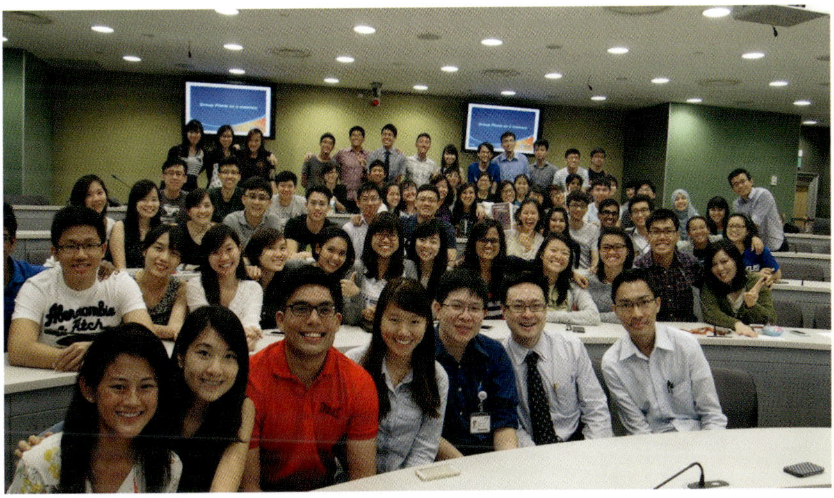

Medical students and their teachers after the revision lecture which was held on the last day of teaching.

Examinations

The end-of-posting examination adopts the latest evaluation methods which consist of multiple choice questions (MCQs), extended matching items (EMIs), short answer questions (SAQs) and objective structured clinical examination (OSCE). The examination covers most of the topics taught during the posting.

The examination format mirrors the Membership examination for the Royal College of Psychiatrists. This will provide an early start to prepare students who are interested to be psychiatrists to be familiar with the format of postgraduate examination. This also ensures high standard of the examination.

The Department of Psychological Medicine, National University of Singapore (NUS) maintains the tradition to disclose and discuss the answers with students after the examination. The education director has to explain and defend the answers as a university culture to encourage medical students to question and challenge with reasons.

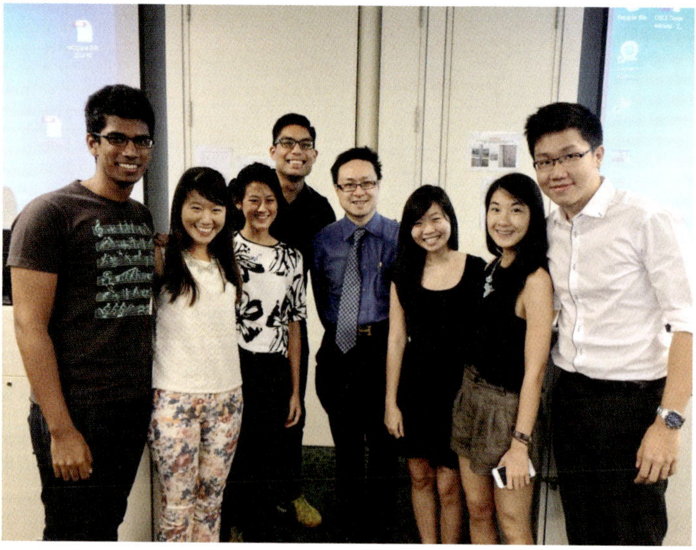

Students with their education director after the written examination and debriefing of answers.

Development

The recent development focuses on applying the stat-of-art technology in medical education. It includes online website who hosts study materials and videos demonstrating clinical skills to elicit psychiatric signs and symptoms. With the funding from the Provost's Office, NUS, we managed to develop a smartphone application which allows students accessing information while they are posted in different hospitals.

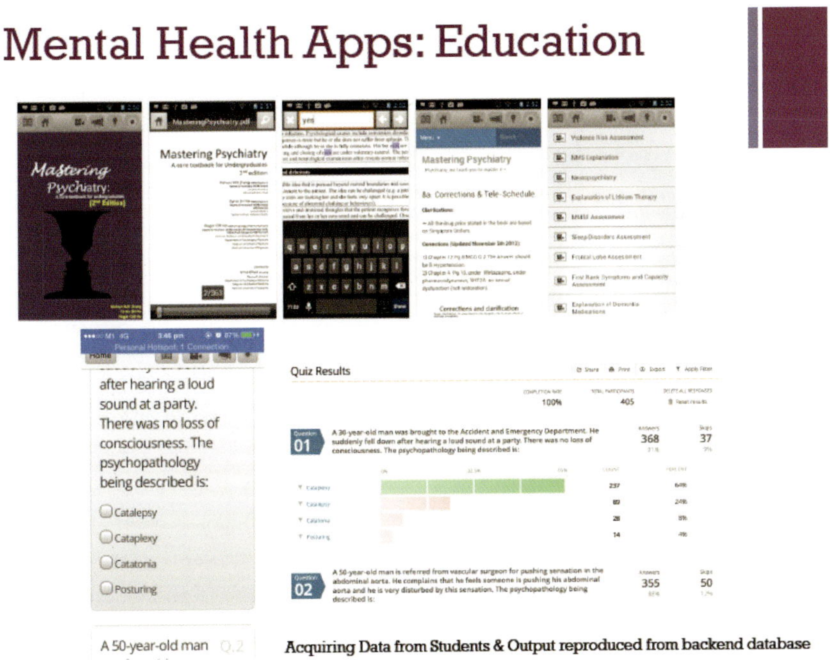
Mental Health Apps: Education
Mastering Psychiatry
Corrections & Tele-Schedule
Corrections and clarification
after hearing a loud sound at a party. There was no loss of consciousness. The psychopathology being described is:
Catalepsy
Cataplexy
Catatonia
Posturing
A 50-year-old man
Quiz Results
100%
405
01
368
37
02
355
50
Acquiring Data from Students & Output reproduced from backend database

Development of education apps to allow medical students to have access to study materials when they are posted to different hospitals.

Teaching performance

With the above development, the teaching performance of undergraduate psychiatric teaching is above national average in academic year 2013/2014.

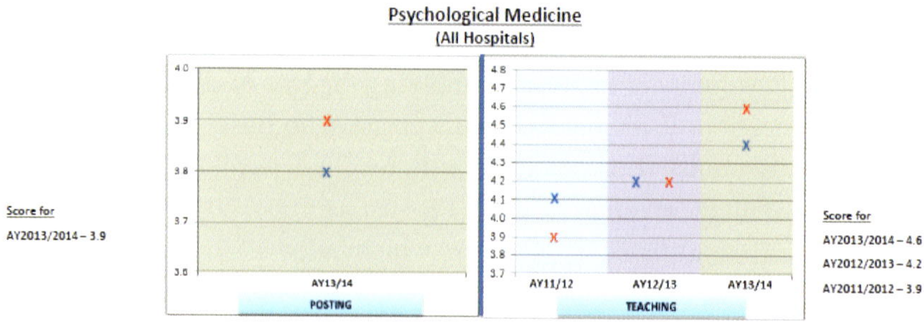

Improvement in teaching scores for psychiatry across all hospitals from academic year 2011 to 2014.

Undergraduate Research Opportunity Programme

This is an account by Dr Melvyn Zhang who graduated in 2011:

'The landscape of teaching in undergraduate psychiatry has evolved and changed significantly in the past decade, ever since the time I did my undergraduate posting in psychiatry, back in academic year 2009/2010. Whilst some might be sceptical about changes, I must say that after speaking to the current batch of undergraduates who are doing their core psychiatry posting in year 4, there had been more changes in the pedagogy and curriculum. Their current experience is a vastly different experience from what I have had experienced previously. Perhaps, let me share my perspectives of how Psychiatry as an undergraduate was like for me, in order for any individual to comprehend how much this field has advanced.

Prior to entering medical school, I did some basic studies in psychology and counselling, and that was why I got myself so interested in this specialty. When I was in my junior medical student years, there were not many opportunities to have a taste of what this specialty was like. Thankfully, I chanced upon the Undergraduate Research Opportunity Programme (UROP) that the School of Medicine offered. The programme was indeed beneficial for me, as it enabled me to explore more into the research aspect of psychiatry. I got to know leading researchers in the local field, such as A/Prof Ng Tze Pin and Dr Roger Ho, who taught me the fundamentals of research, and got me involved and mentored me through various research projects, which included that of clinical research and more advanced research methodologies such as meta-analysis. It was through this mentorship and research programme that enabled me to have opportunities to co-author papers and publish a meta-analysis paper in a moderately high-impact factor journal, even before graduation. But most importantly, the programme taught me valuable skills that I am still using today, as a resident in training. At least for now, I have the knowledge to conduct basic research and write up papers. Undeniably, research is a core aspect of every discipline, and even so in psychiatry, where there are many unknown truths about various mental health disorders.

Apart from early research exposure that my former medical school offered, the Yong Loo Lin School of Medicine also stood out due to the comprehensive undergraduate psychiatric training program that it offered during the clinical years. I have had adequate exposure to patients with different diagnosis throughout the posting, and there are many opportunities for us to interview patients with supervision and guidance from the core faculty. There were several outstanding educators in the field, which did serve to inspire myself and my colleagues today to consider the possibility to pursue an educational track in the later years of residency.

In addition, there was also the opportunity being offered by the medical school for us to plan our electives according to what we wanted to experience more. Definitely for me, it was psychiatry and I am glad that I have had the freedom to plan and the opportunity to rotate through all the subspecialty in the Institute of Mental Health. It offered me a better idea and perspective of what I needed to expect if I were to select this as my future career choice.

Apart from the strengths that Yong Loo Lin School of Medicine offer in terms of early research experience as well as a well devised undergraduate training schedule, the medical school also stands out by having inspiring educators, who are keen to teach and write valuable notes for students to help us clear our respective end of posting examinations. Their dedication, their devotion and commitment to the field inspires us much; and it also demonstrates to us that the field not only offers opportunities (if we chose it as our future career) for research, but also for various other academic achievements such as publishing books.

Listening to what the current batch of undergraduates have shared about their posting, it is heartening to hear that the current programme offers even more, than what I used to have previously. I am confident that the current system would serve to inspire more to embark on psychiatry as a potential career option; or at the bare minimum, ensure that we have competent primary care providers who are capable enough to handle and manage psychiatric disorders.'

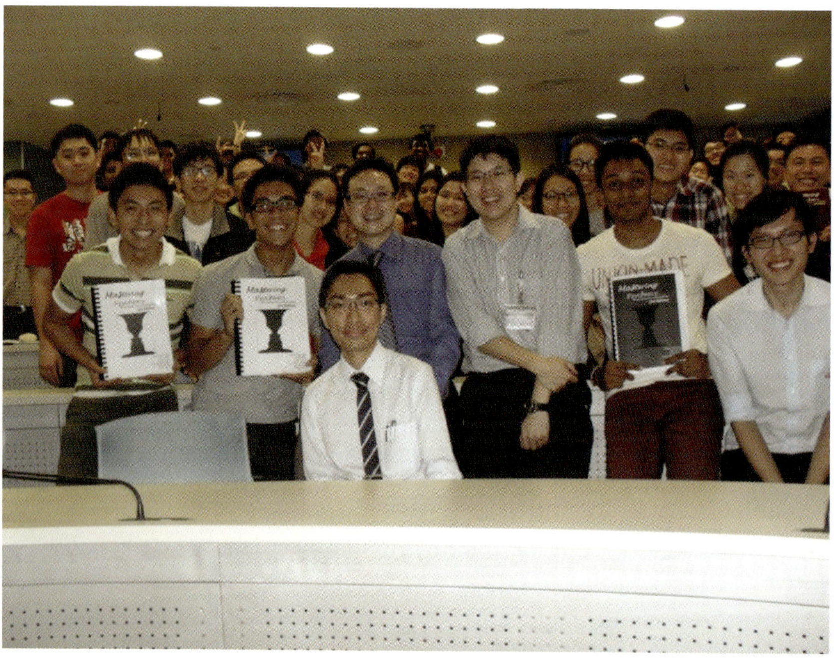

Dr Melvyn Zhang, Dr Cyrus Ho and Dr Roger Ho — authors of an undergraduate reference book, Mastering Psychiatry, with medical students

This is an account of medical students Aaron Tiong and Joel Wong, year 4 medical students (Class 2016):

'Our clinical posting and electives in psychiatry have been an enriching and rewarding experience. We were exposed to patients with problems which we had never encountered before in our previous medical postings. Prior to the posting, psychiatry seemed to be something of an unknown quantity, mostly hidden from view amongst the daily bustle of the medical and surgical wards, with the occasional inpatient referral the closest we were ever exposed to the specialty. It was only after the posting that we came to realise how important the field really was, and the reality of how patients with psychiatric issues are sometimes misunderstood and misrepresented.

Every day, many patients in restructured hospitals are referred to the psychiatric department, and countless more are seen in the outpatient clinics for their various disorders. Whether or not one eventually becomes a psychiatrist, a general practitioner or a doctor in any other specialty, there is a need to have the skills to pick up a psychiatric condition in its early stages and take the appropriate actions to help the patient, rather than dismissing the patient's concerns and complaints as insignificant. In this aspect, we realised that many health professionals and students often do not take enough time to understand the background and the problems that a patient has, apart from his or her immediate medical needs. We were impressed by the doctors, nurses and health care staff working in the psychiatric departments because of their willingness and patience in understanding the patient, and in developing a holistic management plan and communicating these plans to relatives and caregivers.

Our six-week psychiatric posting was well organised and divided into three weeks of postings at the psychiatric unit of a restructured hospital, and two weeks at the Institute of Mental Health. There were also regular lectures at the National University Hospital on Thursdays and Fridays, as well as a revision session during our final week to prepare us for the End of Posting Examination. The curriculum was well planned and our undergraduate education director, Dr Roger Ho had kindly prepared a reference book, *Mastering Psychiatry* for us to read through to learn more about Psychiatry.

At the Institute of Mental Health, we were exposed to patients with severe mental illnesses and were given the opportunity to speak to some of the patients. We remember our first encounter with a patient suffering from schizophrenia who gave us a vivid recount of his life and his past experiences with the disease. Even though the psychiatric history was long and time consuming, it provided us with a full picture of the patient's life and the issues that he was suffering from. Some of the doctors also took some time off to help us with our history taking and taught us the basics of management based on a biopsychosocial model. We also learned important communication skills and had a brush with addiction medicine during our two-week posting at the Institute of Mental Health.

We were posted to the Changi General Hospital during our three-week Psychological Medicine Programme at the restructured hospitals. Throughout the three weeks, we clerked and followed up a patient suffering from obsessive–compulsive disorder. Each of us was also attached to a consultant who acted as our mentor to whom we could turn to if we had any questions during the posting. We also had the opportunity to sit in with some of the allied health professionals during therapy sessions such as occupational therapy. The consultants in the ward and in the clinics also took turns to give us small tutorials about topics in psychiatry. We were also assigned to rounds within the consultation-liaison team. Our best experience was sitting in with the doctors in their outpatient clinics. We were given the opportunity to talk to the patients before they saw the doctor, to present their history, and to discuss the cases shortly after the patients left. I saw a variety of cases in the outpatient clinics ranging from mood disorders to somatisation disorders and even to eating disorders.

Even though the six-week posting did not allow us to cover too many aspects of psychiatry in great detail, we were still able to pick up important skills and pieces of knowledge that will help us in our future careers to help our patients. For instance, there were many opportunities for us to practise our interview, counselling and risk assessment skills, through mock OSCEs and observed clinical interviews between a senior doctor and a patient. The use of videos to augment our learning in lectures and tutorials also exposed us to a wider range of conditions.

As we were interested in pursuing psychiatry as a specialty, we proceeded to do an Eating Disorder Elective at the Singapore General Hospital after having completed our examinations. During our three-week elective, we were exposed to many eating disorder cases at the outpatient clinics and inpatient ward, and also given a chance to participate in the Eating Disorder Intensive Treatment Programme where we observed many different allied health professionals such as dieticians, psychologists and other therapists collaborating with one another. In my subsequent four-week elective at the National University Hospital, we were able to sit in and participate in case management rounds (REACH, child psychiatry team and G-RACE, geriatric psychiatry team) for children and elderly with psychiatric problems. We also clerked patients in the outpatient clinics and did a follow-up and home visit for a patient who was subsequently admitted. We have also attended a volunteer orientation session at the Institute of Mental Health and will be looking forward to interacting with the inpatients on a regular basis.

Our experiences with psychiatry have not only empowered us with knowledge, but also in soft skills in supporting and helping the patient in his or her emotional journey. We would like to thank all the patients, doctors and allied health professionals who have imparted the knowledge of their world with us, and we hope to apply these skills to be a compassionate and patient physician.'

Conclusion

The undergraduate psychiatric education at Yong Loo Lin School of Medicine, NUS and its partner institutions is well received by medical students and has enhanced the competency of future generation of doctors. Through our publication, technology development and collaboration with other universities, the undergraduate psychiatric teaching will be a role model for other universities to follow.

Academic Psychiatry

Rathi MAHENDRAN

Introduction

Academic psychiatry in Singapore has evolved in parallel with the development of mental health services in the country. In the early years much of the academic mantle was borne by the National University of Singapore (NUS)'s Department of Psychological Medicine. However, as new Academic Medical Centres (AMCs) were set up in the country and as the Institute of Mental Health/Woodbridge Hospital (IMH/WH) expanded its research and teaching focus, academic psychiatry has made significant strides in supporting psychiatry education, the growth of psychiatric knowledge through research and the provision of psychiatric services in the country. This is a vast improvement from a time when undergraduate psychiatry training consisted of didactic lectures and postgraduate training was unavailable locally.

Psychiatry Education

In the early years, prior to 1972, undergraduate psychiatry training was of brief duration. The curriculum consisted of just 20 hours of didactic lectures and a hospital visit to WH. Psychiatry for the medical students was taught by psychiatrists at WH until a formal Department of Psychological Medicine was formed in the University of Singapore in September 1979. Between 1972 and 1989, the clinical attachments at WH, and from the eighties at the National University Hospital (NUH), grew from a one week to a four-week posting. The present six-week rotation provides medical students the opportunity to gain clinical experience at IMH/WH as well as the smaller psychological medicine departments in the various restructured hospitals. The students' clinical experience has broadened and ranges from the care of the acutely ill to the chronic mentally ill individuals as well as those with medical conditions and co-morbid psychiatric problems and specialised areas such as Child and Adolescent Psychiatry, Geriatric Psychiatry and subspecialties such as Eating Disorders.

The setting up of the second medical school, Duke-NUS Graduate Medical School in 2007, led to a different psychiatric pedagogy. This was a collaboration between NUS and Duke University in the US. Students are taught psychiatry in a four-week rotation in year two (of a four-year programme). The focus of the teaching is on embedding students with the clinical team. Teachers had to adapt to the new way of delivering the psychiatry curriculum, but the progress in psychiatry teaching in the second medical school has indicated that the clinical teachers were able to quickly adapt. The third medical school, Lee Kong Chian School of Medicine, Nanyang Technological University–Imperial College, a UK collaboration had its first intake in 2013 and will provide undergraduate psychiatry teaching as well. In teaching three different groups of medical students, the three psychiatry training programmes will need to eventually align pedagogy, curriculum and the clinical experience for students to ensure the quality of training. Importantly, clinician educators need to be able to deliver and sustain a high quality in psychiatry education.

The development of postgraduate psychiatry training occurred later. In 1969, NUS started a Division of Graduate Medical Studies (DGMS) which together with the Academy of Medicine, a professional body and the Ministry of Health (MOH), Singapore, established postgraduate training for Singapore doctors. Links with the British Royal Colleges were maintained and assistance was sought in providing a training course and in the conduct of the examination. But it was only in 1983 that the local Master of Medicine (Psychiatry) programme was offered by the University of Singapore.

The introduction of the American-styled Residency programme in 2010, with its own standards and requirements surfaced challenges as there was a transitional arrangement with two parallel programmes (the older British-styled training program and the newer Residency programme). A study amongst trainees and residents in both programmes revealed that while they felt supported and perceived autonomy in their roles, they were critical of the teaching they received (Mahendran *et al.*, 2013). This highlights the issues of the clinician educators. Even as more psychiatrists are called upon to teach the growing number of medical students and provide postgraduate training and supervision, their skills and competencies in this area deserve closer attention. There are increasing opportunities for training in medical education, such as the Teachers of Psychiatry Meeting first organised by the University's Department of Psychological Medicine in 2003 and the yearly Asia Pacific Medical Education Conference (APMEC) by the University's Medical Education Unit, an internationally recognised meeting for training in education. But attention is still required to issues of protected time for teaching and training and academic recognition and promotion.

Research

Research in psychiatry has seen a significant growth with increasingly large population studies to address gaps in knowledge about the incidence and prevalence of psychiatric disorders, but also to understand the needs and unique cultural perspectives of psychiatric disorders in our population. The extensive research work undertaken at IMH/WH is mentioned in the chapter by Prof Chong Siow Ann. Added to this is the work at the Department of Psychological Medicine, NUS; the Gerontology Research Programme includes large community cohort studies with the elderly namely the Singapore Longitudinal Ageing Study which examines the psychosocial, behavioural and biomedical determinants of ageing in our population (Yong Loo Lin School of Medicine, 2013). There are also programmes to improve population health such as the Dementia and Depression Prevention Programme, a community-based project with elderly living in the Jurong area (Wu *et al.*, 2014). The Department also collaborates in multi-centre regional work such as the Research in East Asia of Psychotropic Prescription (REAP) (Chee *et al.*, 2014). These have served to widen expertise and knowledge in areas of psychiatry and drive clinical service development and enhancement.

Clinical Service

The third arm of academic work is of course clinical service. This is where the developments in academic psychiatry are very clear. The provision of psychiatric services across the spectrum and the development of specialised services has been growing over the years but received a significant boost with the National Mental Health Blueprint (NMHB) in 2007 with its particular focus in the areas of community outreach and early detection and psycho-education. It has also supported the expansion of efforts in primary care psychiatry training, an important component of care delivery.

The Growth of Academic Psychiatry

It is worth studying the advances that have driven Academic Psychiatry to what it is today. Psychiatry services are available in all the general hospitals providing the opportunities for teaching at both undergraduate and postgraduate levels. There are numerous advances in psychiatry training in Singapore, the chief of which is that students have the opportunity to experience continuity of care and integration of multidisciplinary care. There is continuity of training from undergraduate to postgraduate levels and doctors need not go overseas for training except for subspecialisation and to gain additional experience at world renowned centres.

Quality assurance in education is in place through curriculum mapping from undergraduate to postgraduate level and ACGME (Accreditation Council for Graduate Medical Education)-I accreditation; NUHS has also achieved JCI (Joint Commission International) accreditation as an AMC. Undergraduate psychiatry training now includes greater opportunities for Elective Study in subspecialty areas such as Child Psychiatry and Geriatric Psychiatry and also in Psychiatry Research. Undergraduate and postgraduate evaluations are both formative and summative and competency based.

Postgraduate sub-specialisation is available in Singapore in well-developed and established areas in Early Psychosis, Child and Adolescent Psychiatry, Geriatric Psychiatry, Addiction Medicine and Community Psychiatry. Overseas training opportunities are available for public-sector psychiatrists through government and hospital funded scholarships for skills development and expertise in niche areas. Training in psychiatry research is available to postgraduate students through sponsored Clinician-Scientist programmes allowing exceptional psychiatry trainees to undertake postgraduate psychiatry training and pursue a Master's degree in Clinical Investigation or a PhD in psychiatry research concurrent with their clinical training.

The NMHB in 2007 established mental health care needs for the population and focused on service development and manpower needs. The initiative estimated the population needed 250 psychiatrists. Not only did this parallel an increase in training positions but also increased training opportunities for allied health professionals. Upskilling of Medical Social Workers with minimum requirements for training in basic counselling skills and for minimum Master's level for Clinical Psychologists rather than those with basic psychology degrees were set in place. Competencies were developed to provide Multidisciplinary Team Care and Community Mental Health Care.

The Future

The demands for mental health services in the country and the drive for community mental health care requires an academic curriculum that is responsive to changing needs. It calls for a review of how some of the psychiatry teaching could be shifted or integrated with the primary care services as many patients with subsyndromal conditions and minor psychiatric morbidity seek help from polyclinics and family physicians. Training opportunities for family physicians which now includes a Graduate Diploma in Mental Health has been a step in the right direction.

The curriculum needs to reflect the new trends of competency-based education and learning theories that highlight transition from 'knowing' to 'doing'. The rapid pace of medical and scientific developments necessitates skills for 'life-long learning'. The psychiatry curriculum should incorporate measures to develop greater independence for learning. Students have to be trained for the shift away from Institutionalisation and Acute Care to Community Care and early Detection and Prevention.

There is a new generation of learners with different learning needs. Whether the learning experience is relevant to their future clinical practice and to what extent new technologies are explored for teaching have to be examined. These are some of the very many tasks ahead for the educators in psychiatry.

Teachers are important mentors who guide students through career choices and pursuit of specialist training and instil values of the profession. At present, much of the training is provided by psychiatrists who are primarily clinicians and excellent in their clinical duties. However, the educator mantle requires much more specific skills and knowledge of pedagogy. We need to pay attention to 'Training the Teachers' as clinician-educators. The various Psychological Medicine Departments that teach and train undergraduate and postgraduate psychiatry students are primarily clinical service driven. They need to develop a culture of learning and where possible interest for research or at least create the opportunities for psychiatry research for their students to enrich and broaden the overall experience in psychiatry.

Effective training in Quality Improvement should be a consideration at the postgraduate level. Psychiatry lends itself well to this as there are many areas such as polypharmacy and patient safety that require attention. The training should encompass didactic education regarding the language and science of improvement and also experiential learning.

Finally, while not elaborated upon here, issues such as professionalism, ethical practice and social responsibility are also within the ambit of academia and require attention.

References

Chee KY, Tripathi A, Avasthi A, Chong MY, Sim K, Yang SY, *et al.* (2015). International study on antidepressant prescription pattern at 40 major psychiatric institutions and hospitals in Asia: A 10 year comparison study. *Asia Pac Psychiatry* **7**(4): 366–374.

Mahendran R, Broekman B, Wong CM, Lai YM, Kua EH (2013). The educational environment: Comparisons of the British and American postgraduate psychiatry training programs in an Asian setting. *Med Teach* **35**(11): 959–961.

Wu D-X, Feng L, Yao S-Q, Tian X-F, R Mahendran, EH Kua (2014). The early dementia prevention programme in Singapore. *Lancet Psychiatry* **1**: 10–11.

Yong Loo Lin School of Medicine (2013). Gerontology Research Programme. Available at: http://medicine.nus.edu.sg/pcm/research/ageing-psychiatry.shtml

Psychiatry Specialist Training

CHIAM Peak Chiang

Introduction

Woodbridge Hospital started providing psychiatry specialist training which leads to a Master of Medicine (MMed) (Psychiatry) degree from the National University of Singapore in 1982. Training included on-the-job-training and a three-week intensive course just before the MMed (Psychiatry) Final Examinations.

Psychiatry Specialist Training in Singapore was well established by 1993. It was then a three-year training programme which included six months of compulsory medicine training and six months of optional neurology training. The trainees sat for Primary and Final Master of Medicine or MMed (Psychiatry) Examinations leading to the issue of the degree. Upon passing the MMed (Psychiatry) Examinations, the trainee medical officers were promoted to registrar grade. In order to be registered as specialists, the registrars needed to publish an article as first author in a psychiatry or medical journal, after which they could be registered on the Roll of Specialists.

In 1997, the cohort of trainees who started their Psychiatry Traineeship in 1994, after completing three years of Basic Specialist Traineeship (BST) and clearing the Final MMed (Psychiatry) Examinations, were the first to have to apply for Advanced Specialist Traineeship (AST). During the AST period, each trainee completed a research project and submitted a 3,000-word thesis. At the end of the AST training, the trainees sat for a half-hour Exit Interview which included journal critique and case scenarios. Successful candidates could then register with the Specialist Accreditation Board (SAB) as a Specialist. In July 2000, Dr Tan Lay Ling, Dr Lee Cheng and Dr Samuel Cheng became the first trainees to successfully sit for, and pass the Psychiatry Exit Interviews.

At that time, doctors who wanted to apply for psychiatry traineeship could not do so until after completing two years as a medical officer. As a result, some of the applicants would already have completed a few psychiatry or medicine postings by the time they applied for traineeship. It was not uncommon then for the trainees to request for pre-traineeship accreditation of the postings which were done prior to traineeship. Up to one year of pre-accreditation was allowed by the Specialist Training Committee (STC), enabling the trainees to shorten their BST by up to a year.

Seamless Training

Under the leadership of A/Prof Rathi Mahendran, who was the STC Chairperson then, the Psychiatry Seamless Specialist Training track was started in 2008, replacing the three-year BST and three-year AST. The medical officers were required to complete 2 to 6 months of psychiatry posting, and six months of medicine posting prior applying for the Seamless Psychiatry Training. This requirement of 2 to 6 months of psychiatry was to ensure that the medical officers had some working experience in psychiatry before deciding on psychiatry as a career. After passing the MMed (Psychiatry) exams, the trainees continued seamlessly into advance training without having to apply for AST training positions. The Exit Requirements were the same as the three-year Advanced Specialist Traineeship.

The Exit Examinations were usually held in July, at the same time as the Final MMed (Psychiatry) Examinations using the same external examiner. The Exit Examinations, which are specialist accreditation examinations, were administered by STC, whereas the MMed (Psychiatry) Examinations, are administered by Division of Graduate Medical Studies (DGMS) with a Chief examiner and an MMed (Psychiatry) Examinations Committee. The MMed (Psychiatry) Examinations are qualification examinations.

Residency Training

In 2009, the Ministry of Health (MOH), after discussions with SAB, recommended that the training be switched from the British-based apprenticeship style of specialist training to the American-style residency programme established by the Accreditation Council for Graduate Medical Education International (ACGME-I). The residency emphasises on structured training and regular formative evaluations for residents to develop core competencies and to enable them to take on progressive graded responsibilities. Institutional resources are made available and core faculty are appointed to plan curriculum, supervise and assess the residents.

In 2010, Psychiatry was one of the eight specialties in the first phase to switch to the ACGME-I residency. Unlike most other specialties which have separate programmes with the three different sponsoring institutions, the psychiatry residency programme is a national programme with National Healthcare Group (NHG) as the sponsoring institution and the Institute of Mental Health (IMH) as the primary training site.

The first NHG Designated Institutional Officer (DIO) was Prof Lim Tock Han, and under his leadership, a working committee comprising A/Prof Nicholas Chew, senior consultant of Tan Tock Seng Hospital (TTSH), A/Prof Chiam Peak Chiang of IMH (and who was later appointed as Programme Director) and Dr Aaron Ang, Dr Ng Beng Yeong, Dr Lai Yew Min, Dr Ong Seh Ong and Dr Peh Lai Huat of TTSH, Singapore General Hospital (SGH), National University Health System (NUHS), Khoo Teck Puat Hospital (KTPH) and Changi General Hospital (CGH), respectively (and who were later appointed as Associate Programme Directors) started planning the new psychiatry curriculum based on ACGME requirements in early 2009. The workgroup benefitted from sessions conducted by ACGME trainers arranged by MOH to familiarise them with the six ACGME core competencies, formative and summative evaluations, policies, data collection systems, faculty development and training for programme coordinators.

As Singapore was the first country outside the US to adopt the ACGME-style residency training, the ACGME-I requirements were written for us. There was a Singapore addendum which spelt out some deviations from the ACGME-I training structure. For example, the residents who are fresh medical school graduates, i.e. postgraduate year 1 (PGY1) are required to complete four months of either general surgery or orthopaedic surgery during their first year for licensing purpose. Instead of four years duration in US, the Singapore Programme spans five years, of which the first four years are accredited by ACGME-I and the fifth year is an elective year, during which the residents also sit for the Exit Examinations.

Postings were six months in duration in the former Seamless and BST/AST training programmes. However, the residency programme has shorter three-month rotations in order to accommodate all the rotations required to be completed in the four-year ACGME-I accredited programme. Another difference is that the psychotherapy is a requirement in residency while it was not in the BST/AST and Seamless programmes.

The first residency intake was in 2010. For the first time, final-year medical students were allowed to apply for residency. The first cohort started with just eight residents, out of which four eventually dropped out. That year, the Seamless Traineeship was still available and several medical officers opted for the Seamless track rather than venturing into residency. The intake increased to 12 the next year, 15 in the following year, after which, the yearly intake has been 16. The table below summarises the acceptance and drop-out rates for cohors from 2010 to 2015.

Year of Intake	Number Accepted	Number Dropped Out
2010	8	4
2011	12	0
2012	15	2
2013	16	0
2014	16	2
2015	16	0

The start month of residency training is July each year, which was not aligned with the Medical Officer Posting Exercise (MOPEX) changeover which occurred in May and November. To solve the problem of residents being out of phase with the medical officer postings, MOPEX postings were lengthened to seven months each, from May to November 2012 and

December 2012 to June 2013. By July 2013, MOPEX was aligned with residency start date.

Evolving Specialist Training

The STC was closed in 14 September 2011 and a new Psychiatry Resident Advisory Committee chaired by A/Prof Chua Hong Choon was formed. The first ACGME-I site visit was in in October 2010, and the programme was successfully accredited for two years. The only citation was that the Programme Letters of Agreement (LPA) did not indicate how residents would regularly participate in the programme's required didactics when at a participating site. In response to this, an addendum was added to the LPA which includes a clause stating that residents are to be released to participate in the programme's required didactics. With the second ACGME-I site visit in November 2012, the programme was re-accredited for four years. The only citation was that at the time of the site, residents were not routinely entering their cases into the ACGME-I resident Case Log System.

The first cohort of residents sat for the local version of the American Board of Psychiatry and Neurology (ABPN) examinations in August 2014 where 20% of the multiple choice questions were contributed by our local examiners. In April 2015, Dr Janine Kee and Dr Lim Wen Phei became the first residents to successfully clear the Exit Examinations.

In July 2015, A/Prof Sim Kang took over from A/Prof Chiam Peak Chiang as the psychiatry residency Programme Director. Together with his team of Associate Programme Directors, he has continued to oversee and improve on the psychiatry residency programme.

Reference

Lim BL (2013). Residency programmes in Singapore — challenges ahead. *Ann Acad Med Singapore* **42**: 265–266.

Mental Health Research

CHONG Siow Ann

Definition of Research

Research is the means by which we generate knowledge that will change the way we think about mental illnesses, about the way we deliver care, or has the potential to yield a 'seminal' observation — one that creates truly new knowledge, leads to new ways of thinking, and lays the foundation for further research in the field. That is, in fact, our stated vision for research in the Institute of Mental Health (IMH) which is: *to change the way we think about mental health and changes the way that we treat those with mental illnesses.*

Development of Research in IMH

The Research Division of IMH was established in 2000 with an Institutional Block Grant (IBG) from the National Medical Research Council (NMRC). With the restructuring of IMH in October 2000, there was a sea change in the emphasis on research. Previously, research was done ad hoc without any tangible support; however once IMH secured the IBG and continued to do so on a yearly basis, it has enabled the Institute to lay the foundation of a research infrastructure and culture.

We also had a simple strategy which was to leverage and focus on our strengths as the single national tertiary mental health treatment centre with a wide range of clinical expertise serving a huge patient population.

In the years that followed, there were assiduous efforts made to build such an infrastructure and to expand the research portfolio. The Research Division was initially co-located with the Department of Early Psychosis Intervention (EPI). With the progressive expansion of our research activities and funding, the Research Division had to be relocated a number of times, and more recently to its present site with well-furnished cubicles, meeting rooms and assessment rooms, including facilities for blood sampling and processing.

At its onset in 2000, there was an appointed Research Director who was a full time clinical psychiatrist, a Research Assistant and an Administrative Assistant. From that humble beginning, we are now a Division comprising 50 staff from multiple fields and disciplines, working at various levels and on different projects.

An early focus of research was tardive dyskinesia which is a common and severe movement disorder that is consequent to treatment with conventional antipsychotics. Through a series of studies, we established the high prevalence of this disorder among our population of patients with schizophrenia — including among the Malay population for which there were no previously published data — and demonstrated that contrary to common belief, this disorder was not of lower prevalence among the Chinese; and that it was associated with a higher mortality rate. The research team also uncovered a number of novel findings — among others, the association of a particular genetic mutation which has been replicated in an international collaboration. This has led to further collaborations with groups in Israel, India and China involving thousands of patients.

The focus of our research has remained constant throughout the years and the focus is to do relevant and meaningful research that serves those with mental illness. An example of this has been the incorporation of a research programme with a clinical one: the Early Psychosis Intervention Programme was set up to address the issues of long duration of psychosis and lack of awareness of sources of help among those with psychosis. The subsequent research has emphasised the need for early detection in mental illnesses — a concept which has hitherto not been the focus in the local mental healthcare scene — and it is now a key facet of the National Mental Health Blueprint (NMHB). The research work in this area was recognised with the prestigious World Health Organisation (WHO), State Of Kuwait Prize for Research in Health Promotion in 2006; and the inaugural National Clinical Excellence Team Award in 2008.

The body of clinical and research from this programme has led to the Translational and Clinical Research in Neuroscience Flagship Programme which is a five-year, SGD 25-million-dollar study funded by the National Research Foundation (NRF). This is an international consortium which includes leading researchers and clinicians in Singapore, US, Australia and Hong Kong in a cutting-edge research programme to identify the biomarkers for schizophrenia and related psychosis.

Cognition and Biomarkers

The programme has now extended to include research in neurocognition and biomarkers, and a Clinical Trial Unit. Dr Jimmy Lee also leads a team which focuses on biological and cognitive subtypes in psychosis, as well as clinical issues such as cardio-metabolic risks and the development of treatment resistance in schizophrenia.

On a related and parallel track, is a focus of neuroimaging studies which has been principally been under the direction of A/Prof Sim Kang. He has built up a neuroimaging program employing structural magnetic resonance imaging (MRI) and diffusion tensor imaging (DTI) and with his team have been investigating the macroscopic and microstructural brain grey and white matter anomalies found in schizophrenia and bipolar disorder (BD) with the aim of identifying potential markers of illness, possible mechanisms of pathophysiology and plausible targets for intervention in the future. Their findings have been published in high-impact journals and won a number of research awards.

Mental Health Policy

Another game-changing development is our Programme for Mental Health Policy Research which is committed to generate the relevant research findings to stakeholders including the policy makers, research administrators, patients and general public to enable better service development, allocation of resources and patient outcomes. This programme has its origins in the work done with the Department of Early Intervention in Psychosis, and subsequently with a number of commissioned studies from external service providers and policy makers including those from various Ministries. This programme is led by Associate Professsor Mythily Subramaniam and under her leadership it has greatly improved its research capabilities, expertise and range of studies. These include qualitative studies and large scale population based studies like the landmark Singapore Mental Health Study (which has also developed a culturally valid instrument to measure the level of positive mental health in our local population) and the Well-Being Study of the Elderly — both these studies have assessed the mental health status of the general population in Singapore.

Our Department of Nursing Administration started its research journey in the year 1999 with a group of enthusiastic nursing leaders and was further enhanced with the introduction of evidence-based practice in 2008. In succession, our nurse-researchers won a string of Research Grants, went on to forge international partnerships that contributed to the development and maintenance of quality healthcare globally with the establishment of Joanna Briggs Institute (JBI)–IMH (Singapore) Centre for Evidence-Based Practices in Mental Health Care in 2010. This is the first collaboration between JBI, an internationally recognised leader in evidence-based practice, and a mental health institution in the world. To date, the Centre has produced numerous systematic reviews and evidence from research studies that enables IMH to develop clinical services, policies and treatment guidelines.

Addictions

The National Addictions Management Service (NAMS) research team, established in 2009, was initially tasked to design and implement a treatment outcome monitoring system to establish the effectiveness of treatment for individuals with substance or behavioural addictions, as well as a study examining predictors of outcome for pathological gamblers. In 2010, the team conducted a series of neuropsychological studies examining attention, memory and executive functioning in patients diagnosed with alcohol dependence undergoing inpatient detoxification or pathological gamblers attending the outpatient clinic. The findings revealed the presence of significant cognitive impairment among alcohol dependent patients that can limit patient engagement and response to psychological treatment interventions during detoxification and thus increase vulnerability to relapse. The team soon expanded to six full-time researchers and secured funding for a study to validate a screening instrument to detect cognitive impairment in substance misusers. In 2012, the team embarked on its first drug trial: a double-blind, randomised, controlled trial examining lofexidine as an alternative pharmacotherapy to diazepam to reduce the opiate withdrawal syndrome during inpatient detoxification from heroin. The NAMS research team is also involved in examining patient responses to acupuncture as an adjunct treatment in the recently opened clinic. Meanwhile, NAMS researchers continue to seek opportunities to establish studies on effective ways of identifying, treating and reducing harm from addiction.

Children and Adolescents

The Research Unit in the Department of Child and Adolescent Psychiatry (DCAP) was established in 2008. Prior to that, research was conducted sporadically by individual clinicians with little support. Its first major undertaking was to support a large scale randomised controlled trial (RCT) investigating the effectiveness of social skills training and omega-3 intake in children and adolescents with Disruptive Behaviour Disorders (DBD). Since then, this budding team of researchers has expanded into a dynamic multidisciplinary team of psychiatrists, allied health specialists and research staff with vast areas of research interests. These include research on alternative treatment with two major trials looking at non-medicated treatment on Attention-Deficit/Hyperactivity Disorder (ADHD) and other Disruptive Behaviour Disorders (DBD). Besides the omega-3 and social skills training trial, the other trial looked at the use of a Traditional Chinese Medicine (TCM) herbal compound as an alternative to conventional stimulant medication. Other current research areas are the exploration of a brain–computer interface (BCI) intervention that targets the inattentive symptoms of ADHD children, one of the first large-scale RCTs, and the use of an interactive web-based game that could help children and adolescents with DBD manage their aggression. The research team has secured many grants and rewards and has established collaborations with various foreign and local institutions including the Nanyang Technological University (NTU), A*Star, Duke-NUS Graduate Medical School and the University of Pennsylvania.

Ethics

Research on people with mental illness can be fraught with difficulties as the effects of certain mental illnesses impair decisional capacity that makes them a 'vulnerable' population. With this ever in mind, we had set up a Hospital Ethics Committee and when the ethical review and approval process was taken over by NHG's Domain-Specific Boards, this committee was transformed to the IMH Clinical Research Committee (CRC). This was an additional layer of protection and standard setting we have insisted on having, and I think is a demonstration of our commitment to research of the highest scientific and ethical standard.

At the same time, the push forward in scientific inquiry should be accompanied by further elucidation of certain ethical issues. In this aspect, we have forged an ongoing collaboration with the Centre for Biomedical Ethics at the Yong Loo Lin School of Medicine to do research in factors affecting decisional capacity in clinical practice and research, understanding of risks and benefits (during the SARS epidemic, we have published our analysis of its impact on ongoing research involving human participants), prodromal and high-risk research, psychiatric genetic research, and other dilemmas encountered in psychiatric practice.

Notable Achievements

If you look at what has been done since 2000, it will be abundantly clear that we have come a long way. Before 2000, this Institute was almost wholly a hospital that provides clinical care and some teaching; whatever studies done were usually small projects, the sum of which did not amount to any significant body of work in any particular area. There was hardly any collaboration with external researchers.

But since we had made that initial determined start in 2000, we have to date garnered more than SGD *70* million in extramural funding, published extensively and won many awards, and forged numerous and extensive collaboration with local and overseas research centres.

What has been notable is the change in the attitude towards research. I think we have succeeded in creating a culture for research where none had existed. A sense of the importance and relevance of research has penetrated the awareness of everyone in the Institute. This is evident in the number of people engaged in research, the exponential growth in the number of research projects and papers published, the high ethical standard that we have upheld, and the various mechanisms that are in place to facilitate research.

One of our key achievements is that we have now a coterie of committed and senior-level researchers who drive their own respective research programme: Associate Professor Mythily Subramaniam who is also our Director of Research (psychiatric epidemiology), Associate Professor Sim Kang (neuroimaging), Dr Jimmy Lee (Schizophrenia and related psychosis), Dr Lim Choon Guan and Dr Sung Min (child and adolescent psychiatry), Associate Professor Swapna Verma (first episode psychosis) and Ms Janhavi Vaingankar. I have just named these few, but there are others including those in other clinical departments, in NAMS, nursing, occupational therapy, case management, and other allied health who are actively engaged in research.

What has often been overlooked is the importance of the administrative support for research and it is often not appreciated that this is a highly specialised area which spans personnel, capital, contractual, budgetary and intellectual property issues. In the years, we have painstakingly built this structure. Credit goes to Associate Professor Mythily and Ms Jenny Tay for putting in place (and through hard work over many years) a very professional and responsive support structure without which we would not be able to do all these research.

But what is ultimately the most important goal for our research is whether we have achieved what we have stated to be our Vision. I think the answer is yes. We have contributed significantly to the body of knowledge through the publications of some of the novel findings. We can also expect more significant finding from the Flagship Translational Clinical Research Programme. We have definitely made a difference in how the public has come to view mental illness and mental health, improve the clinical outcome of young people with first episode psychosis as shown by the research done in this area, and influence policies and service development through the landmark Singapore Mental Health Study.

When the first NHMB was implemented in 2007, there was an emphasis on the need to build up research and there were key initiatives that have been identified. These include establishing a platform for the inter-disciplinary collaboration, and doing research in population-based epidemiological studies, genetics of mental disorders, brain imaging and neuro-biological basis of mental disorders, health service research, and clinical trials. We have done all that.

Acknowledgements

The author wishes to thank Mythily Subramaniam, Jenny Tay, Jimmy Lee, Guo Song, Lim Choon Guan, Sim Kang for their contributions to the chapter.

Developing a National Mental Health Blueprint

Daniel FUNG and CHUA Hong Choon

Mental and behavioural disorders are found in people of all ages, ethnicities and socio-economic groups. According to estimates from the World Health Organisation (WHO)'s World Health Report 2001, about 450 million people worldwide suffer from mental disorders. One person in four will develop one or more mental or behavioural disorders during their lifetime. Mental and behavioural disorders are present at any point in time in about 5 to 10% of the adult population worldwide.

Mental and neurological disorders have also been estimated to account for 12.3% of the total Disability-Adjusted Life Years (DALYs) lost due to all diseases and injuries in the world. Five of the 10 leading causes of disability worldwide are mental disorders, including depression, alcohol use, schizophrenia and obsessive–compulsive disorder. Projections estimate that by the year 2020 neuropsychiatric conditions will account for 15% of disability worldwide, with unipolar depression alone accounting for 5.7% of DALYs. In the addition, the cost of poor mental health extends beyond direct treatment costs. Indirect costs include the burden on care-givers, lost productivity and employment and increased risks of developing physical health problems. The costs of poor mental health have been estimated at that time to be at 3–4% of the gross national product (GNP) in Europe and 2.5% of the GNP in the US. Singapore's mental health manpower was also significantly lower than most developed countries (WHO, 2005). For example, there is an acute shortage of psychiatrists: the number of registered psychiatrists as of 15 May 2006 is 108; based on current requirements, Singapore needs at least 200 psychiatrists, or 4.76

per 100,000 population, which is still lower than corresponding figures for many Western developed countries (Table 1).

Table 1: International Comparison of Psychiatrists and Psychiatric Nurses.

Country	Psychiatrists (Per 100,000 Population)	Psychiatric Nurses (Per 100,000 Population)
United States	13.7	6.5
United Kingdom	11	104
Germany	11.8	52
France	22	98
Denmark	16	59
Belgium	18	—
Sweden	20	32
Australia	14	53
New Zealand	6.6	74
Japan	9.4	59
Singapore	2.3	10.4
Thailand	0.6	2.7
Malaysia	0.6	0.5
South Korea	3.5	10.1
Hong Kong	2	46.4
Macau	2.2	8.5

At the turn of the new millennium, Singapore's suicide rates were showing signs of concern, particularly among the young. In 2000/2001, we had the second highest rate of adolescent suicide. Prevalence studies up till that point showed that we had comparable rates for mental health disorders. Singapore's population structure is expected to age progressively in the next 10 to 15 years. Mental well-being and dementia in the elderly will be important challenges. Other social changes such as increasing divorce rates, changing family structures and economic pressures will also pose mental well-being challenges for Singaporeans.

These national trends along with WHO reports on the impact that mental health disorders and their burden are likely to make in the next decades prompted the Government of Singapore to embark on developing a national mental health policy. Such policy has long-term consequences on the mental health of the population. A good policy can improve accessibility, organisation and quality of services as well as the participation and integration into the community of persons with mental illness and their caregivers. This process is a delicate one involving the complex body of health, welfare and general social policies. A comprehensive approach to mental health is to establish a policy that covers the entire spectrum of the community: the mentally healthy, those at risk of a mental disorder, those with minor psychiatric morbidity, those with mental disorders and finally those who succumb to suicide and death. Such an approach demands the establishment of a stronger relationship between mental health services and the wider health sector and the consideration of the social and physical environment in which people live. It is also necessary to ensure inter-agency collaboration to ensure adequate consideration of the impact to mental health when education programmes and community services, housing, welfare and employment policies, the maintenance of law and order, and policies specifically addressing the young and the old are being planned or implemented.

The Ministry of Health (MOH) formed the National Mental Health Committee in 2005 led by the then Chairman of the Medical Board of the Institute of Medical Health (IMH), Professor Wong Kim Eng. The terms of reference were to review the ongoing efforts in the area of mental health and propose a blueprint of initiatives from 2007 to 2011. She formed a main committee which had 10 subcommittees that formulated the strategies. The national committee took the lead to develop this national policy based on the following principles:

1. **Mental health encompasses both mental well-being and the absence of mental disorder.**
   To be mentally healthy is not simply to be free of mental disorders; it is also to possess a sense of mental well-being and the resilience to overcome life stressors.

2. **Mental health is indivisible from general health.**
   Physical illness can precipitate mental disorders. Persons with mental illness are also more likely to suffer from other disorders. They are more likely to have behavioural factors that put them at risk. Persons with mental illness may be less likely to access medical care for physical illness. It is important to view mental health as an intrinsic component of overall health. Mental health promotion and the delivery of mental health care cannot be considered in isolation from other health promotion and care services.

3. **Mental health promotion and care must be evidence-based and cost-effective.**
   Resources are limited. It is essential that services are based on the best scientific evidence. The cost-effectiveness of services is also important given that there are multiple competing healthcare needs for the financial resources available.

4. **Persons with mental illness should be provided with appropriate services, preferably within the community.**
   Internationally, provision of mental healthcare has shifted away from being centralised in large psychiatric hospitals into community-based care. This is based on evidence that such forms of care are associated with better outcomes, when supported by well-planned community programmes and facilities. Services provided to persons with mental illness should be commensurate with their needs.

5. **Services should be accessible to all people.**
   Mental health promotion and services should be based on the principle of equality. Vulnerable and difficult-to-reach groups such as the poorly educated and the low-income should be targeted to improve their access to services.

6. **Persons with mental illness should not be discriminated against.** There is great stigma associated with mental disorders. This has resulted in limited employment opportunities, discriminatory health insurance coverage and poor social integration.

7. **The views and needs of persons with mental illness and their caregivers should be considered when planning, delivering and evaluating services.** This will enable the provision of services that are appropriate, culturally sensitive and effective.

8. **Mental health care and promotion is a multi-sectoral effort** There is a close relationship between mental health and social factors. Social factors can predispose to, precipitate and prolong mental disorders. Promoting mental health and delivering mental health services require an inter-sectoral approach and should involve the collaboration and participation of all relevant stakeholders.

With these principles in mind, the new mental health policy has as its vision for Singapore to be an emotionally resilient and mentally healthy community with access to community-based, comprehensive and cost-effective mental health services. It aims to i) promote mental health and, where possible, prevent the development of mental health problems and mental disorders; and ii) reduce the impact of mental disorders.

Strategic Initiatives

Singapore's mental health services in 2006 consisted of a system of hospital-centric services of outpatient ambulatory care with more than 90% of psychiatric beds at IMH and an increasing network of outpatient psychiatric services at the general hospitals. Community care was largely focused on a hospital centric community nursing support as well as a small number of voluntary welfare organisations (VWOs) focused on helping the most severe mental illnesses. Treatment for mental disorders is mostly provided by IMH which had both general and specialist psychiatric inpatient and outpatient services. Psychiatric treatment is available in all the general hospitals, as well as in the Singapore Armed Forces (SAF) and some private hospitals. Mental health promotion is principally spearheaded by the Health Promotion Board (HPB), which runs the 'Mind Your Mind' programme targeted at the general public. The Ministry of Education (MOE) promotes mental resilience and health through pastoral programmes and life skills packages for schoolchildren. The Ministry of Manpower (MOM) and then Ministry of Community Development Youth and Sports (MCYS) support mental well-being in the working population by promoting work-life balance. VWOs also provide mental health promotion services. Social support and rehabilitation services for vulnerable populations, including persons with mental illnesses, are provided by MCYS and various VWOs.

The National Mental Health Blueprint (NMHB) formulated by the National Committee for Mental Health and endorsed by the then Minister of Health, Mr Khaw Boon Wan was developed with this backdrop in mind. It focused on five main areas that would address the greatest gaps in our system and to meet the challenges for the future. This was then operationalised into 10 strategic initiatives which was to be rolled out over 3 to 5 years with specific leads and outcomes for measurement.

Focus Area 1: Primary Prevention and Health Promotion

The evidence of prevention of mental illness is not as strong as that for health promotion. It was then decided that mental health prevention and promotion should be focused on: i) maintenance of mental well-being;

ii) children and adolescents; iii) at the workplace; iv) the elderly; and v) destigmatisation of mental disorders. Initiatives include:

Engaging family physicians in the care of mental health disorders

i) Increase training of family physicians in psychiatry;
ii) Enhance collaboration/develop partnership programmes between family physicians and tertiary service providers; and
iii) Review the use of Mediave to pay for follow-up of specific chronic psychiatric conditions at family physician clinics.

Promoting positive mental well-being

Mental health promotion should focus on positive mental health:

i) Mental health promotion will embrace a variety of channels to communicate its messages;
ii) Efforts to promote mental well-being in the elderly should be expanded and enhanced;
iii) MOH should play a key role in coordination of mental health promotion efforts at the national level; and
iv) Efforts to destigmatise and to create awareness of mental disorders in the general population should be continued.

Focus Area 2: Provision and Coordination of Services

Provision and co-ordination of services should be improved in areas where gaps were apparent and easier to reach targets. Based on this, the following areas were identified: i) community-based programmes and facilities should be developed so as to manage persons with mental illness within the community; ii) inter-sectoral collaboration should be enhanced to reduce fragmentation and duplication of services; iii) right-siting of care should be emphasised to optimise healthcare resources; iv) mental health services for children and adolescents should be enhanced; v) mental health services for the elderly should be enhanced; vi) services for the management of addiction disorders should be further developed; and vii) services for the offenders with mental illness should be developed and coordinated. Initiatives include:

Improving the provision and co-ordination of mental health services for children and adolescents

i) Establish an interdisciplinary committee for the mental health of children and adolescents;
ii) Establish multidisciplinary community mental health teams; and
iii) Provide better training for mental health professionals.

Improving the management of persons with mental illness in the community

i) Establish community-based psychiatric services for private and general hospital patients;
ii) Develop a range of community-based care services, such as residential and employment services;
iii) Establish an interdisciplinary committee on community psychiatry, which should explore, among other issues, the feasibility of using Medisave for outpatient treatment, raising the cap for inpatient treatment, and providing insurance coverage for psychiatric disorders; and
iv) Review the applicability of Community Treatment Orders after community resources for mental health care have been enhanced.

Improving the provision and coordination of mental health services for the elderly

i) Implement an 'Area Psychogeriatric Service Framework'; and
ii) Enhance collaboration with existing eldercare services.

Improving the provision and coordination of services for patients with addiction disorders

i) Establish the National Addiction Medicine Service (NAMS), and under it, develop specialised services to treat youths with addictions and/or high-risk behaviour, specialised services for women and the elderly and community-based services and residential facilities to provide continuum of care. This was initially conceptualised as a separate institution which eventually it became obvious that it should be part of the Buangkok campus; and
ii) Set up an inter-ministry committee for addiction services.

Improving the provision and coordination of services for offenders with mental illness

i) Improve forensic nursing manpower;
ii) Introduce psychosocial rehabilitation;
iii) Introduce community forensic services and case management;
iv) Develop training modules in basic Forensic Mental Health for prison wardens, police, MCYS officers and nurses; and
v) Improve Prisons psychiatric services.

Focus Area 3: Mental Health Professionals

The mental health workforce is under resourced in Singapore and should be expanded; i) the number of psychiatrists should be increased to meet current shortage and the projected future increase in demand; ii) training of family physicians to recognise and manage mental disorders should be improved; iii) training standards for clinical psychologists should be set, and the implementation of a registration system should be explored; and iv) training and subspecialisation of allied mental health professionals (such as occupational therapists, medical social workers and psychiatric nurses) should be developed.

Initiatives include:

i) Start mandatory registration for clinical psychologists;
ii) Encourage voluntary certification of medical social workers and occupational therapists;
iii) Increase the number of psychiatrists, registered mental health nurses, Advanced Practice Nurses (Mental Health) and clinical psychologists; and
iv) Enhance training opportunities by starting a degree programme in occupational therapy, providing short courses for medical social workers and developing a Diploma in Mental Health for family physicians.

Focus Area 4: Monitoring

Monitoring of the quality of mental health services should be improved so that i) global indicators of mental health are developed; ii) care pathways should be developed and utilised for common mental disorders; and iii) quality audit indicators for specific mental disorders should be developed with relevant targets. Initiatives include:

Improving the monitoring of the quality of mental health services

i) Conduct regular mental health surveys of the population;
ii) Develop appropriate audit criteria to measure the quality of psychiatric services at general hospitals, IMH and community-based services; and
iii) Enhance indicators for the National Disease Control Plan for Mental Health.

Focus Area 5: Research

Funding for mental health research in i) development of appropriate and cost-effective mental health services; and ii) clinical research.

Cost of Initiatives

A fund of over SGD 70 million dollars was set aside of which 58.7% was focused on the integrated mental healthcare, 24.5% on mental health promotion and prevention, 13.3% on developing mental health manpower and 3.5% on mental health research.

Indicators and Targets Used

A combination of lead and lag indicators were used. Leading indicators include:

Mental health promotion

i) Health promotion outreach to employees annually
ii) Proportion of Singaporeans aged 18–65 years who
   a. are aware of positive ways to maintain mental health
   b. engage in appropriate activities to maintain good mental health
iii) Proportion of children/adolescents who are
   a. aware of coping strategies to facilitate the achievement of mental wellness
   b. engage in appropriate activities to maintain good mental health
iv) Proportion of Singaporeans aged 18–65 who are willing to seek help if symptoms of mental illness are present

Integrated mental health care

i) Train General Practitioners (GPs) to participate in the GP partnership programme which allows flow of chronic patients to primary care
ii) Enrol GPs in a mental health skills-based course to upgrade their capability in managing stable chronic mental health conditions

Mental health manpower

i) Improve the numbers of registered psychiatrists
ii) Improve the numbers of clinical psychologists and Advance Practice Nurses in Psychiatry

iii) Development of a degree programme in occupational therapy
iv) Evaluation of registration of clinical psychologists

Mental health research

i) Enrol and train clinician scientists and investigators
ii) Recruit expert clinical scientists and investigators
iii) Conduct regular national mental health surveys
iv) Develop research collaborations with renowned centres
v) Develop pilot projects for mental health promotion
vi) Develop clinical research programmes in specified areas

Lagging indicators which represent overall indicators of performance include:

i) Reduce prevalence of adult mild mental health conditions
ii) Reduce rates of attempted suicides
iii) Reduce overall suicide rates
iv) Reduce annual readmission rates for serious mental health disorders such as schizophrenia, depression and bipolar disorders
v) Reduce occurrence of depression
vi) Reduce length of stay for acute schizophrenia, and bipolar disorders

Conclusions

The NMHB provided the first steps in paving the way towards improving mental health care and service delivery in Singapore. A variety of initiatives with an emphasis on improving awareness of mental health and shifting the existing system from a largely hospital-based model towards a community-based model of care. The Blueprint helped to galvanise the development of community-based programmes with the establishment of community mental health teams for patients of all ages.

Moving Ahead

From 2012, the Blueprint provided the basis for expansion of community-based psychiatric services and capabilities in the community and increasing accessibility to care to fully support de-institutionalisation efforts. One major challenge ahead for government and the community is to ensure that mental illness is treated like any other physical health issue, as well as ensure that appropriate community services are in place to address the unique disabling effects that can be associated with the illness. It was with these challenges that, a community mental health masterplan was proposed to integrate care and services outside of our healthcare system. This included physician-led multidisciplinary teams to assess and manage patients for acute mild mental health conditions which then can be discharged back to their primary care physicians. The primary care doctors are supported by psychotherapy and counselling services for service coordination and continuity of care. At the same time, social agencies will be equipped to conduct outreach activities to educate residents on common types of mental illnesses and avenues to seek help and support. All of these will be supported by a network of helplines and case management systems to provide surveillance and support.

As Singapore celebrates the jubilee of its independence, it will also need to look at a new mental health plan that can build on the foundations of the blueprint and fill the gaps that have emerged. The principles for this new plan will involve integrating physical and mental health care, integrating mental health and social health, avoiding over-medicalisation of mental health issues activating and empowering patients and caregivers, re-designing systems, not creating more services/programmes, moving from transactional to relationship based care, whole-of-government, multi-agency approach including involvement and support of community groups and achieving more with the finite resources.

References

Comtois KA (2002). A review of interventions to reduce the prevalence of parasuicide. *Psychiatr Serv* **53**: 1138–1144.

Department of Health, UK. The Health of the Nation benchmarked to the target set under 1992.

Fisher WH, Barreira PJ, Geller JL, White AW, Lincoln AK, Sudders M (2001). Long-stay patients in state psychiatric hospitals at the end of the 20th century. *Psychiatr Serv* **52**: 1051–1056.

Harman JS, Cuffel BJ, Kelleher KJ (2004). Profiling hospitals for length of stay for treatment of psychiatric disorders. *J Behav Health Serv Res* **31**(1): 66–74.

Hickie IB, Davenport T, Luscombe GM, Groom GL, McGorry PD (2005). Australian mental health reform: Time for real outcomes. *Med J Aust* **182**(8): 401–406.

Institute of Mental Health (2007). National Mental Health Blueprint Singapore. 2007–2012. Available at: https://www.imh.com.sg/uploadedFiles/Publications/IMH%20National%20Mental%20Health%20Blueprint.pdf

World Health Organisation, WHO (2005). Mental Health Atlas. Available at: http://www.who.int/mental_health/evidence/atlas/

Samaritans of Singapore

Arnab Kumar GHOSH, KHOO Hui Leng and Christine WONG

Introduction

Samaritans of Singapore (SOS) is a secular non-profit suicide prevention centre which provides 24-hour confidential emotional support to people with difficulty coping during a crisis, contemplating suicide or affected by suicide. Since its establishment on 1 December 1969, SOS has developed into a professionally run organisation.

Its vision is to be the premier organisation in suicide prevention. Armed with a mission to be an available lifeline to anyone in crisis, it works with a holistic approach; focusing on prevention, intervention and postvention.

It is a member of Singapore's National Council of Social Service (NCSS) and is supported by the Community Chest. It has affiliations with the American Association of Suicidology (AAS), International Association for Suicide Prevention (IASP), Befrienders Worldwide (BW) and International Federation of Telephonic Emergency Services (IFOTES). (More details can be found here: https://sos.org.sg/)

History

Singapore underwent rapid urbanisation in the 1960s. Kampongs and communal livings were replaced by high-rise buildings within a short span of time. There were rising concerns about increased pace of living and stress levels. In 1966 the Churches' Counselling Centre (later renamed Counselling and Care Centre) (CCC) was launched by the Methodist and Anglican Churches. SOS was established by the CCC in 1969. Rev Dr Gunnar J. Teilmann Jr, an American Methodist missionary pastor was the founding director. Even though SOS' cause was strongly supported by the churches, there was a clear rule that no Samaritan was to take the opportunity in SOS to preach about his or her religion (Wong, 2009).

Key Milestones

On 1 December 1969, SOS launched its suicide prevention telephone hotline number 96544 from an office at the YWCA Centre, 254 Outram Road. Subsequently in1973, another telephone line was added and the number was changed to 91444. SOS eventually moved to its own premises at 591A New Bridge Road in 1976 and its hotline number was changed to 221 4444.

In 1986, SOS installed a special emergency line for referring agencies, SOS leaders and clients in crisis. In 1989, the SOS office shifted to Block 18, #03-21 at Outram Park, which offered more room for operations and training. With the introduction of toll-free lines for callers, the SOS Hotline number was changed to 1800-221-4444 in 1991.

Later in 1992, in line with its suicide prevention work, SOS and NCSS jointly organised a two-day Suicide Intervention Workshop. SOS also conducted two Suicide Intervention Workshops at the Association of Psychological and Educational Counselors of Asia (APECA) 9th Biennial Conference in Indonesia and another one at the Women Crisis Centre (Pusat Krisis Anita) in Penang, Malaysia.

SOS organised its first annual Suicide Prevention Week (thereafter renamed Suicide Awareness Week) in 1993. In the same year SOS published the book '*The Wish to Die: Suicidal Behavior in Singapore*' by Kok Lee Peng, Tsoi Wing-Foo and Maureen Fung.

The SOS office relocated to Block 10 Cantonment Close and was officially opened on 12 January 2002 by Mr Mah Bow Tan, then Minister for National Development and Patron of SOS in the presence of His Excellency S. R. Nathan, then President of the Republic of Singapore.

In 2003, SOS started the Email Befriending service and the first suicide bereavement support group in Singapore, called '*The Healing Bridge*'. The following year, a new Community Gatekeepers Training Programme was launched together with the Emotional First-Aid workshop targeting youths.

The Local Outreach to Suicide Survivor (LOSS) Programme was officially launched island-wide in 2006. SOS also started to conduct training in suicide postvention.

SOS received the Non-Profit Organisation Award for Volunteer Management during the National Volunteerism and Philanthropy Awards in 2008. In the same year, SOS published Yin's '*Why? When Both My Parents Took their Lives*', the first book in Singapore to relate the story of an individual affected by suicide (commonly referred to as suicide survivor). The book provides invaluable insight into the journey of a grieving suicide survivor in Singapore and seeks to impart hope and comfort to other survivors.

In 2010, SOS held a two-day conference in conjunction with the Suicide Awareness Week and in celebration of its 40th anniversary. The conference was attended by local professionals as well as delegates from various Befrienders Worldwide member centres. Prof Graham Martin, National advisor on suicide prevention to the Australian Government, was the keynote speaker.

In 2011, a new training programme, called Youth Support Youth (YSY), was developed as part of a collaborative effort between SOS, the Health Promotion Board (HPB), the Institute of Mental Health's Community Health Assessment Team (CHAT) and Silver Ribbon (Singapore).

In 2013, the SOS constitution was revised to better reflect the organisation's vision, mission and structure. The Board of Management developed a three-year strategic plan to review and enhance its services and programmes.

In the same year, SOS published the book '*Letters to Aly: Surviving my BFF's Suicide*' by Lee-Ann in conjunction with World Suicide Prevention Day. It is a compilation of diary entries of a local teenage suicide survivor about losing her best friend to suicide and her journey to recovery.

In 2014, SOS commemorated the International Survivors of Suicide Loss (ISOS Loss) day for the first time.

24-Hour Hotline Service

The SOS hotline, 1800-221 4444, is available round-the-clock. Calls are received by trained volunteers from diverse backgrounds. As of 31 March

2014, SOS had a total of 183 full-fledged volunteers and 24 provisional volunteers (undergoing pre-service training). SOS professional staffs are also available to provide consultation and support to the volunteers, as well as follow-up on critical cases.

During the period of April 2013 to March 2014, SOS hotline handled a total of 37,462 incoming calls with an average of 103 per day. The 'Suicide Question' was posted in 52% of the incoming calls. Callers expressed suicide ideation or plans in 36% of calls where 'Suicide Question' was asked. Of the calls with suicide risk, 828 incoming calls were assessed to be of high and medium risk.

The hotline has also been attending to repeat callers with poor social support. During this period, about 41% of total incoming calls were from such regular callers. A variety of problems were presented in the calls, with relationship and social problems among the top. 50% of the suicidal callers below the age of 30 spoke about their difficulties with family relationships (SOS, 2014).

The hotline witnessed a surge of crisis calls from April 2008 to March 2009 corresponding with the global financial crisis. The total number of crisis calls has decreased since then but the number of calls with suicidal risk still remains high. (SOS, 2005–2014) (Graph 1).

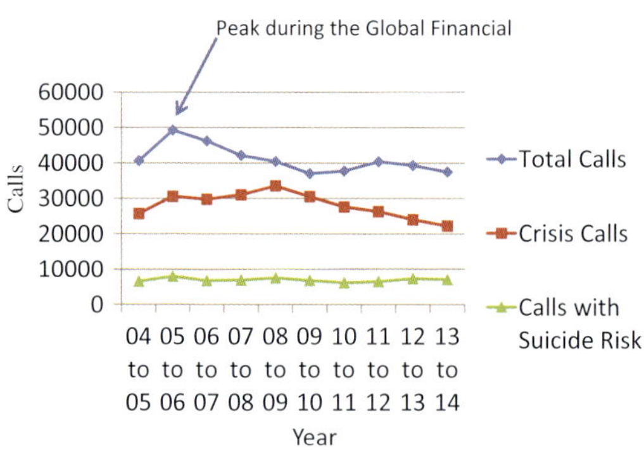

Graph 1: SOS Hotline call trends in recent years.

Email Befriending

With the digital revolution, internet use became widespread in the 2000s. SOS set up the Email Befriending service in 2003 to provide an alternate platform for people in crisis to seek emotional support. It is not a round the clock service and the response time is usually within two working days. The email address is pat@sos.org.sg.

Both the number of clients using this service and number of emails exchanged have increased rapidly over last few years. SOS handled 993 clients from April 2013 to March 2014 as compared to 276 from April 2009 to March 2010. In 2013/2014, out of the 420 clients who disclosed their age, close to 80% were aged 30 and below.

About 63% of the clients who wrote to Pat during this period felt suicidal at some point in time. Many of these suicidal clients cited having multiple stressors, with common stressors being relationship difficulties with family members, depression and stress over studies and exams (SOS, 2014).

Specialist Counselling

SOS has adopted a holistic approach to crisis work. It offers face-to-face counselling sessions to clients who need professional support and intervention to cope with their suicide-related crises. These counselling sessions are conducted by professional staffs who are counsellors, psychologists and social workers. In 2013/2014, 168 clients were attended to and a total of 408 sessions were conducted. Out of the 168 clients, 115 clients presented with personal crises due to various reasons and were at risk of suicide. The remaining 53 clients (32%) were suicide survivors and were seen for grief counselling. More than half of the suicide survivors who went through grief counselling had suicidal ideation themselves (SOS, 2014).

Local Outreach to Suicide Survivors (LOSS)

LOSS is the only local outreach programme providing information and emotional support to people affected by suicide death. SOS has been partnering with Singapore Police Force and other partners since the inception of the LOSS in 1 June 2006. In some cases, the team gets activated to a suicide site, mortuary or residence to make the first contact with grieving families. SOS professional staff follow up with the grieving family and friends through phone, emails, and SMSes. In 2013/2014, there were 133 LOSS cases in total. A LOSS team was activated in 77 cases.

As a part of outreach, care cards are sent to clients prior to the anniversary of their loss or festive periods, which are known to be particularly difficult times. A total of 116 care cards were sent in 2013/2014 (SOS, 2014).

Healing Bridge

Healing bridge is a suicide bereavement support group co-facilitated by staffs professionally trained in grief work and experienced survivors. Members meet at SOS to share experiences, talk about their feelings and receive positive encouragement from others who have suffered similar losses.

A total of 30 survivors attended at least one Healing Bridge session in 2013/2014. About one-third of the Healing Bridge members were foreigners from countries such as India, Malaysia, China and the UK (SOS, 2014).

Crisis Support

In some cases, professional staff follow up with suicidal clients to continue crisis support. This is done via outgoing calls, emails and SMSes. Face-to-face counselling can be arranged as well. This service is also extended to clients referred by the police and concerned others. When SOS receives a referral from a community partner or concerned party, SOS initiates contact with the person-at-risk to offer support.

In 2013/2014, 4,159 calls were made by professional staff to clients in crisis. Some 413 emails were initiated to follow up on clients with suicide risk. The years 2013/2014 saw an increase in the use of SMS as a way to contact clients. There were 2,507 SMSes sent from April 2013 to March 2014 compared to 2,059 in April 2012 to March 2013. SMSes also serve as a visual reminder of the hotline number (SOS, 2014).

Referral and Case Consultations

SOS has been working closely with the Singapore Police Force (SPF) and various other community partners. In 2013/2014, SOS received 691 referrals among which 396 were from SPF. In recent years, referrals from non-official sources such as from family, friends and other concerned third parties have increased, indicating greater community awareness about suicide and available community resources. Such referrals made up 37% of the referrals received in that year (SOS, 2014).

SOS provides consultation on cases related to suicide crises or deaths and other related topics to other voluntary welfare organisations (VWOs) and agencies. This can be done by phone or email. Upon request, SOS can also arrange small group sessions where social workers, counsellors or psychologists can consult our professional staff on ongoing or past cases. For example, a group consultation session was organized for the Ministry of Education (MOE)'s school counsellors in 2013. Twenty participants attended the consultation session entitled 'A Conversation with SOS — Teen Suicide Attempters', and consulted on related cases they handled in their respective schools.

Professional Training

SOS believes that suicide prevention, intervention and postvention require the combined efforts of many, and try to achieve this through sharing knowledge and skills that can be applied in different settings. Professional training programs by SOS like the Suicide Intervention Skills Workshop

(SISW), Suicide Postvention Skills Workshop (SPSW) and Clinical Skills in Suicide Work (CSSW) are recognised by the Singapore Association for Social Workers (SASW) and Singapore Association for Counsellors (SAC) as continuing professional education (CPE) courses. The workshops generally comprise of lectures, video clips, simulation exercises and small-group discussions. All courses are conducted by SOS staff, comprising trained practitioners with local hands-on experience of working with suicidal clients and suicide survivors.

SOS has also been conducting a range of training programmes for schools and even the general public. Besides the standardised training programmes, SOS also runs various customised workshops to suit the needs of different groups and institutions.

In 2013/2014, SOS conducted a total of 13 workshops for 304 professionals in the social service, medical and educational sectors. SOS held 24 sessions for 333 students from different educational institutions ranging from the secondary to the tertiary level as it believes in the importance of training young people to engage and reach out to their peers at risk. In an effort to bridge the gap in service, SOS also initiated suicide prevention talks and workshops in Mandarin (SOS, 2014).

Community Awareness and Outreach

SOS organises talks and sharing sessions regarding suicide prevention to heighten community awareness and surveillance. In 2013, SOS produced postcards and notebooks using award-winning artworks, to spread awareness in community and promote help seeking behaviour. It has published numerous books and articles and participated in various conferences and forums to spread its message (SOS, 2014).

Conclusion

Since its inception in 1960s as a hotline manned by volunteers, SOS has evolved as a professionally run organisation with a holistic approach.

Over the years, SOS has established itself as a leading suicide prevention centre in Singapore. With its innovative ways to reach out to the community it has been successful in meaningfully engaging and rallying the community in suicide prevention. The increasingly demanding nature of the hotline work poses a considerable challenge to SOS in recruiting volunteers to keep its 24-hour volunteer-run hotline going (*The Straits Times*, 2015).

References

Samaritans of Singapore, SOS (2006). Annual Report 2005–2006.

Samaritans of Singapore, SOS (2007). Annual Report 2006–2007.

Samaritans of Singapore, SOS (2008). Annual Report 2007–2008.

Samaritans of Singapore, SOS (2009). Annual Report 2008–2009.

Samaritans of Singapore, SOS (2010). Annual Report 2009–2010. Available at: https://sos.org.sg/images/AR/SOS%20Annual%20Report%2009-10.pdf

Samaritans of Singapore, SOS (2011). Annual Report 2010–2011. Available at: https://sos.org.sg/images/AR/SOS%20Annual%20Report%2010-11.pdf

Samaritans of Singapore, SOS (2012). Annual Report 2011–2012. Available at: https://sos.org.sg/images/AR/SOS%20AR%20FY2011-2012.pdf

Samaritans of Singapore, SOS (2013). Annual Report 2012–2013. Available at: https://sos.org.sg/images/AR/AR2013.pdf

Samaritans of Singapore, SOS (2014). Annual Report 2013–2014. Available at: https://sos.org.sg/images/AR/AR2014.pdf

The Straits Times, 18 May 2015. 'Up to 30% more volunteers needed to help those in distress', Available at: http://www.todayonline.com/singapore/30-more-volunteers-needed-help-those-distress?page=1

Wong C (2009). Hello, Samaritans of Singapore, can I help you? *Methodist Message* **111**(3): 19–20.

The Development of Mental Health Services by VWOs (1993–2013)

TAN Weng Mooi and Elaine SOH

'Since the 1950s, due to increased focus on the human rights of individuals with mental disorders, their long-term placements in mental asylums, many of which provided poor living conditions, were considered less than ideal. The development of new and effective medications has enabled patients with severe mental illness to live safely within the community. The move towards the deinstitutionalisation of mental state hospital patients was emphasised in many developed countries, and most of the large state mental hospitals were either downsized or closed.' (Goldman *et al.*, 1983)

Moving from Custodial Care to Community Support Care

In 1975, Singapore set up a secondary institution named View Road Hospital to meet the high demand of the inpatient population at Woodbridge Hospital. At that point in time, the inpatient population at Woodbridge Hospital reached a peak of 2,654 for average daily occupancy while the bed capacity was only 2,029 (Ng, 1993).

At that point in time, the model of care provided was pretty much custodial and authoritarian where the institution confined raging individuals who were deemed dangerous to themselves and a nuisance to others. The objective then was to keep all mentally ill patients away from the community and the patients were made to conform to the rules and regulation of institutionalisation. Mechanical restraints played a large role in 'treatment'. Camisoles, restraint-chains and waist-belts were used to gain the necessary submission and respect of the patients.

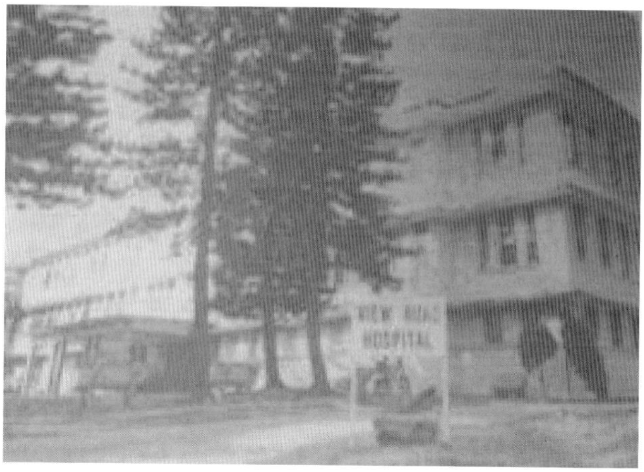

View Road Hospital providing institutionalised care.

As the population boomed, the hospital facility was unable to cope with the increased intake of patients. Thus, the hospital attempted to release the more stable patients back into the community. However, the patients were sent back to the hospital as there were no community support resources for the patients and their families. Often, the families were at a lost, not knowing how to cope and manage their loved ones in the community. As such, the hospital set up the Community Psychiatric Nursing team in 1988 and psychiatric nurses conducted home visits to provide care, support and follow-up for patients within the community.

However, with the increasing focus on holistic therapeutic care and growing patients with mental illness, the government saw the need to change the model of care. In 1984, the Ministry of Health (MOH) mooted the idea of a new psychiatric hospital to evolve from a largely custodial care model to one of community care for the benefit of the people. The prevention, early treatment and rehabilitation of clients with mental conditions would actively operate within the community as opposed to late treatment within an institution that would isolate them from everyday life and make it much harder for them to reintegrate into the community.

A couple of voluntary welfare organisations (VWOs) were set up in the 1980s and 1990s as they saw the need to provide support resources for the mentally ill patients in the community. They include the Singapore Anglican Community Services (SACS), then known as the Singapore Anglican Welfare Council till 2005, and Caregivers' Association of the Mentally Ill (CAMI). Existing VWOs such as the Singapore Association for Mental Health (SAMH) also felt the need to expand their services, in order to better support persons with mental illness to be reintegrated into the community.

However, as the hospital and VWOs were focused on developing their own work in different niches, they were pretty much operating in silos with little coordination, cooperation and communication.

Community Support Care

'It is paradoxical that the community provides hospitals for the care and treatment of the mentally ill person so that he may recover and resume his place in the community. But what happens! When he returns from the hospital to the community, he is shunned by society and cut off into a social isolation with little or no help in getting him back on his feet...the formation of a mental health association will not only deal with the rehabilitation of the mentally ill patient but shall include the prevention of mental illness and the promotion of mental health in its widest implication.' Dr Paul W. Ngui, former President of SAMH at the Inaugural Meeting (SAMH, 2010)

Seeing the need to ensure that persons with mental illness receive support in the community, SAMH set up the Oasis Club in 1969, the first Social Rehabilitation Programme for persons with psychiatric conditions to focus on developing self-respect, social skills and friendships. Members learnt to socialise and build relationships with one another, helping them to reintegrate back into the community. As part of the rehabilitative process, SAMH set up a Half-Way House at Rochester Park for women recovering from mental illness in 1977 and in 1981, they also provided counselling services for the community to allow early identification of mental health issues and promote mental wellness.

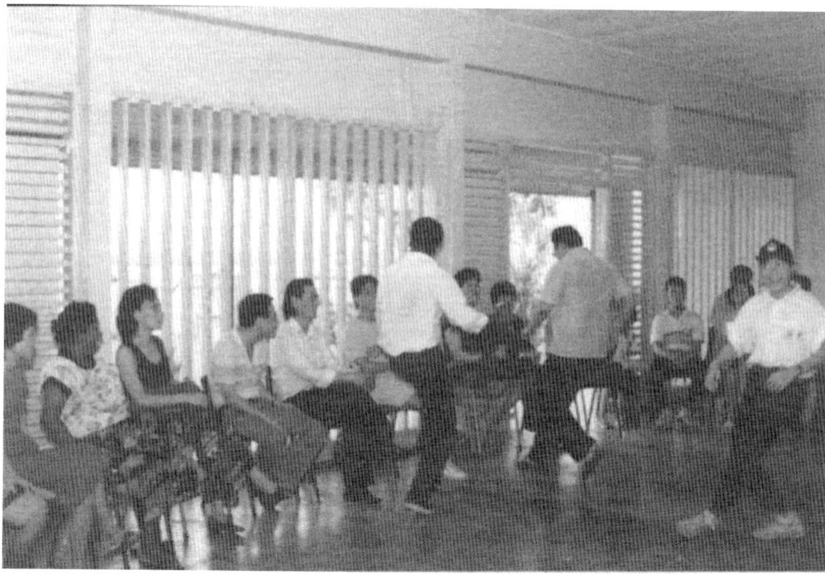

Members of the Oasis Club engaged in social activities.

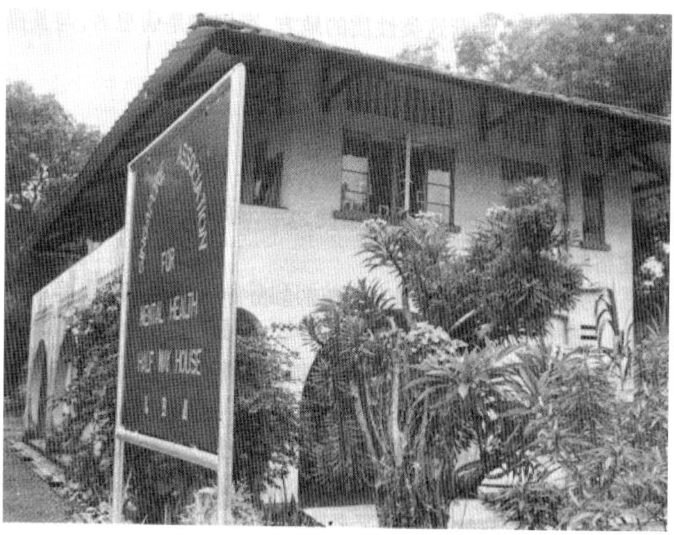

Half-Way House for recovering women.

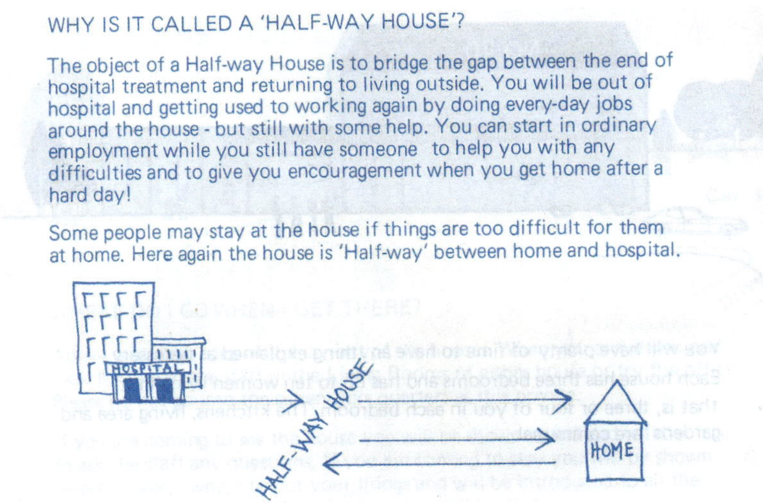

WHY IS IT CALLED A 'HALF-WAY HOUSE'?

The object of a Half-way House is to bridge the gap between the end of hospital treatment and returning to living outside. You will be out of hospital and getting used to working again by doing every-day jobs around the house - but still with some help. You can start in ordinary employment while you still have someone to help you with any difficulties and to give you encouragement when you get home after a hard day!

Some people may stay at the house if things are too difficult for them at home. Here again the house is 'Half-way' between home and hospital.

With the increasing need to reach out to those in need of the services, the SAMH Insight Centre and Oasis Day Centre were set up in 1994. The Insight Centre provides counselling, community mental health education programmes and support services such as Oasis Club and support groups, while the Oasis Day Centre provides psychosocial rehabilitation for clients who attend programmes at the centre which aims at helping them reintegrate into the community. In addition, SAMH set up the Bukit Gombak Group Homes (BGGH) in 1995, providing normalisation with residential services for clients within the common HDB community. Vocational and psychosocial rehabilitation are provided at BGGH to assist in their recovery, living, working, social and learning goals. All of these services are based in the community, thereby assisting clients in experiencing true community integration in the heartlands.

One other VWO who provided community services in the 1980s is the Singapore Anglican Community Services (SACS), then known as the Singapore Anglican Welfare Council till 2005. SACS has been providing community services since 1986 starting off with counselling services for victims of domestic violence who started showing mental health issues. As such, a day care centre for psychiatric clients was set up at the

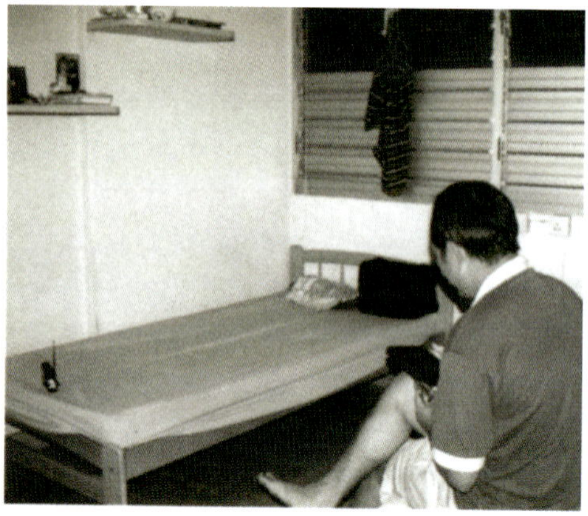

The first step to living within the community — Bukit Gombak Group Homes.

Whampoa Care Centre which started seeing more and more psychiatric clients instead. With this new need, SACS set up the Elliot Road Care Centre in 1992 for women with psychiatric conditions and subsequently the East Coast Care Centre for men. All three centres provided residential and day rehabilitation services within the community, and saw increasing demand in terms of caseload.

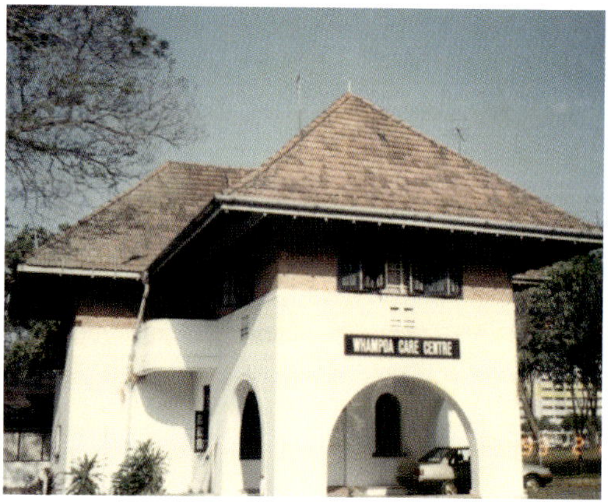

Whampoa Care Centre.

Paradigm Shift to Community Therapeutic Care

While the VWOs focused on developing community-based support services for mental health clients, the government saw the need to develop a new model of care towards right-siting where health care is dispensed to the appropriate site, which is not always going to be a hospital. The vision is to move away from a largely acute illness-centred, institutionalisation-based healthcare delivery system towards a community based model of psychiatric care. In order to achieve this, the government turned to existing VWOs who had been providing community mental health services and boosted their capability and capacity to provide better care. With the new move, View Road Hospital ceased operations in 2001. Where did the patients move to then?

The government recognised the capability of SACS' care centres in their management of patients with mental illnesses and thus boosted the capacity of SACS by setting up Hougang Care Centre (HCC) in 2002 and Simei Care Centre (SCC) in 2004. The patients from View Road Hospital were subsequently transferred to HCC.

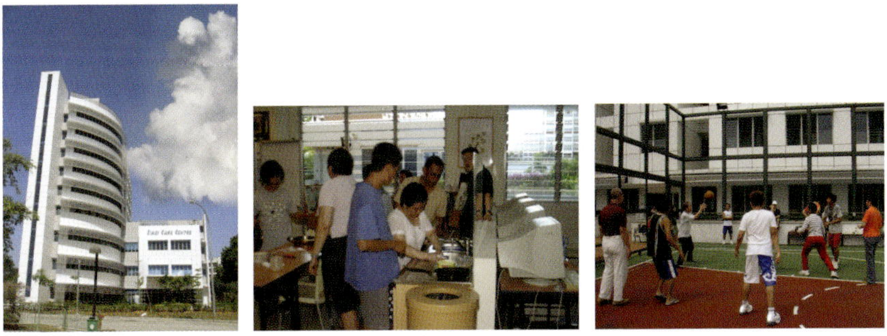

The new Simei Care Centre which simulates communal living and work place conditions.

The models of care provided in HCC and SCC are different. HCC is based on the Clubhouse model of psychosocial rehabilitation. This model focuses on the strengths, interests and talents of the individuals. It offers opportunities for clients to engage in meaningful activities that will help them develop confidence, life skills and social skills through working side by side with staff and volunteers in their journey towards recovery. SCC adopts the social enterprise model which provides skills-based training with the clients receiving remuneration for the work they put in.

How did SACS develop the various models of psychiatric rehabilitation? Back in the 1980s and 1990s, the types of psychiatric rehabilitation services provided was minimal and the key objective was purely to keep the patients occupied. Examples of psychiatric rehabilitation included farming and manual work. Recognising that these are not enough, SACS visited other countries to learn from them and adopted their models of care.

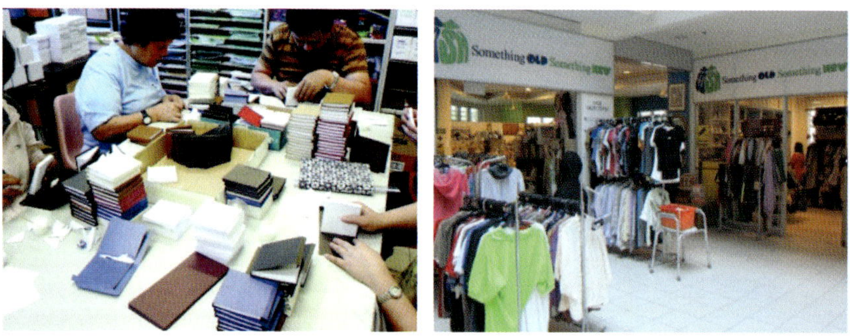

Rehabilitation workshops and Social Enterprises creating employment opportunities for the clients.

Recognising the importance of providing quality psychiatric rehabilitation services, the Association for Psychiatric Rehabilitation (Singapore), APRS, was set up in 2003 by mental health professionals from SACS, SAMH and IMH. It trained many professionals in CPRP (or Certified Psychiatric Rehabilitation Practitioners) and boosted the delivery of quality community-oriented rehabilitation services in Singapore.

Notwithstanding the existing community involvement, SACS is moving towards further community-based work who believe that everyone can recover and be reintegrated into society. As part of the holistic approach, SACS have also developed the Employment Support Services which was started with funds from Temasek Cares which prepares and trains our clients for long-term employment in the community. Again the collaborative approach is adopted and they also work with employers to better prepare them to hire the clients.

SACS never stopped reviewing their services and constantly look for new care models to better serve the clients' needs. Community Rehabilitation Support and Service (CRSS) was naturally set up in 2006 to move closer to the community, providing services in the clients' homes, helping them feel supported. To date, SACS has never denied care for those who cannot afford it. Their motto is 'To Counsel, to Restore and to Equip' — they believe that everyone can recover and be reintegrated into society. As part of their holistic approach, they set up the Employment Support Services which prepares and trains their clients for long-term employment in the community by working closely with the employers.

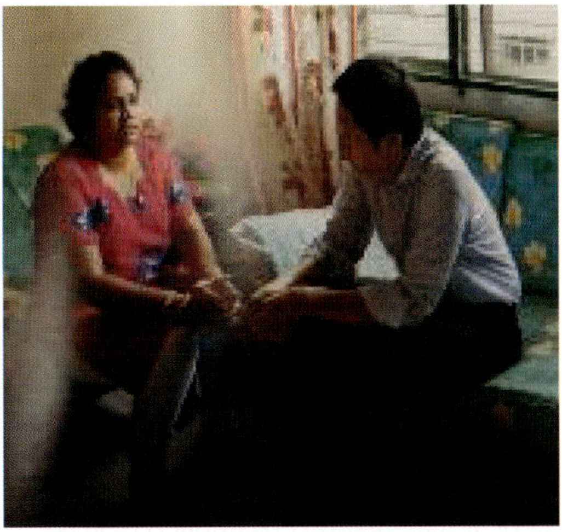

Home visits conducted by the CRSS team.

While SACS focused on rehabilitation and home visits for clients with mental illnesses, over the years, SAMH developed new innovative programmes and services to meet the needs of the clients and their caregivers. These include the Activity Hub@Pelangi Village, Club 3R, Family Link Programme (FLP), Illness Management and Recovery Programme (IMR) and Job Connect and Creative Hub. The Creative Hub was developed in 2011 based on the belief that people can heal and grow through creative expression, as such visual arts, music and dance which are utilised in a supportive environment to promote recovery and mental wellness and at the same time reduce stigmatisation. Together, SACs and SAMH serve as pioneers providing mental health services to a range of patients.

SAMH also identified the growing needs of youths which have not been catered to. In response to service gap resulting from the increased referrals from Child Guidance Clinic (CGC) and realising more young people were taking leave from school or had stopped schooling due to mental illness, the Oasis Day Centre thus expanded their services to reach out to the youth group aged between 14 and 18 years old. It was subsequently developed into the YouthReach Programme, catering to youths below 18 years old. The Programme included a mentorship component, interventions such as case management, counselling and various activities, as well as a 24-hour helpline to help the youths develop their maximum potential and be reintegrated with their family and the community. Family members and caregivers are also taught to understand and manage the youth's mental illness. Ensuring that the youth's needs are being met holistically, SAMH will be setting up the YouthReach Residence, a step-down facility from hospital inpatient care providing respite that addresses the recovery of youth identified with a mental illness.

Caregivers' Mental Well-Being Is Equally Important as the Clients'

While SACS provides rehabilitation for their clients, they understand that to ensure fast recovery for the clients, services are not the only factor.

There is a need to involve the caregivers in the recovery process. Caregivers often did not know how to care for their loved ones with mental illnesses and this created a need for education, training and support for caregivers. HCC and SCC had started running courses for the caregivers but both centres were unable to cope with the growing demand. Thus, in concurrence with some of the caregivers, SACS initiated the set-up of the Caregivers' Association of the Mentally Ill (CAMI) in 2005.

In short, CAMI is an association for caregivers by the caregivers. The caregivers come together to share common challenges and experiences. Other than providing workshops and support groups, CAMI also provides a helpline for caregivers to seek help. Due to limited resources, the helpline was manned by passionate board members who saw the need to journey with the caregivers to support them in their daily living.

A little girl and her father were crossing a bridge. The father was feeling scared so he asked his little daughter, 'Sweetheart, please hold my hand so that you don't fall into the river.'

The little girl said, 'No, Dad. You hold my hand.'
'What's the difference?' Asked the puzzled father.
'There's a big difference,' replied the little girl.

'If I hold your hand and something happens to me, chances are that I may let your hand go. But if you hold my hand, I know for sure that no matter what happens, you will never let my hand go.'

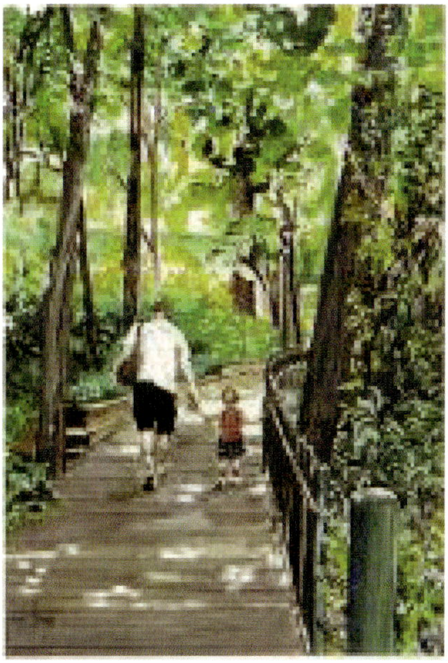

The mentally ill one is just like the little girl. The caregiver being the father will have to journey and provide them the assurance.

Caregivers often have to cope with issues such as emotional stress, lack of knowledge about the condition, lack of social support networks and neglecting personal health. While we aim to keep the clients within the community, there is a need to help the caregivers manage their loved ones to prevent the revolving door syndrome.

The Caregivers Alliance Limited (CAL) was set up in 2002 to provide training and support for caregivers. Instead of engaging professionals to conduct training, CAL adopted the National Alliance on Mental Illness (NAMI) model by identifying and developing caregiver leaders who are able to provide training and support to other caregivers. Other than providing caregiver support, CAL saw the need to provide outreach and training to caregivers regarding mental illness and the care of their loved ones through quality training. CAL aims to improve the lives of family and caregivers of persons with mental illness through education, outreach, referral and support.

Destigmatisation

In order to reduce institutionalisation and allow the patients to better re-integrate into the community, there is a need to change the public mindset thinking all mentally ill patients are dangerous. To combat mental health stigma, several VWOs were set up to encourage early treatment and facilitate integration of people with mental illness within the society through innovative means of promoting mental health literacy. They include Silver Ribbon (Singapore), the Action Group for Mental Illness (AGMI) and the Lejia Society.

To combat mental health stigma and encourage early treatment, Silver Ribbon (Singapore) organises at least two mental health events monthly and commemorates World Mental Health Day annually, collaborating with local and overseas mental health organisations, consumers, caregivers, government agencies, grassroots organisations, religious groups, school institutions, VWOs and the media to reach out to the community of all age groups through innovative means.

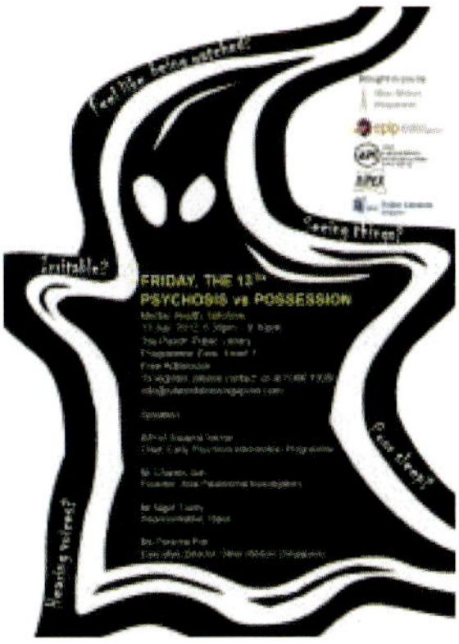

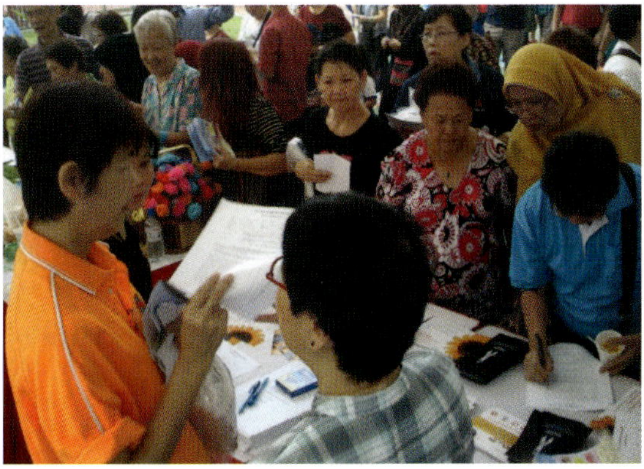

World Mental Health Day and outreach events.

Not Forgetting Development of Support for Dementia Clients and Caregivers

While community-based specialised services and support for psychiatric clients were developed by SACS and SAMH, the Alzheimer's Disease Association (ADA) was formed in the 1990s to provide support for elderly with dementia and their family members. The first Dementia Day Care Centre, named New Horizon Centre was set up by ADA in Toa Payoh to handle the increasing number of elderly with dementia. This was followed by three other centres.

> *'As Singapore's population ages, the number of people suffering from dementia is expected to rise. Based on our estimates, we currently have about 28,000 elderly aged 60 years and above with dementia, and this is expected to more than double to 80,000 by 2030'*
>
> Mr Gan Kim Yong, Minister for Health,
> at the 3rd Singapore International Neurocognitive Symposium,
> 5 April 2013

ADA was formed to increase the support and quality of care for persons with dementia. At the same time, it also wanted to enhance the ability of the caregivers and families to cope with and provide continual care for their loved ones with dementia. Although the set-up of the day care centres help the caregivers take care of their loved ones during the day, caregivers needed help to care for their loved ones when they are home. This eventually led to ADA's development of the Caregiver Support Groups and specialised Caregiver Support Centres.

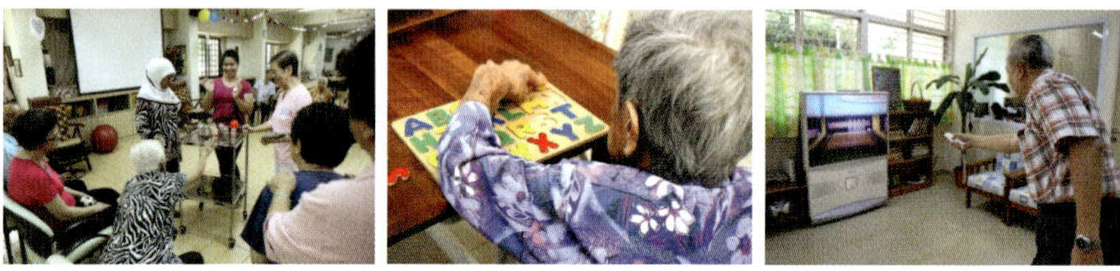

Activities at the Dementia Day Care Centres.

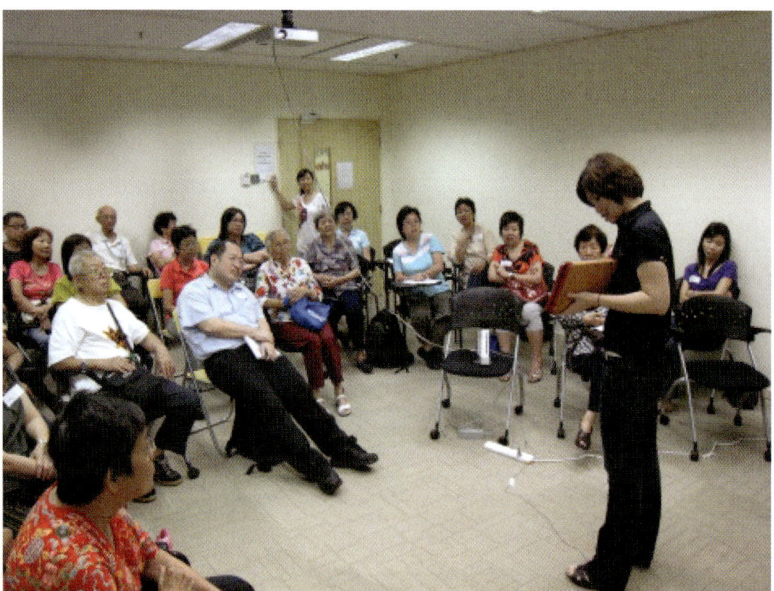

Caregivers attending support group session.

Positioning itself as the National Dementia Support Advocate, ADA would like to see itself in an advisory role — supporting other organisations providing dementia services instead of competing with them.

> *'ADA has come a long way since its inception in 1990 and although we have grown significantly since then, I believe there is still so much more that can be done to expand our services and presence in Singapore. This includes opening more day care centres, increasing our home-based services, starting a dementia resource and training centre and possibly looking into residential care.'*
>
> – Jason Foo, CEO of ADA

National Mental Health Blueprint

A National Mental Health Survey was conducted in 2004 which reported a lifetime prevalence of depression amongst adults as 5.6% (Chua *et al.*, 2004) and that of dementia amongst the elderly as 5.2% (Chiam *et al.*, 2004). Not only do more people in Singapore die from suicide than from road traffic accidents every year, but conditions like schizophrenia, major depression, and alcohol-use disorders significantly increase the risk of early mortality (Bruce *et al.*, 1994).

The results highlighted the need for more mental-health programmes and in 2005, MOH convened a committee of psychiatrists, medical administrators, other mental health professionals and representatives from non-governmental organisations to draw up a National Mental Health Blueprint (2007–2011) for the country, focussing on four strategic areas (Chong *et al.*, 2008):

- Mental health education and promotion;
- Integrating mental health care — through community-based mental health programmes and integration of psychiatric services in general hospitals;
- Developing mental health professionals; and
- Developing mental health research.

With the Blueprint, we made significant progress by improving mental health awareness, enhancing early detection and increasing access to treatment. The Blueprint also increased outreach from acute hospitals to the community for patients with mental illness, and thereby improved their clinical outcomes and quality of life.

However, the Singapore Mental Health Survey 2010 showed that more than half of those with mental disorders do not come forward for treatment which further illustrated the need for a community safety network.

Community Mental Health Masterplan Towards a Community-Based Population Health Approach

With the outcomes of the survey and the ending of the National Mental Health Blueprint, MOH decided to develop a Community Mental Health Masterplan (2012–2016) focusing on the following key areas:

- General Community Mental Health (CMH) Services;
- Dementia Care; and
- Psychiatric Intermediate and Long-Term Care (ILTC) Services.

In particular, for the General CMH Services, MOH had appointed the Agency for Integrated Care (AIC) as the programme manager to oversee and coordinate the development and implementation efforts on the ground. AIC is also tasked to look at integration across the various sectors such as the social and health care and provide navigation for the community to enable them to provide better support for the people with mental illness and their caregivers.

The goal of the General CMH Services can be achieved via the following strategic key thrusts:

- Empowerment through capability building in the community;

- Improve accessibility through capacity building and community support mechanism; and
- Destigmatisation and reintegration through targeted communications and outreach programmes.

Each network consists of stakeholders from the health and social care sectors integrating services through multi-layered community support network. Each network will be riding on the Regional Health System (RHS) with the objectives of:

- Integrating physical health and mental health;
- Integrating health and social care; and
- Adapting according to population needs, dovetailing on the strengths of the local community partners.

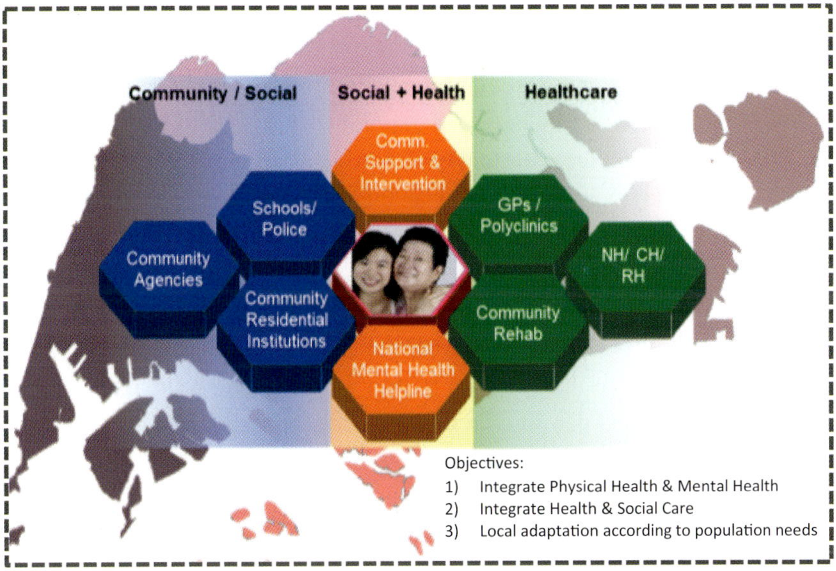

Integrating health and social care according to population needs.

Three focus areas of the General CMH Services were thus identified:

Capability building

Most people in the community will prefer to see General Practitioners (GPs) instead of a specialist psychiatrist in the hospital. According to research study, GPs were the most commonly preferred caregivers and were used by 41.1% of those who sought help (Ng *et al.*, 2003). Also, GPs are consulted more frequently as the sole provider of mental health care than the counsellors (Chong *et al.*, 2012). Thus, there is a need to partner more GPs and empower them by boosting their capability to manage the patients within the community.

The Community Intervention Team (COMIT) works hand-in-hand with the GPs where the GPs remain as the primary provider of care while COMIT provides additional support to the GPs. COMIT is a community-based allied health-led team which presents a holistic service and focuses on improving the clients' and caregivers' quality of life, equipping them with information to make informed decisions for the management of their condition and supporting social re-integration. COMIT is offered by O'Joy Care Services and Clarity Singapore.

O'Joy Care Services started gerontological counselling in 2004 for elderly clients at their homes and at their centre. With their extensive experience and network, they became a natural partner for COMIT as part of the iCommunity@North network in early 2012. To empower their staff to better manage the clients with dementia and depression, O'Joy worked closely with the Khoo Teck Puat Hospital (KTPH) who provided training in the use of various assessment scales. In addition, KTPH also refer discharged cases to O'Joy and facilitate weekly case discussions to ensure all discharged patients are carefully managed in the community. In June 2012, O'Joy also started their services in the central region, working closely with the Institute of Mental Health (IMH).

Another COMIT provider, Clarity Singapore, was launched in 2010 with the vision of assisting persons struggling with or recovering from mental illness to find hope and acceptance, to help and guide them so that they can overcome their difficulties and to develop their abilities. Clarity is an ideal partner for the COMIT programme as they are already providing specialised counselling, psychotherapy, art therapy, support group, mental health workshops and public education.

Besides counsellors, working hand in hand with the GPs are the Assessment and Shared Care Team (ASCAT). ASCAT are physician-led multidisciplinary teams situated in the community to manage patients for short interim period until they are stabilised and can be discharged back to their GPs for continual management. At the same time, GPs can also refer patients to see ASCAT to assess the need for upstream referral to the Specialist Outpatient Clinics (SOCs) in the hospitals. To date, there are ASCATs in Ang Mo Kio Polyclinic and KTPH and these two teams have helped around 400 patients as of March 2013. A total of six ASCAT teams across Singapore will be set up by 2016 to support up to 9,500 patients at any point in time.

Communication building

While we move towards developing and strengthening care and support in the community, engagement and communications is an important element which we cannot miss out. These include prevention and education programmes to destigmatise and build acceptance so that people with mental illnesses faces less resistance to stay within the community and can integrate smoothly into the society.

One key initiative is the Integrated Champions for Community Mental Health (iCHAMPs) which targets to create a network of advocates to enhance mental health awareness and support people at risk within their community through their existing relationships, with the ultimate aim to reduce stigmatisation.

Capacity building

As we intensify efforts to boost mental healthcare and support in the community, it is also important to put in place the infrastructure required to support it. We need a balanced, integrated and person-centred care model through multi-layered support network. There is a need to integrate the current community psychiatric facilities such as the Psychiatric

Nursing Homes and Day Care Centres with the acute hospitals to tighten workflow and referral processes to ensure people with mental illnesses are receiving right treatment at appropriate settings in a seamless manner.

While we boost capacity, there is a need to enhance the community support mechanism with new initiatives as below:

Mental Health Helpline and Community Support Team

Social service agencies such as Family Service Centres (FSCs), Senior Activity Centres (SACs), town councils and VWOs often face difficulty in managing clients who shows signs of mental illness. In order to empower them to better manage their clients, they can now tap on the existing Mental Health Helpline provided by IMH. The helpline acts as a lifeline for community groups to get immediate support as they extend help to people in the community with mental health issues.

The Community Support Team supports the helpline as a response team, conducting home visits and assessments for clients and caregivers who may need help and support. The service providers providing this services are Silver Ribbon (Singapore) and SACS. Together with the helpline, both initiatives aim to support the community in early detection and intervention for people with mental health issues and provide accessibility to appropriate mental health support.

Community Resource, Engagement and Support Team

The Community Resource, Engagement and Support Team, or CREST, is embedded in the community such as the SACS as the 'linking point' between residents and the appropriate mental health care and social support networks. This service model aims to provide basic emotional support, service linkages, early recognition and awareness, and community engagement and networking in the community. It also seeks to promote early recognition of signs and symptoms of depression and to encourage early diagnosis and intervention. In collaboration with the Ministry of Social and Family Development (MSF) and MOH, AIC is working with

Thye Hua Kwan Moral Charities and GoodLife!@South East to provide the services.

Eldersitter and Home Intervention Team

> *'In dementia care, we always try to avoid hospitalisation because an acute hospital ward can be a malignant environment for the person with dementia. People with dementia are generally more secure in familiar places and comfortable with set routines, so they are best in their own homes.'*
>
> – Dr Philip Yap Lin Kiat, Senior Consultant Geriatrician, KTPH

Recognising the needs to keep our dementia clients at home, the Eldersitter Programme is designed to provide respite for caregivers of people living with dementia while promoting cognitive stimulation for clients with dementia. The clients with dementia will be engaged by eldersitters in meaningful and therapeutic activities to maintain their cognitive functioning through activities that are designed to meet their interests and abilities. For clients who demonstrate behavioural and psychological systems of dementia which the caregivers are unable to cope with, the Home Intervention Team provides education and support by equipping the caregivers with effective management skills. With their specialisation in dementia, ADA had enhanced their existing programmes and boosted their capacity to take on the role for both programmes.

With HEART, We Can Achieve 'Integrated Community Living, Ageing in Place'

All VWOs have grown over the years and expanded their services to close the service gaps within the community, ensuring all clients' and caregivers' needs are being met and managing clients within the community. How did the VWOs manage to do so? The key factor is HEART. This is not an easy journey but they succeeded because they all have the heart to care and they have compassion, patience, resilience and perseverance. It may not be easy for the clinical and social professionals to collaborate and work out respective principles and approaches but we all have a common goal — 'Integrated Community Living, Ageing in Place'.

References

Bruce ML, Leaf PJ, Florio L, Hoff RA (1994). Psychiatric status and 9-year mortality data in the New Haven Epidemiologic Catchment Area study. *Am J Psychiatry* **151**: 716–721.

Chiam PC, Ng TP, Tan LL, Ong PS, Ang A, Kua EH (2004). Prevalence of dementia in Singapore — results of the National Mental Health Survey of the Elderly 2003. *Ann Acad Med Singapore* **33**(Suppl. 5): S14–S16.

Chong SA, Abdin E, Vaingakar JA, Kwok KW, Subramaniam M (2012). Help-seeking pattern of the mentally ill. *Ann Acad Med* **41**(4): 154–160.

Chong SA, Subramaniam M, Deurenberg-Yap M, Verma S, Swartz M (2008). Performance measures for mental healthcare in Singapore. *Ann Acad Med Singapore* **37**: 791–796.

Chua HC, Lim L, Ng TP, Lee T, Mahendran R, Fones C, *et al.* (2004). The prevalence of psychiatric disorders in Singapore adults. *Ann Acad Med Singapore* **33**(Suppl. 5): S102.

Goldman HH, Adams NH, Taube CA (1983). Deinstitutionalisation: The data demythologized. *Hosp Community Psychiatry* **4**: 129–134.

Ng BY (2000). Service provision and further developments. In: Ng BY, ed. *Till the Break of Day: A History of Mental Health Services in Singapore, 1841–1993*. Singapore University Press, Singapore, p. 206.

Ng TP, Fones CSL, Kua EH (2003). Preference, need and utilization of mental health services, Singapore National Mental Health Survey. *Aust N Z J Psychiatry* **37**: 613–619.

Singapore Association for Mental Health, SAMH (2010). *Touching Hearts, Reaching Minds — Celebrating 40 Years of Community Wellness*. SAMH, Singapore.